INNOVATIVE RHEUMATOLOGY

Edited by **Hiroaki Matsuno**

Innovative Rheumatology
http://dx.doi.org/10.5772/55641
Edited by Hiroaki Matsuno

Contributors

Wahid Ali Khan, Mohd. Wajid Ali Khan, Mohd Wajid Khan, Andrew B Lemmey, Stevan Stojanović, Branislav Predrag Belić, Rafael Burgos, María A. Hidalgo, Juan L. Hancke, Juan C. Bertoglio, Giovanni Ciancio, Uta Schurigt, Michał Gajewski, Przemyslaw Rzodkiewicz, Koichiro Komiya, Maria Das Graças Henriques, Hiroaki Matsuno, Katarzyna Romanowska-Prochnicka, Marzena Olesinska, Chenqi Zhao

Published by InTech
Janeza Trdine 9, 51000 Rijeka, Croatia

Publishing Process Manager Danijela Duric
Technical Editor InTech DTP team
Cover InTech Design team

Additional hard copies can be obtained from orders@intechopen.com

Innovative Rheumatology, Edited by Hiroaki Matsuno
p. cm.
ISBN 978-953-51-0916-7

For EU product safety concerns:
IN TECH d.o.o., Prolaz Marije Krucifikse Kozulić 3, 51000 Rijeka, Croatia,
info@intechopen.com or visit our website at intechopen.com.

Meet the editor

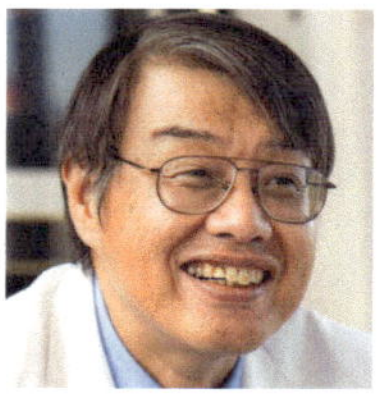

2005-present Director of Matsuno Clinic for Rheumatic disease (Toyama, Japan). 2003-2005 Professor of the Department of Biomedical Engineering, Toin Yokohama University (Kanagawa, Japan). 2003-2005 Chief of Outpatient Clinic in the Department of Rheumatology, Japanese Red Cross Hospital. 2000 Visiting researcher in the Department of Rheumatology, London University (UK). 2000-present Associate Professor in the Department of Orthopedic Surgery, Toyama Medical and Pharmaceutical University. 2000 American Orthopedic Surgery Traveling Fellowship (in the Department of Orthopedic Surgery, University of California, Harvard Medical School, and Lenox Hill Hospital). 2000 Ministry of Education consignment abroad research worker, Exchange foreign Medical Doctor of Japan Rheumatoid Association 1992-2000 Lecturer in the Department of Orthopedic Surgery, Toyama Medical and Pharmaceutical University (Toyama, Japan). 1991 Received a Ph.D. in Toyama Medical and Pharmaceutical University. 1989-1992 Teaching fellow in the Department of Orthopedic Surgery, Toyama Medical and Pharmaceutical University. 1988 Staff doctor in the Department of Orthopedic Surgery, Toyama Medical and Pharmaceutical University. 1987-1988 Staff doctor in the Department of Orthopedic Surgery, Yokohama Higashi National Hospital (Kanagawa, Japan). 1986-1987 Staff doctor in the Department of Orthopedic Surgery , Chiba Rosai Hospital (Chiba, Japan). 1985-1986 Staff doctor in the Department of Orthopedic Surgery, Kawatetsu Chiba Hospital (Kanagawa, Japan). 1984-1985 Resident in the Department of Orthopedic Surgery, Chiba University (Chiba, Japan). 1978-1984 Undergraduate studies in Kinki University Faculty of Medicine (Osaka, Japan).

Contents

Preface

First of all, we are delighted to be able to provide the "Innovative Rheumatology" to everyone involved in the treatment and research of rheumatoid arthritis. In recent years, the treatment of Rheumatoid Arthritis has undergone tremendous changes due to methotrexate and biologics in large part. Until a decade ago, avoiding joint destruction in rheumatoid arthritis was not realistic for rheumatologist. However, prevention of joint deterioration is now possible, and the quality of life of patients with rheumatoid arthritis in long-term has been able to improve by advances in treatment. However, there are still many problems to be overcome before achieving the treatment of rheumatoid arthritis. All of review articles presented on this book are explaining treatment, basic research, and patient care of rheumatoid arthritis with innovative perspective and ideas. I hope that the ideas that have been described in these articles help the reader to resolve the outstanding issues in rheumatoid arthritis. Finally, the editor would like to thank the wonderful authors for their contribution to this book. Furthermore, I would like to thank Mr. Danijela Duric and Ms. Silvia Valsa of InTech's for their unfailing help.

Hiroaki Matsuno
Director,
Matsuno Clinic for Rheumatic Diseases,
Toyama, Japan

Section 1

Basic Science

Chapter 1

Sphingosine-1-Phosphate and Rheumatoid Arthritis: Pathological Implications and Potential Therapeutic Targets

Zhiyi Zhang and Chenqi Zhao

Additional information is available at the end of the chapter

http://dx.doi.org/10.5772/53308

1. Introduction

Rheumatoid arthritis (RA) is a chronic autoimmune disease that affects approximately 1% of the population worldwide. RA mainly targets the synovial tissues of the small joints of the hands and feet, although larger joints are also affected. The disease is characterized by 1) proliferation of synovial fibroblasts, leading to synovial hyperplasia; 2) recruitment of inflammatory cells into joint tissue, resulting in tissue destruction; and 3) excessive secretion of pro-inflammatory cytokines/chemokines, contributing directly to synovium inflammation. While the etiology of RA remains unknown, inflammatory mediators appear to drive the evolution of the disease. In particular, TNF-α together with proinflammatory cytokines, including IL-1β and IL-6, have been shown to be pivotal in promoting cytokine, chemokine and matrix metalloproteinase production within the RA synovium, along with cellular activation and joint erosion [1,2]. Given the complexity of the inflammatory cascade in the RA synovium, it is of great importance to identify novel biochemical signalling moieties that have the potential to constitute intracellular molecular checkpoints within the cell.

Sphingosine-1-phosphate (S1P) is a bioactive sphingolipid metabolite which is formed from sphingosine by sphingosine kinases (SphKs) and degraded by S1P phosphatases (SPPs) and S1P lyase (SPL). S1P is critically involved in both physiological and pathological processes. The lipid is implicated in many cellular processes including proliferation, apoptosis and migration via binding to and activation of its G protein-coupled cell surface receptors. Alterations in S1P signalling as well as in the enzymes involved in its synthesis and metabolism have been observed in many types of pathological situations such as angiogenesis, metastasis, and autoimmunity. Accumulating evidence now suggests a role for S1P in various aspects of RA biology. This can involve, for example, activation of SphKs [3] and an elevated level of S1P [4] in the synovium and synovial fluids of patients with RA, as well as alterations in S1P signalling that lead to synovial fibroblast migration, proliferation, survival and production of proinflammatory cytokines/chemokines [4,5]. This review will highlight how S1P is involved in RA pathology and the mechanisms of its action. In addition, the therapeutic potential of drugs that alter S1P actions will be examined with reference to RA.

2. S1P biology

Sphingolipids are a class of complex, structurally-related compounds derived from sphingoid bases, with hundreds of known class members; they represent a major class of lipids that are ubiquitously expressed in eukaryotic cell membranes. Apart from their structural functions, sphingolipids have emerged as the source of important signalling molecules; these sphingolipid metabolites have important roles in stimulus/agonist-mediated signalling which regulate many cellular processes including inflammation, cell proliferation, apoptosis, angiogenesis, and transformation [6]. Sphingolipid-mediated signalling also influences the pathophysiology of many diseases including cancer, and autoimmune and inflammatory diseases.

S1P is one of the most important sphingolipid metabolites. It was first identified as a potent second messenger in the early 1990s [7,8]. Since then, S1P has been shown to be involved in many important cell signalling pathways and physiological processes such as angiogenesis, cell migration and movement, cell survival and proliferation, cellular architecture, cellular contacts and adhesions, heart development, vascular development, atherogenesis, acute lung injury and acute respiratory distress, tumorogenicity and metastasis, and inflammation and immunity (reviewed in [9,10]). New tools, such as specific agonists and antagonists and the generation of targeted knockouts, have led to a surge of interest in the role of S1P in numerous diseases. Recent studies have shown, for example, that it modulates the pathophysiological consequences of various autoimmune diseases, such as Sjogren's syndrome [11] and systemic sclerosis [12].

2.1. S1P metabolism

S1P is present at submicromolar concentrations in various biological fluids and tissues [13]. It is predominantly present in the platelets and erythrocytes in the blood, at concentrations of 100 nM to 4 μM [14], because the platelets lack the S1P degradation enzyme SPL [15]. Human serum is also a rich source of S1P with concentrations ranging from 340 nM to 1 μM [16,17]. Moreover, the erythrocytes appear to be the cells mostly responsible for the storage and constant supply of plasma S1P [14].

S1P is produced intracellularly by a series of enzymatic reactions (Figure 1); all cells are able to generate it during the normal physiologic metabolism of sphingolipids. Sphingomyelin hydrolysis is considered to be the first step in the pathway generating S1P. The reaction is catalyzed by sphingomyelinases yielding ceramide. Ceramide is the central step in sphingolipid metabolism and can be also synthesized de novo from serine and palmitate by the action of ceramide synthase [18]. Ceramide is, in turn, deacylated by ceramidase to release sphingosine, which is then phosphorylated either by SphK1 or SphK2 to yield S1P. While both SphK1 and SphK2 can phosphorylate sphingosine, SphK1 produces most of the S1P [19]. SphKs can be activated by a large variety of agonists, such as TNF-α (reviewed in [20-22]). Activation of SphK1 leads to its translocation to the plasma membrane where its substrate sphingosine is located, resulting in the production of S1P [23,24]. S1P, in turn, activates specific S1P receptors present on the surface of the same cell or on nearby cells in autocrine and/or paracrine manners [20]. This "inside-out" signaling of intracellularly generated S1P is crucial for many of its functions [25]. S1P is degraded through two distinct mechanisms, the reversible dephosphorylation into sphingosine by SPPs, and the irreversible degradation by SPL to hexadecenal and ethanolamine phosphate [26,27]. Consequently, the cellular levels of S1P are tightly regulated by its formation from sphingosine through the activity of SphKs and its degradation through the activity of SPPs and SPL. In the basal state, the balance between S1P generation and degradation results in low cellular levels of S1P [28,29].

The mechanism by which S1P is exported to the outside of cells after synthesis is not fully understood. Several studies suggested the involvement of the ATP-binding cassette (ABC) family of transporters in S1P secretion [30-32]. It has been shown that its release from mast cells is regulated by ABCC1 [31] while the ABCA1 transporter is critical for release of S1P from astrocytes [32]. Altogether, these studies suggested that members of the family of ABC transporters may be important for the transport of S1P out of cells.

2.2. S1P receptors and S1P receptor-mediated signalling

S1P exerts diverse biological activities under physiological and pathological conditions via both intracellular and extracellular signalling pathways, but mostly the latter. To date, five cell surface G protein-coupled S1P receptors (S1P1-5), belonging to the endothelial differentiating gene (EDG) family, have been identified [13]. S1P receptors exhibit variable tissue distribution: S1P1, S1P2, and S1P3 are widely expressed in various tissues, whereas the expression of S1P4 and S1P5 is more restricted to cells of the immune system and nervous system, respectively (reviewed in [33]). Each S1P receptor couples to a specific heterotrimeric G protein: $G_{i/o}$, G_q and $G_{12/13}$. When activated, the G protein dissociates into its α and $\beta\gamma$ subunits and transduces signals toward the downstream pathways. In particular, S1P1 is coupled predominantly to $G_{i/o}$, through which it activates signalling known to be essential for embryonic blood vessel development as the murine S1P1 knockout is lethal at the embryonic stage, as a result of hemorrhage [34]. In addition, plasma S1P has been shown to elicit egress of lymphocytes into the blood in an S1P1-dependent manner [35] and to regulate basal and inflammation-induced vascular leak *in vivo* [36]. S1P2 and S1P3 are linked predominantly to G_q and $G_{12/13}$; knockout of both receptors in mice decreases litter size and survival rates [37]. S1P4 and S1P5 are the least studied receptors, although it is known that S1P4 is involved in T-cell proliferation [38] and S1P5 is required in natural killer cell trafficking [39]. More detailed information on the various signalling pathways triggered by S1P receptor activation can be found in previous reviews [40,41]. The five known S1P receptors can lead to activation of different downstream targets, such as Rac, ERK, PI3K, adenylyl cyclase, phospholipase-C, Rho or JNK, resulting in the abovementioned cellular responses [42]. The extracellular pathways mediated by each S1P-specific receptor are common; however, given the existence of agonists and antagonists that exhibit receptor specificity, it is probable that the S1P receptors are not totally redundant [43]. Upon binding to one of the five known cell surface receptors, S1P initiates signal transduction leading to various cellular responses.

S1P also exerts its action as a second messenger via intracellular pathways. For example, it intracellularly targets the histone deacetylases HDACs, regulating specific and contextual chromatin states that impact gene transcription [44]. S1P has been shown to promote growth and survival, independently from its G protein-coupled receptors, in mouse embryonic fibroblasts devoid of S1P receptors [35]. There is also evidence supporting a role for intracellular S1P in calcium mobilization [45].

3. Alteration of S1P in rheumatoid arthritis

TNF-α is the predominant proinflammatory cytokine in RA. TNF-α can activate SphK, which leads to the production of S1P [46]. Indeed, SphK1, SphK2 [3,47] and S1P levels [48] are elevated in the synovium of patients with RA. Moreover, administration of S1P to RA synovial fibroblasts causes their proliferation, survival, and migration, as well as cytokine/chemokine and other proinflammatory mediator production [4,5]. The findings suggest that S1P may play a role in RA pathology (Figure 2).

3.1. SphK activity and S1P levels in RA synovium

Activated SphKs and elevated S1P levels are associated to RA (Table 1). For instance, increased SphK1 expression and activity was found in RA B lymphoblastoid cell lines, and identified as the underlying mechanism of impaired Fas-mediated death signalling in RA [47]. More recently, SphK2 has been shown to be strongly expressed in RA synovial fibroblasts *in vivo* and *in vitro*, which is associated with upregulation of S1P [3]. Suppression of SphK2 by siRNA results in a more aggressive disease and greater secretion of proinflammatory cytokines, such as IL-6, TNF-α and IFN-γ in a murine collagen-induced arthritis (CIA) model [49]. Of more interest, in a murine CIA model, administration of a pharmacological SphK inhibitor, *N,N*-dimethylsphingosine (DMS), and an siRNA approach to knockdown SphK1 isoform markedly suppressed joint pathologies such as adjacent cartilage and bone erosion, synovial hyperplasia, and inflammatory infiltration into the joint compartment [49].

At present, evidence for roles in RA of other S1P metabolic enzymes, such as SPPs and SPL, is limited. However, up-regulation of SPP2 was detected in samples of skin lesions from patients with psoriasis, a chronic inflammatory skin disease [50]. Interestingly, an elevated mRNA expression of SPP1 and SPL was observed in RA synovial fibroblasts, as compared to non-arthritic synovial fibroblasts (Zhao et al., unpublished data).

http://dx.doi.org/10.5772/53308

S1P is widely expressed in RA synovium. Elevated levels were detected in both synovial tissue and synovial fluids from patients with RA [4,48]. Moreover, the S1P content in synovial fluids from patients with RA was compared to that from patients with osteoarthritis (OA), a degenerative joint disease [4]. S1P levels were shown to be much higher in synovial fluids of RA patients than in those of OA patients. In that study, the S1P level in RA synovial fluids was even higher than those in serum or plasma from normal donors. A similar experiment was performed with a different experimental strategy, in which the S1P level in RA synovial fluids was five fold higher than that in OA synovial fluids [48]. Peripheral blood B lymphoblastoid cell lines from patients with RA exhibited a high level of S1P level as well [47]. This increase in S1P level could be responsible for the recruitment and retention of the immune infiltrates in the synovium.

	RA	OA	Normal	Experimental Strategy	Reference
S1P content in synovial fluids	17.51±4.23 μM	3.45±0.85 μM	N/A	Competitive ELISA	[48]
	1,078.92 p*M*/ml	765.01 p*M*/ml	N/A	HPLC	[4]
S1P intracellular level in synovial cells	Increased level in LDLs compared to normal control cells	N/A		Chromatography	[47]
SphK activity in synovial cells	Markedly increased enzymatic activity in LDLs compared to normal control cells	N/A		Sphk enzymatic activity assay	[47]
SphK expression in synovial fibroblasts	More SphK2 positive cells than those in OA	Weakly positive	N/A	Immunofluorescence	[3]
S1P1 receptor expression in synovial tissue	Markedly enhanced expression than that in OA	Weak expression	Weak expression	immunostaining	[4]

N/A: not applicable or not available

Table 1. SphK expression/activity, S1P levels, and S1P receptor expression in synovium of RA, OA, and normal donors.

3.2. S1P receptor expression in synovial fibroblasts

Synovial fibroblasts or fibroblast-like synovial synoviocytes (FLS) are key contributors to RA chronic inflammation due to their abnormal growth and erosive activity. During RA disease progression, these cells become hyperplastic, closely interact with infiltrated immune cells to form the aggressive pannus tissue that invades and degrades the cartilage and bone and eventually promotes joint destruction (reviewed in [51]). Synovial fibroblasts also contribute to the local production of cytokines/chemokines, small molecule mediators of inflammation, and proteolytic enzymes that degrade the extracellular matrix [52].

RA synovial fibroblasts have been reported to express three of five known S1P receptors, S1P1-3 [4,5,53]. Expression of S1P1 in RA inflamed synovial tissue is significantly higher than that in OA synovial tissue [4]. Of more interest, pretreatment of RA synovial fibroblasts with TNF-α, the cytokine well-recognized to be critical in RA, results in up-regulation of S1P3 receptor expression in synovial fibroblasts, which likely contributes to the synergistic production of inflammatory cytokines/chemokines, migration (or invasion) and survival of these cells upon subsequent exposure to S1P [5]. Thus, it seems that the elevated TNF-α levels observed in the synovial fluid of RA patients could make synovial fibroblasts more responsive to increases of S1P in RA synovium; in turn, the enhanced responsiveness to S1P through the S1P3 receptor could increase synovial fibroblast survival, migration and production of cytokines/chemokines, processes that all likely contribute to the pathology of RA.

3.3. Influence of S1P on the secretion of proinflammatory cytokines/chemokines and other proinflammatory mediators by synovial fibroblasts

One key feature of RA is the large amounts of pro-inflammatory cytokines and chemokines produced by activated synovial cells. These cytokines/chemokines may directly contribute to cartilage and bone erosion by promoting matrix metalloproteinase (MMP) production and chondrocyte/osteoclast destruction function [51]. S1P can stimulate synovial fibroblasts to release various inflammatory mediators, including cytokines, chemokines, and prostaglandin E2 (PGE2) [4,5]. S1P administration notably stimulates the synovial fibroblast secretion of IL-8, IL-6, MCP-1 and RANTES via S1P2 and S1P3 receptors and through modulation of p38, ERK, and Rho kinase activities [5]. The S1P-induced cytokine/chemokine secretion and S1P receptor-mediated signalling pathways were further suggested as the driving force for synovial fibroblast invasion into the surrounding tissue [5]. Moreover, inhibition of S1P production by a potent SphK1 inhibitor, DMS, significantly suppresses production of these cytokines [48]. The effect of S1P on cytokine secretion is further amplified by TNF-α [5], suggesting that the cytokine-rich environment of the inflamed synovium may synergize with S1P signalling to exacerbate the disease process [5].

In addition, S1P has been found to indirectly stimulate IL-17 secretion by activating T-cell receptor-activated CD4 T cells [54]. IL-17 is produced by cultured peripheral blood mononuclear cells (PBMC) and synovial membrane cells, and elevated levels of IL-17 are detected in the synovial fluid of RA patients [54,55]. It was reported that IL-17-deficient mice showed resistance to CIA [56]. Furthermore, IL-17 was demonstrated to contribute to the severity of synovial inflammation and bone destruction in RA by stimulating the production of proinflammatory cytokines and chemokines such as TNF-α, IL-1β, IL-6, MMPs, and receptor activator of NF-κB ligand (RANKL) [57,58].

S1P is able to stimulate the production of other inflammatory mediators, such as PGE2, and of its metabolic enzymes cyclooxygenases (COXs) in RA synovial fibroblasts [4,53]. PGE2 is an autocrine lipid mediator derived from arachidonic acid metabolism by COX-1 or COX-2 [59]. The inflammation characteristic of RA is actually closely associated to the production of PGE2 by synovial fibroblasts, as PGE2 stimulates angiogenesis in rheumatoid synovium [60] and triggers bone resorption by osteoclasts [61]. Thus, S1P may aggravate synovial hyperplasia, inflammation and angiogenesis through the induction of COX-2 and PGE2 in RA synovial tissues.

3.4. Upregulation of immune cell recruitment and retention by S1P in the RA synovium

Recruitment and retention of inflammatory cells, such as neutrophils, monocytes and T lymphocytes, are other fundamental features of RA synovitis. This process is coordinated by the presence of chemo-attractant proteins at the site of inflammation, assisted by the expression of adhesion molecules. Chemokines and other small chemo-attractant molecules are abundant in the RA synovium and can be produced by synovial fibroblasts in the intimal lining. S1P, as a chemo-attractant, plays a pivotal role in the immune cell egression. S1P1, for example, is essential for lymphocyte recirculation since it regulates lymphocyte egress from both thymus and peripheral lymphoid organs [62,63]. As S1P exists at lower levels in tissues and higher levels in the blood and lymph, it is suggested that the S1P gradient between tissues and the blood/lymph drives such a migration. Likewise, the elevated S1P levels in the synovial fluid of RA patients [48] could be responsible for the recruitment and retention of the immune infiltrates in the RA synovium. Indeed, inhibition of S1P1 down-regulated inflammatory cell accumulation in an adjuvant-induced arthritis (AIA) animal model [64].

S1P may also contribute indirectly to the recruitment and retention of inflammatory cells into RA synovium by stimulating the secretion of other chemo-attractants. In RA, the recruitment of immune cells into the synovium may be due to the large amount of CC and CXC chemokines produced by activated cells of the synovial lining. In particular, IL-8 exhibits selective chemotactic activity for neutrophils, whereas MCP-1, MIP-1α, -1β and RANTES primarily attract monocytes. RA synovial fibroblasts do not secrete detectable levels of cytokines or chemokines, except for low amounts of MCP-1 in the resting state; upon treatment with S1P, however, the secretion of IL-8, IL-6, MCP-1 and RANTES is strongly induced, indicating S1P contribution to and/or amplification of the secretion of chemokines by cells of the inflamed synovium [5]. Since immune cells express a wide repertoire of chemokine receptors, including those of IL-8, MCP-1, SDF-1α, IP-10 and RANTES [65], S1P may indirectly drive the recruitment and retention of inflammatory cells in RA by this chemokine secretion. Indeed, a bioactive lipid structurally-related to S1P, lysophosphatidic acid (LPA), is able to recruit leukocytes into an *in vivo* inflammatory site by stimulating inflammatory cytokine/chemokine secretion [66].

3.5. Promotion of proliferation and/or survival of synovial fibroblasts, B lymphocytes, and chondrocytes by S1P in the RA synovium

Abnormal growth of synovial fibroblasts and chondrocytes has been suggested to contribute directly to hyperplasia of the rheumatoid synovium [67]. The growth in RA of the synovial fibroblast population is likely attributable to an imbalance between cell proliferation, survival, and death. In fact, synovial fibroblast proliferation is difficult to demonstrate in RA. Nonetheless, limited numbers of mitotic figures or cells expressing cell cycle markers suggest that synovial fibroblast DNA synthesis is not a major influence [68,69]. Instead, the RA synovial environment promotes survival of these cells and discourages their depletion through apoptosis. S1P, through S1P1, protects synovial fibroblasts from apoptosis [5]. Thus, the ability of S1P to promote synovial fibroblasts survival, whether or not this agent can also increase cell proliferation, could contribute to RA pannus hyperplasia [70].

B lymphocytes play an important role in the pathogenesis of RA. B-cell accumulation and maturation in the inflamed synovium can form ectopic germinal centers [71-73] and activate T cells [74]. Moreover, mature plasma cells secrete autoantibodies, such as the rheumatoid factor, which are key features of RA [75]. The importance of B cells in RA is illustrated by the success obtained when targeting CD-20-positive B cells with the chimeric monoclonal anti-CD20 antibody, rituximab [76]. In that study, a single short course of rituximab, either alone or in combination with cyclophosphamide or continuing methotrexate, provided patients with significant improvements in disease symptoms, a reduction in B-cell numbers, rheumatoid factors, and total immunoglobulin levels. S1P appears capable of increasing cell survival and inhibiting apoptosis of B lymphocytes derived from RA patients, as these cells are uniquely resistant to Fas-mediated apoptosis [47]. This effect is due to an increased activity of SphK1 and an overproduction of S1P. In a murine experimental arthritis model, administration of SphK inhibitor, DMS, and of SphK1 siRNA significantly decreased the production of anticollagen IgG2a in the mouse serum [48,49].

S1P was also reported to induce chondrocyte proliferation through stimulation of COX-2 and PGE2 production and via activation of ERK [77,78], and was thus suggested to be able to modulate cartilage homeostasis.

3.6. Contribution of S1P to osteoclastogenesis

Pathologic bone loss is a common feature of RA in which progressive destruction of bone is associated with joint inflammation. Focal bone erosion occurs at the pannus-bone interface and in the immediate subchondral bone early in RA, and is associated over time with significant morbidity for patients [79]. Bone-resorbing osteoclasts have been identified as important effector cells in inflammation-induced bone loss in both experimental animal models and human RA. Osteoclasts are derived from hematopoietic precursor cells of the myeloid lineage [80,81]. In normal skeletal remodelling, the balance between bone resorption by osteoclasts and bone formation by osteoblasts is critically regulated [82-84] and osteoclast differentiation is dependent on the presence of two key factors, RANKL and colony-stimulating factor-1(CSF-1), provided by cells of the osteoblast lineage [81,85,86]. In experimental animal models of arthritis, osteoclasts have been observed at sites of focal bone erosion [87,88]. In addition to the RANK/RANKL pathway, many cytokines (such as TNF-α, IL-6, and IL-17) and growth factors elaborated by inflamed synovial tissues may contribute to osteoclast differentiation and activation in RA [89].

S1P has been found to induce chemotaxis of osteoclast precursors and osteoclastogenesis *in vitro* [90] and *in vivo* [91]. In a bone marrow-derived macrophage and osteoblast coculture system, for instance, S1P addition greatly increased osteoclastogenesis by increasing RANKL in osteoblasts via cyclooxygenase-2 and PGE2 regulation [90]. S1P also chemoattracted osteoblasts and enhanced their survival [90]. Moreover, S1P controls the migratory behaviour of osteoclast precursors between bone tissues and the blood stream, dynamically regulating bone mineral homeostasis via S1P receptors. Cells with the properties of osteoclast precursors indeed express functional S1P1 receptors and exhibit positive chemotaxis along an S1P gradient *in vitro* [92]. On the other hand, S1P2 requires a higher concentration of S1P for activation and induces negative chemotactic responses to S1P gradients [91]. S1P2 activation causes cells to move from the bloodstream into bone marrow cavities [91].

3.7. SphKs and S1P in experimental arthritis

Both CIA and AIA are well-established models for studying RA. Administration of the S1P receptor agonist FYT720, which down-regulates S1P receptors, in rat CIA and AIA models inhibits rat hind paw oedema and joint destruction and decreases lymphocyte invasion into the joints [93,94]. In addition to receptor modulation, non-specific inhibition of SphK with DMS in a murine CIA model has been shown to significantly reduce adjacent cartilage and bone erosion, synovial hyperplasia, and inflammatory infiltration into the joint compartment [48,49]. Moreover, suppression of SphK1 via siRNA knockdown results in similar reduction in joint pathology, serum levels of IL-6, TNF-α, IFN-γ and S1P, and the *in vitro* production of these proinflammatory mediators in response to collagen [48,49]. In another murine arthritis model, the transgenic human TNF-α model that develops spontaneous erosive arthritis, Sphk1-deficient mice exhibit significantly less synovial inflammation and joint pathology than the wild-type mice [95].

Interestingly, SphK isoforms may play different roles in RA. In a murine CIA model, down-regulating SphK1 via specific small interfering RNA (siRNA) significantly reduced the incidence, disease severity, and articular inflammation. Treatment with SphK1 siRNA also down-regulated serum levels of S1P, IL-6, TNF-α, IFN-γ, and IgG2a anticollagen antibody [49]. On the other hand, mice receiving SphK2 siRNA developed a more aggressive disease, and higher serum levels of IL-6, TNF-α, and IFN-γ, when compared with control siRNA recipients. These results suggest distinct immunomodulatory roles for SphK1 and SphK2 in the development of inflammatory arthritis via the regulation of the release of proinflammatory cytokines and T cell responses.

S1P metabolism and SphK/S1P/S1P receptor axis-mediated signalling pathways in rheumatoid arthritis synovium and the potential role of S1P in RA pathogenesis are illustrated in Figure 1 and Figure 2, respectively.

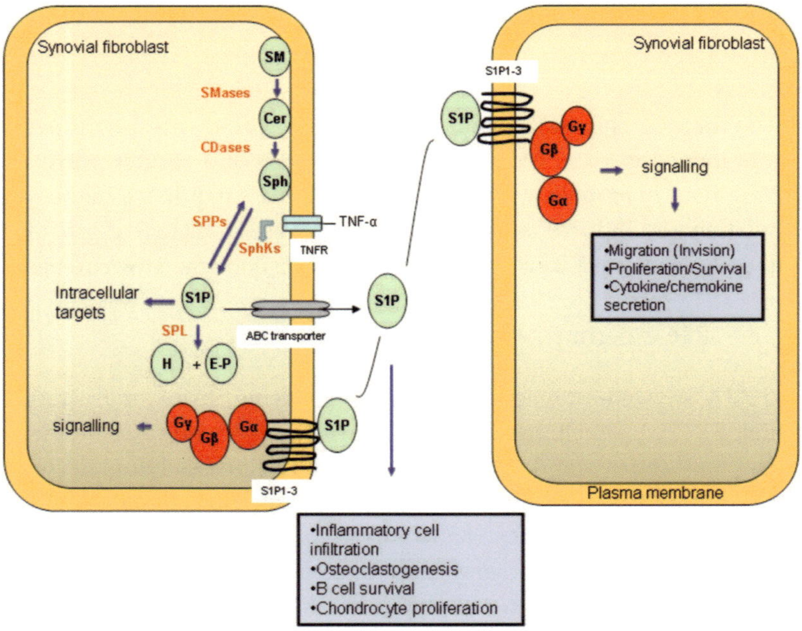

Figure 1. S1P metabolism and SphK/S1P/S1P receptor axis-mediated signalling pathways in RA synovium. S1P homeostasis is tightly regulated by the balance between its synthesis and degradation via three enzyme families: (1) Sphks (SphK1 and SphK2), which generate S1P through phosphorylation of its precursor, sphingosine (Sph), (2) SPPs (SPP1 and SPP2), which reversibly convert S1P back to Sph, and (3) SPL, which irreversibly degrades S1P to generate ethanolamine phosphate and hexadecenal. In the inflamed RA synovium, the specific binding of agonists, such as TNF-α, to their receptors (TNFR) induces the expression of SphKs, which in turn converts the membrane-bound Sph into S1P in synovial fibroblasts. The generated S1P then exits the cell through the ATP binding cassette (ABC) transporter and exerts its action through the G-protein coupled S1P receptors in an autocrine and/or paracrine fashion, activating specific S1P receptors presenting on the surface of the same cell or on nearby cells. Each S1P receptor couples to a specific heterotrimeric G protein. When activated, the G protein dissociates into its α and βγ subunits and transduces signals toward the downstream pathways to regulate cell proliferation, growth, migration, apoptosis, etc. Extracellular S1P can stimulate the infiltration of immune cells, the proliferation and/or survival of synovial fibroblasts, B lymphoblastoid cells, and chondrocytes, as well as the osteoclastogenesis in the synovium. S1P also exerts its action as a second messenger via intracellular pathways, regulating chromatin states that impact gene transcription, cell growth and survival, and calcium mobilization independent of its G protein-coupled receptors. SM, sphingomyelin; Cer, ceramide; H, hexadecenal; E-P, ethanolamine phosphate; SMases, sphingomyelinases; CDases, ceramidases.

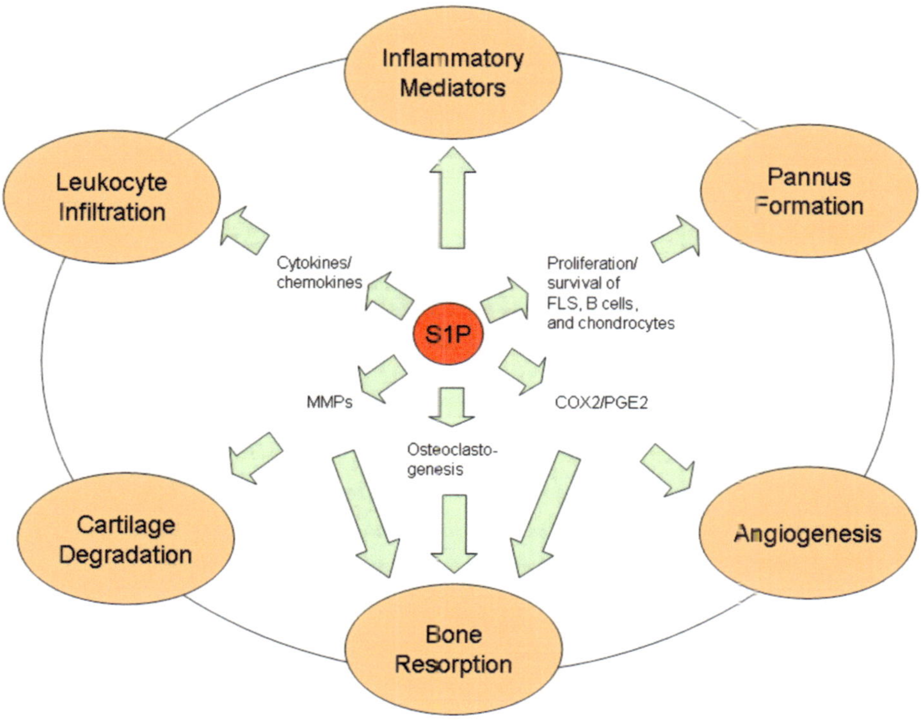

Figure 2. Potential role of S1P in the pathogenesis of RA.

4. Therapeutic POTENTIAL of S1P in rheumatoid arthritis

The introduction of novel biological therapies in the mid-1990s markedly improved clinical outcomes in RA. Cytokine antagonists, such as biologic agents that inhibit TNF-α, IL-6, or IL-1β, decrease inflammation and joint destruction [96]. The impressive efficacy of these biologic agents, however, is only seen in about half of the patients. Similarly, B cell depletion and T cell co-stimulation blockers [96] are beneficial only in non- or partially-overlapping subsets of patients. There is undoubtedly a necessity to develop therapies that target other pathways. As S1P modulates RA pathogenesis in many aspects, manipulation of endogenous amounts of bioactive S1P and/or its receptor activation may be beneficial for joint inflammation and destruction.

4.1. Targeting S1P levels

Decreasing S1P level by inhibiting SphK1 activity may represent a therapeutic approach against RA. Blockage of SphK1 activity in an animal arthritis model indeed significantly suppressed articular inflammation and joint destruction, reduced disease severity, and down-regulated proinflammatory cytokine production and inflammatory cell infiltration into the synovium [49]. In fact, inhibition of S1P synthesis by blocking SphK activity has proven useful as an anti-inflammation strategy in cancer therapy [97-101].

Depleting S1P level by utilizing S1P-blocking agents, such as specific antibodies, may also have therapeutic implications for RA. Indeed, anti-S1P antibodies have been developed and are currently tested in clinical studies for treatment of cancer, fibrosis, inflammation, macular degeneration, diabetic retinopathy, glaucoma, and other diseases or symptoms (reviewed in [102]). These antibodies bind to and inactivate S1P, reducing the extracellular pool of bioactive S1P and inhibiting its stimulating activity [103]. A preclinical study using blocking S1P antibodies to prevent tumour progression, for example, was recently reported [104]. In that study, a specific anti-S1P monoclonal antibody reduced, and in some cases completely eliminated, tumour formation and accompanying tumour angiogenesis. These results suggest that antibody-mediated inhibition of S1P signalling may be developed as a strategy for inhibiting pannus formation and angiogenesis in RA.

SPL, the major S1P-degrading enzyme, catalyzes the irreversible degradation of intracellular S1P. Inhibition of SPL leads to the accumulation of S1P in tissues, including lymphoid tissues [105], and induces premature internalization of the exit-signal-sensing S1P1 receptor on lymphocytes, rendering them unresponsive to S1P and preventing their egress from thymus and lymph nodes [106]. One physiological outcome of this systemic redistribution of lymphocytes is potent immunosuppression, which offers new opportunities for developing immunoregulatory agents to treat autoimmune and inflammatory diseases [107-111]. In fact, SPL-deficient mice showed resistance to various inflammatory and autoimmune challenges [112-114]. Early studies are undergoing on the application of SPL inhibitors to RA treatment. The evaluation of a synthetic SPL inhibitor, LX2931, is currently in phase-II clinical trials in patients with active RA [112]. There are also studies on the SPL inhibitor, LX 3305, which inhibits lymphocyte migration, concerning its potential for RA clinical treatment [115].

4.2. Targeting S1P receptors: S1P receptor agonist FTY720

FTY720 (generic name fingolimod) is a synthetic sphingosine analog (2-amino-2-[2-(4-octylphenyl)ethyl]propane-1,3-diol) that can be phosphorylated by SphKs. The designation FTY-P is used for the phosphorylated compound. FTY720 acts as an agonist with high affinity for all S1P receptors except S1P2 [109], and very effectively down-regulates S1P receptor expression [63,102]. It very actively induces the internalization, ubiquitylation and subsequent degradation of S1P receptors, consequently rendering cells unresponsive to S1P [63]. Compared to FTY720, S1P is much less effective at inducing receptor degradation [116,117].

FTY720 has emerged as a clinically promising novel immunosuppressive drug that presumably acts by limiting effector lymphocyte egress from lymph nodes [118,119]. It rapidly induces lymphopenia through the sequestration of lymphocytes in lymph nodes and by blocking the emigration of mature thymocytes from the thymus through receptor down-modulation [116,117,120]. It differentially affects the sequestration of regulatory T-cells and increases their suppressive activity [121]. It is also reported to display anti-angiogenic activity and to potently diminish angiogenesis and tumor vascularization *in vivo* in growth factor implants and corneal models [122] and via the S1P1 receptor [123].

FTY720 has been proven effective in the treatment of multiple sclerosis (MS). MS and RA are both autoimmune diseases with similar clinical inflammatory characterization, such as the infiltration of immune cells into the inflammatory sites, with RA affecting the joints, while MS affecting the brain and spinal cord. In MS, the most relevant effect of FTY720-P relates to its interaction with S1P1 receptor. After binding with the drug, S1P1 is internalized for several days. This receptor internalization, reduces the number of available S1P1 receptors and subsequently renders T lymphocytes unresponsive to S1P signals, which would otherwise mediate their migration from the thymus and lymph nodes to the peripheral blood and from there to the brain. This way, FTY720 prevents lymphocytes from recirculating to peripheral sites of inflammation [124]. Treatment of human patients with relapsing-remitting MS with considerably low doses of FTY720 has proven to be beneficial [125,126].The results of a phase-II clinical trial, evaluating the efficacy and safety of FTY-720 for treating relapsing MS, showed that the annualized relapse rate of the FTY-720 group was significantly lower [126]. More recently, two large-scale, phase-III clinical trials conducted on relapsing-remitting MS patients demonstrated that FTY720 reduces relapse rates by more than 50%, as compared with the control groups [127,128]. FTY720, which can be taken orally [129], is therefore a highly promising immunomodulatory drug for MS. In fact, FTY720 has been approved by the US Food and Drug Administration for the treatment of relapsing forms of MS.

The therapeutic effect of FTY720 on RA was recently examined in animal models. FTY720 administration suppresses the progression of laminarin-induced arthritis in the SKG mice [130]. FTY720 treatment decreases IL-6 and TNF-α expression in synovial fibroblasts and inflammatory cells, as well as bone destruction. The numbers of CD4+ and CD8+ T cells were significantly increased in the thymus and decreased in the spleen in FTY720-treated SKG mice. FTY720 enhanced IL-4 production by CD4+ T cells stimulated by allogeneic spleen cells and inhibited PGE2 production by a TNF-α-stimulated synovial fibroblast cell line. The anti-arthritic effect of FTY720 was also evaluated in AIA rats [131]. In that study, FTY720 treatment inhibited the incidence of arthritis, hind paw oedema and bone destruction. In addition, it markedly decreased the number of peripheral blood lymphocytes. In a separate study, ovariectomized mice were injected with an arthrogenic anti-collagen II antibodies cocktail and then with lipopolysaccharide (LPS), so that they developed arthritis in their paws [132]. These mice thus exhibit both arthritis and osteoporosis and can be regarded as a model of elderly female RA patients. Results from this study showed that FTY720 was as potent as corticosteroid for suppressing arthritis. In addition, it induced recovery of the ovariectomy-induced bone density loss. These results clearly suggest that S1P-targeted therapy, such as S1P receptor agonists, would be beneficial for treating RA patients with both immunological and bone resorptive disorders.

5. Conclusion

In summary, S1P, via SphK1/S1P/S1P-receptor signalling, appears to play an essential role in modulating RA pathogenesis since activated SphK1 and elevated level of S1P are detected in RA synovium. Moreover, S1P receptor expression is upregulated in inflamed synovium. S1P can stimulate proinflammatory cytokines/chemokines secretion, drive immune cell recruitment into inflammatory sites, and promote the proliferation and/or survival of synovial fibroblasts, B lymphoblastoid cells, and chondrocytes. Although the mechanism of its effect in RA remains unclear, S1P represents an exploitable target for the development of a novel therapeutic approach for RA.

6. Key Points

- S1P plays an important role in rheumatoid arthritis pathogenesis. Proofs are:
  - Levels of S1P and its synthetic enzymes SphKs are elevated in RA synovium;
  - RA synovial fibroblasts are more responsive to S1P;
  - S1P stimulates the production of proinflammatory cytokines/chemokines by RA synovial fibroblasts;
  - S1P drives recruitment and retention of immune cells in RA synovium;
  - S1P promotes RA proliferation and/or survival of synovial fibroblasts, B cells, and chondrocytes;
  - S1P induces osteoclastogenesis in RA synovium; etc.
- S1P represents a potential therapeutic target for rheumatoid arthritis. Evidences are:
  - Decreasing S1P level by inhibiting SphK1 activity reduces RA disease severity in animal models of arthritis;
  - Depleting S1P level by utilizing S1P-blocking agents inhibits the growth of tumours, which is relevant to pannus formation in RA;
  - The strategy of inhibiting SPL activity – with the aim of rendering immune cells unresponsive to S1P and thus decreasing immune cells infiltration– is undergoing in phase-III clinical trials in patients with active RA;
  - Blocking S1P receptor activity by utilizing S1P receptor agonist FTY720 suppresses arthritis in animal models of RA; FTY720 has been approved by the US Food and Drug Administration for the treatment of relapsing forms of another chronic inflammatory disease multiple sclerosis.

http://dx.doi.org/10.5772/53308

Author details

Zhiyi Zhang[1] and Chenqi Zhao[2]

*Address all correspondence to: zhangzhiyi@medmail.com.cn

1 Department of Rheumatology and Immunology, The First Affiliated Hospital of Harbin Medical University, Harbin, China

2 Rheumatology and Immunology Research Center, CHUQ-CHUL Research Center and Faculty of Medicine, Laval University, Quebec, Canada

References

[1] Brennan FM, McInnes IB. Evidence that cytokines play a role in rheumatoid arthritis. J Clin Invest 2008;118:3537-3545.

[2] McInnes IB, O'Dell JR. State-of-the-art: rheumatoid arthritis. Ann Rheum Dis 2010;69:1898-1906.

[3] Kamada K, Arita N, Tsubaki T, Takubo N, Fujino T, Soga Y, Miyazaki T, Yamamoto H, Nose M. Expression of sphingosine kinase 2 in synovial fibroblasts of rheumatoid arthritis contributing to apoptosis by a sphingosine analogue, FTY720. Pathol Int 2009;59:382-389.

[4] Kitano M, Hla T, Sekiguchi M, Kawahito Y, Yoshimura R, Miyazawa K, Iwasaki T, Sano H, Saba JD, Tam YY. Sphingosine 1-phosphate/sphingosine 1-phosphate receptor 1 signaling in rheumatoid synovium: regulation of synovial proliferation and inflammatory gene expression. Arthritis Rheum 2006;54:742-753.

[5] Zhao C, Fernandes MJ, Turgeon M, Tancrede S, Di Battista J, Poubelle PE, Bourgoin SG. Specific and overlapping sphingosine-1-phosphate receptor functions in human synoviocytes: impact of TNF-alpha. J Lipid Res 2008;49:2323-2337.

[6] Bartke N, Hannun YA. Bioactive sphingolipids: metabolism and function. J Lipid Res 2009;50 Suppl:S91-96.

[7] Olivera A, Spiegel S. Sphingosine-1-phosphate as second messenger in cell proliferation induced by PDGF and FCS mitogens. Nature 1993;365:557-560.

[8] Zhang H, Desai NN, Olivera A, Seki T, Brooker G, Spiegel S. Sphingosine-1-phosphate, a novel lipid, involved in cellular proliferation. J Cell Biol 1991;114:155-167.

[9] Alemany R, van Koppen CJ, Danneberg K, Ter Braak M, Meyer Zu Heringdorf D. Regulation and functional roles of sphingosine kinases. Naunyn Schmiedebergs Arch Pharmacol 2007;374:413-428.

[10] Hait NC, Oskeritzian CA, Paugh SW, Milstien S, Spiegel S. Sphingosine kinases, sphingosine 1-phosphate, apoptosis and diseases. Biochim Biophys Acta 2006;1758:2016-2026.

[11] Sekiguchi M, Iwasaki T, Kitano M, Kuno H, Hashimoto N, Kawahito Y, Azuma M, Hla T, Sano H. Role of sphingosine 1-phosphate in the pathogenesis of Sjogren's syndrome. J Immunol 2008;180:1921-1928.

[12] Tokumura A, Carbone LD, Yoshioka Y, Morishige J, Kikuchi M, Postlethwaite A, Watsky MA. Elevated serum levels of arachidonoyl-lysophosphatidic acid and sphingosine 1-phosphate in systemic sclerosis. Int J Med Sci 2009;6:168-176.

[13] Ishii I, Fukushima N, Ye X, Chun J. Lysophospholipid receptors: signaling and biology. Annu Rev Biochem 2004;73:321-354.

[14] Hanel P, Andreani P, Graler MH. Erythrocytes store and release sphingosine 1-phosphate in blood. FASEB J 2007;21:1202-1209.

[15] Ito K, Anada Y, Tani M, Ikeda M, Sano T, Kihara A, Igarashi Y. Lack of sphingosine 1-phosphate-degrading enzymes in erythrocytes. Biochem Biophys Res Commun 2007;357:212-217.

[16] Murata N, Sato K, Kon J, Tomura H, Okajima F. Quantitative measurement of sphingosine 1-phosphate by radioreceptor-binding assay. Anal Biochem 2000;282:115-120.

[17] Murata N, Sato K, Kon J, Tomura H, Yanagita M, Kuwabara A, Ui M, Okajima F. Interaction of sphingosine 1-phosphate with plasma components, including lipoproteins, regulates the lipid receptor-mediated actions. Biochem J 2000;352 Pt 3:809-815.

[18] Marchesini N, Hannun YA. Acid and neutral sphingomyelinases: roles and mechanisms of regulation. Biochem Cell Biol 2004;82:27-44.

[19] Kohama T, Olivera A, Edsall L, Nagiec MM, Dickson R, Spiegel S. Molecular cloning and functional characterization of murine sphingosine kinase. J Biol Chem 1998;273:23722-23728.

[20] Alvarez SE, Milstien S, Spiegel S. Autocrine and paracrine roles of sphingosine-1-phosphate. Trends Endocrinol Metab 2007;18:300-307.

[21] Spiegel S, Milstien S. Sphingosine-1-phosphate: an enigmatic signalling lipid. Nat Rev Mol Cell Biol 2003;4:397-407.

[22] Taha TA, Hannun YA, Obeid LM. Sphingosine kinase: biochemical and cellular regulation and role in disease. J Biochem Mol Biol 2006;39:113-131.

[23] Johnson KR, Becker KP, Facchinetti MM, Hannun YA, Obeid LM. PKC-dependent activation of sphingosine kinase 1 and translocation to the plasma membrane. Extracellular release of sphingosine-1-phosphate induced by phorbol 12-myristate 13-acetate (PMA). J Biol Chem 2002;277:35257-35262.

[24] Pitson SM, Xia P, Leclercq TM, Moretti PA, Zebol JR, Lynn HE, Wattenberg BW, Vadas MA. Phosphorylation-dependent translocation of sphingosine kinase to the plasma membrane drives its oncogenic signalling. J Exp Med 2005;201:49-54.

[25] Takabe K, Paugh SW, Milstien S, Spiegel S. "Inside-out" signaling of sphingosine-1-phosphate: therapeutic targets. Pharmacol Rev 2008;60:181-195.

[26] Le Stunff H, Peterson C, Liu H, Milstien S, Spiegel S. Sphingosine-1-phosphate and lipid phosphohydrolases. Biochim Biophys Acta 2002;1582:8-17.

[27] Le Stunff H, Peterson C, Thornton R, Milstien S, Mandala SM, Spiegel S. Characterization of murine sphingosine-1-phosphate phosphohydrolase. J Biol Chem 2002;277:8920-8927.

[28] Hannun YA, Luberto C, Argraves KM. Enzymes of sphingolipid metabolism: from modular to integrative signaling. Biochemistry 2001;40:4893-4903.

[29] Sandhoff K, Kolter T. Biosynthesis and degradation of mammalian glycosphingolipids. Philos Trans R Soc Lond B Biol Sci 2003;358:847-861.

[30] Kobayashi N, Nishi T, Hirata T, Kihara A, Sano T, Igarashi Y, Yamaguchi A. Sphingosine 1-phosphate is released from the cytosol of rat platelets in a carrier-mediated manner. J Lipid Res 2006;47:614-621.

[31] Mitra P, Oskeritzian CA, Payne SG, Beaven MA, Milstien S, Spiegel S. Role of ABCC1 in export of sphingosine-1-phosphate from mast cells. Proc Natl Acad Sci U S A 2006;103:16394-16399.

[32] Sato K, Malchinkhuu E, Horiuchi Y, Mogi C, Tomura H, Tosaka M, Yoshimoto Y, Kuwabara A, Okajima F. Critical role of ABCA1 transporter in sphingosine 1-phosphate release from astrocytes. J Neurochem 2007;103:2610-2619.

[33] Sanchez T, Hla T. Structural and functional characteristics of S1P receptors. J Cell Biochem 2004;92:913-922.

[34] Liu Y, Wada R, Yamashita T, Mi Y, Deng CX, Hobson JP, Rosenfeldt HM, Nava VE, Chae SS, Lee MJ, Liu CH, Hla T, Spiegel S, Proia RL. Edg-1, the G protein-coupled receptor for sphingosine-1-phosphate, is essential for vascular maturation. J Clin Invest 2000;106:951-961.

[35] Pappu R, Schwab SR, Cornelissen I, Pereira JP, Regard JB, Xu Y, Camerer E, Zheng YW, Huang Y, Cyster JG, Coughlin SR. Promotion of lymphocyte egress into blood and lymph by distinct sources of sphingosine-1-phosphate. Science 2007;316:295-298.

[36] Camerer E, Regard JB, Cornelissen I, Srinivasan Y, Duong DN, Palmer D, Pham TH, Wong JS, Pappu R, Coughlin SR. Sphingosine-1-phosphate in the plasma compartment regulates basal and inflammation-induced vascular leak in mice. J Clin Invest 2009;119:1871-1879.

[37] Ishii I, Ye X, Friedman B, Kawamura S, Contos JJ, Kingsbury MA, Yang AH, Zhang G, Brown JH, Chun J. Marked perinatal lethality and cellular signaling deficits in

mice null for the two sphingosine 1-phosphate (S1P) receptors, S1P(2)/LP(B2)/EDG-5 and S1P(3)/LP(B3)/EDG-3. J Biol Chem 2002;277:25152-25159.

[38] Wang W, Graeler MH, Goetzl EJ. Type 4 sphingosine 1-phosphate G protein-coupled receptor (S1P4) transduces S1P effects on T cell proliferation and cytokine secretion without signaling migration. FASEB J 2005;19:1731-1733.

[39] Walzer T, Chiossone L, Chaix J, Calver A, Carozzo C, Garrigue-Antar L, Jacques Y, Baratin M, Tomasello E, Vivier E. Natural killer cell trafficking in vivo requires a dedicated sphingosine 1-phosphate receptor. Nat Immunol 2007;8:1337-1344.

[40] Choi JW, Lee CW, Chun J. Biological roles of lysophospholipid receptors revealed by genetic null mice: an update. Biochim Biophys Acta 2008;1781:531-539.

[41] Rosen H, Gonzalez-Cabrera PJ, Sanna MG, Brown S. Sphingosine 1-phosphate receptor signaling. Annu Rev Biochem 2009;78:743-768.

[42] Olivera A, Rosenfeldt HM, Bektas M, Wang F, Ishii I, Chun J, Milstien S, Spiegel S. Sphingosine kinase type 1 induces G12/13-mediated stress fiber formation, yet promotes growth and survival independent of G protein-coupled receptors. J Biol Chem 2003;278:46452-46460.

[43] Taha TA, Argraves KM, Obeid LM. Sphingosine-1-phosphate receptors: receptor specificity versus functional redundancy. Biochim Biophys Acta 2004;1682:48-55.

[44] Hait NC, Allegood J, Maceyka M, Strub GM, Harikumar KB, Singh SK, Luo C, Marmorstein R, Kordula T, Milstien S, Spiegel S. Regulation of histone acetylation in the nucleus by sphingosine-1-phosphate. Science 2009;325:1254-1257.

[45] van Koppen CJ, Meyer zu Heringdorf D, Alemany R, Jakobs KH. Sphingosine kinase-mediated calcium signaling by muscarinic acetylcholine receptors. Life Sci 2001;68:2535-2540.

[46] Xia P, Wang L, Gamble JR, Vadas MA. Activation of sphingosine kinase by tumor necrosis factor-alpha inhibits apoptosis in human endothelial cells. J Biol Chem 1999;274:34499-34505.

[47] Pi X, Tan SY, Hayes M, Xiao L, Shayman JA, Ling S, Holoshitz J. Sphingosine kinase 1-mediated inhibition of Fas death signaling in rheumatoid arthritis B lymphoblastoid cells. Arthritis Rheum 2006;54:754-764.

[48] Lai WQ, Irwan AW, Goh HH, Howe HS, Yu DT, Valle-Onate R, McInnes IB, Melendez AJ, Leung BP. Anti-inflammatory effects of sphingosine kinase modulation in inflammatory arthritis. J Immunol 2008;181:8010-8017.

[49] Lai WQ, Irwan AW, Goh HH, Melendez AJ, McInnes IB, Leung BP. Distinct roles of sphingosine kinase 1 and 2 in murine collagen-induced arthritis. J Immunol 2009;183:2097-2103.

[50] Mechtcheriakova D, Wlachos A, Sobanov J, Kopp T, Reuschel R, Bornancin F, Cai R, Zemann B, Urtz N, Stingl G, Zlabinger G, Woisetschlager M, Baumruker T, Billich A.

Sphingosine 1-phosphate phosphatase 2 is induced during inflammatory responses. Cell Signal 2007;19:748-760.

[51] Feldmann M, Brennan FM, Maini RN. Role of cytokines in rheumatoid arthritis. Annu Rev Immunol 1996;14:397-440.

[52] Bartok B, Firestein GS. Fibroblast-like synoviocytes: key effector cells in rheumatoid arthritis. Immunol Rev 2010;233:233-255.

[53] Nochi H, Tomura H, Tobo M, Tanaka N, Sato K, Shinozaki T, Kobayashi T, Takagishi K, Ohta H, Okajima F, Tamoto K. Stimulatory role of lysophosphatidic acid in cyclooxygenase-2 induction by synovial fluid of patients with rheumatoid arthritis in fibroblast-like synovial cells. J Immunol 2008;181:5111-5119.

[54] Huang MC, Watson SR, Liao JJ, Goetzl EJ. Th17 augmentation in OTII TCR plus T cell-selective type 1 sphingosine 1-phosphate receptor double transgenic mice. J Immunol 2007;178:6806-6813.

[55] Raza K, Falciani F, Curnow SJ, Ross EJ, Lee CY, Akbar AN, Lord JM, Gordon C, Buckley CD, Salmon M. Early rheumatoid arthritis is characterized by a distinct and transient synovial fluid cytokine profile of T cell and stromal cell origin. Arthritis Res Ther 2005;7:R784-795.

[56] Nakae S, Nambu A, Sudo K, Iwakura Y. Suppression of immune induction of collagen-induced arthritis in IL-17-deficient mice. J Immunol 2003;171:6173-6177.

[57] Jovanovic DV, Di Battista JA, Martel-Pelletier J, Jolicoeur FC, He Y, Zhang M, Mineau F, Pelletier JP. IL-17 stimulates the production and expression of proinflammatory cytokines, IL-beta and TNF-alpha, by human macrophages. J Immunol 1998;160:3513-3521.

[58] Hwang SY, Kim HY. Expression of IL-17 homologs and their receptors in the synovial cells of rheumatoid arthritis patients. Mol Cells 2005;19:180-184.

[59] Ghosh M, Stewart A, Tucker DE, Bonventre JV, Murphy RC, Leslie CC. Role of cytosolic phospholipase A(2) in prostaglandin E(2) production by lung fibroblasts. Am J Respir Cell Mol Biol 2004;30:91-100.

[60] Ben-Av P, Crofford LJ, Wilder RL, Hla T. Induction of vascular endothelial growth factor expression in synovial fibroblasts by prostaglandin E and interleukin-1: a potential mechanism for inflammatory angiogenesis. FEBS Lett 1995;372:83-87.

[61] Mino T, Sugiyama E, Taki H, Kuroda A, Yamashita N, Maruyama M, Kobayashi M. Interleukin-1alpha and tumor necrosis factor alpha synergistically stimulate prostaglandin E2-dependent production of interleukin-11 in rheumatoid synovial fibroblasts. Arthritis Rheum 1998;41:2004-2013.

[62] Allende ML, Dreier JL, Mandala S, Proia RL. Expression of the sphingosine 1-phosphate receptor, S1P1, on T-cells controls thymic emigration. J Biol Chem 2004;279:15396-15401.

[63] Matloubian M, Lo CG, Cinamon G, Lesneski MJ, Xu Y, Brinkmann V, Allende ML, Proia RL, Cyster JG. Lymphocyte egress from thymus and peripheral lymphoid organs is dependent on S1P receptor 1. Nature 2004;427:355-360.

[64] Piali L, Froidevaux S, Hess P, Nayler O, Bolli MH, Schlosser E, Kohl C, Steiner B, Clozel M. The selective sphingosine 1-phosphate receptor 1 agonist ponesimod protects against lymphocyte-mediated tissue inflammation. J Pharmacol Exp Ther 2011;337:547-556.

[65] Chen X, Oppenheim JJ, Howard OM. Chemokines and chemokine receptors as novel therapeutic targets in rheumatoid arthritis (RA): inhibitory effects of traditional Chinese medicinal components. Cell Mol Immunol 2004;1:336-342.

[66] Zhao C, Sardella A, Chun J, Poubelle PE, Fernandes MJ, Bourgoin SG. TNF-alpha promotes LPA1- and LPA3-mediated recruitment of leukocytes in vivo through CXCR2 ligand chemokines. J Lipid Res 2011;52:1307-1318.

[67] Ospelt C, Neidhart M, Gay RE, Gay S. Synovial activation in rheumatoid arthritis. Front Biosci 2004;9:2323-2334.

[68] Firestein GS. Etiology and pathogenesis of rheumatoid arthritis. In: Firestein, GS; Budd, RC; Harris, T; McInnes, IB; Ruddy, S; Sergent, JS, editors Kelly's Textbook of Rheumatology 8. Philadelphia, PA: Saunders Elsevier; 2009:1035-1086.

[69] Pap TG, S. Fibroblasts and fibroblast-like synoviocytes. In: Firestein, GS; Budd, RC; Harris, T; McInnes, IB; Ruddy, S; Sergent, JS, editors Kelly's Textbook of Rheumatology 8 Philadelphia, PA: Saunders Elsevier; 2009:201-214.

[70] Knedla A, Neumann E, Muller-Ladner U. Developments in the synovial biology field 2006. Arthritis Res Ther 2007;9:209.

[71] Dechanet J, Merville P, Durand I, Banchereau J, Miossec P. The ability of synoviocytes to support terminal differentiation of activated B cells may explain plasma cell accumulation in rheumatoid synovium. J Clin Invest 1995;95:456-463.

[72] Hayashida K, Shimaoka Y, Ochi T, Lipsky PE. Rheumatoid arthritis synovial stromal cells inhibit apoptosis and up-regulate Bcl-xL expression by B cells in a CD49/CD29-CD106-dependent mechanism. J Immunol 2000;164:1110-1116.

[73] Schroder AE, Greiner A, Seyfert C, Berek C. Differentiation of B cells in the nonlymphoid tissue of the synovial membrane of patients with rheumatoid arthritis. Proc Natl Acad Sci U S A 1996;93:221-225.

[74] Takemura S, Klimiuk PA, Braun A, Goronzy JJ, Weyand CM. T cell activation in rheumatoid synovium is B cell dependent. J Immunol 2001;167:4710-4718.

[75] Steiner G, Smolen J. Autoantibodies in rheumatoid arthritis and their clinical significance. Arthritis Res 2002;4 Suppl 2:S1-5.

[76] Edwards JC, Szczepanski L, Szechinski J, Filipowicz-Sosnowska A, Emery P, Close DR, Stevens RM, Shaw T. Efficacy of B-cell-targeted therapy with rituximab in patients with rheumatoid arthritis. N Engl J Med 2004;350:2572-2581.

[77] Kim MK, Lee HY, Kwak JY, Park JI, Yun J, Bae YS. Sphingosine-1-phosphate stimulates rat primary chondrocyte proliferation. Biochem Biophys Res Commun 2006;345:67-73.

[78] Masuko K, Murata M, Nakamura H, Yudoh K, Nishioka K, Kato T. Sphingosine-1-phosphate attenuates proteoglycan aggrecan expression via production of prostaglandin E2 from human articular chondrocytes. BMC Musculoskelet Disord 2007;8:29.

[79] Scott DL. Prognostic factors in early rheumatoid arthritis. Rheumatology (Oxford) 2000;39 Suppl 1:24-29.

[80] Takahashi N, Akatsu T, Udagawa N, Sasaki T, Yamaguchi A, Moseley JM, Martin TJ, Suda T. Osteoblastic cells are involved in osteoclast formation. Endocrinology 1988;123:2600-2602.

[81] Tanaka S, Takahashi N, Udagawa N, Tamura T, Akatsu T, Stanley ER, Kurokawa T, Suda T. Macrophage colony-stimulating factor is indispensable for both proliferation and differentiation of osteoclast progenitors. J Clin Invest 1993;91:257-263.

[82] Harada S, Rodan GA. Control of osteoblast function and regulation of bone mass. Nature 2003;423:349-355.

[83] Teitelbaum SL, Ross FP. Genetic regulation of osteoclast development and function. Nat Rev Genet 2003;4:638-649.

[84] Wada T, Nakashima T, Hiroshi N, Penninger JM. RANKL-RANK signaling in osteoclastogenesis and bone disease. Trends Mol Med 2006;12:17-25.

[85] Kong YY, Yoshida H, Sarosi I, Tan HL, Timms E, Capparelli C, Morony S, Oliveira-dos-Santos AJ, Van G, Itie A, Khoo W, Wakeham A, Dunstan CR, Lacey DL, Mak TW, Boyle WJ, Penninger JM. OPGL is a key regulator of osteoclastogenesis, lymphocyte development and lymph-node organogenesis. Nature 1999;397:315-323.

[86] Lacey DL, Timms E, Tan HL, Kelley MJ, Dunstan CR, Burgess T, Elliott R, Colombero A, Elliott G, Scully S, Hsu H, Sullivan J, Hawkins N, Davy E, Capparelli C, Eli A, Qian YX, Kaufman S, Sarosi I, Shalhoub V, Senaldi G, Guo J, Delaney J, Boyle WJ. Osteoprotegerin ligand is a cytokine that regulates osteoclast differentiation and activation. Cell 1998;93:165-176.

[87] Kuratani T, Nagata K, Kukita T, Hotokebuchi T, Nakasima A, Iijima T. Induction of abundant osteoclast-like multinucleated giant cells in adjuvant arthritic rats with accompanying disordered high bone turnover. Histol Histopathol 1998;13:751-759.

[88] Suzuki Y, Nishikaku F, Nakatuka M, Koga Y. Osteoclast-like cells in murine collagen induced arthritis. J Rheumatol 1998;25:1154-1160.

[89] Walsh NC, Gravallese EM. Bone loss in inflammatory arthritis: mechanisms and treatment strategies. Curr Opin Rheumatol 2004;16:419-427.

[90] Ryu J, Kim HJ, Chang EJ, Huang H, Banno Y, Kim HH. Sphingosine 1-phosphate as a regulator of osteoclast differentiation and osteoclast-osteoblast coupling. EMBO J 2006;25:5840-5851.

[91] Ishii M, Kikuta J, Shimazu Y, Meier-Schellersheim M, Germain RN. Chemorepulsion by blood S1P regulates osteoclast precursor mobilization and bone remodeling in vivo. J Exp Med 2010; 207:2793-2798.

[92] Ishii M, Egen JG, Klauschen F, Meier-Schellersheim M, Saeki Y, Vacher J, Proia RL, Germain RN. Sphingosine-1-phosphate mobilizes osteoclast precursors and regulates bone homeostasis. Nature 2009;458:524-528.

[93] Matsuura M, Imayoshi T, Okumoto T. Effect of FTY720, a novel immunosuppressant, on adjuvant- and collagen-induced arthritis in rats. Int J Immunopharmacol 2000;22:323-331.

[94] Wang F, Tan W, Guo D, He S. Reduction of CD4 positive T cells and improvement of pathological changes of collagen-induced arthritis by FTY720. Eur J Pharmacol 2007;573:230-240.

[95] Baker DA, Barth J, Chang R, Obeid LM, Gilkeson GS. Genetic sphingosine kinase 1 deficiency significantly decreases synovial inflammation and joint erosions in murine TNF-alpha-induced arthritis. J Immunol 2010;185:2570-2579.

[96] Bingham CO, 3rd. Emerging therapeutics for rheumatoid arthritis. Bull NYU Hosp Jt Dis 2008;66:210-215.

[97] Billich A, Bornancin F, Mechtcheriakova D, Natt F, Huesken D, Baumruker T. Basal and induced sphingosine kinase 1 activity in A549 carcinoma cells: function in cell survival and IL-1beta and TNF-alpha induced production of inflammatory mediators. Cell Signal 2005;17:1203-1217.

[98] Bonhoure E, Pchejetski D, Aouali N, Morjani H, Levade T, Kohama T, Cuvillier O. Overcoming MDR-associated chemoresistance in HL-60 acute myeloid leukemia cells by targeting sphingosine kinase-1. Leukemia 2006;20:95-102.

[99] French KJ, Upson JJ, Keller SN, Zhuang Y, Yun JK, Smith CD. Antitumor activity of sphingosine kinase inhibitors. J Pharmacol Exp Ther 2006;318:596-603.

[100] Gamble JR, Xia P, Hahn CN, Drew JJ, Drogemuller CJ, Brown D, Vadas MA. Phenoxodiol, an experimental anticancer drug, shows potent antiangiogenic properties in addition to its antitumour effects. Int J Cancer 2006;118:2412-2420.

[101] Leroux ME, Auzenne E, Evans R, Hail N, Jr., Spohn W, Ghosh SC, Farquhar D, McDonnell T, Klostergaard J. Sphingolipids and the sphingosine kinase inhibitor, SKI II, induce BCL-2-independent apoptosis in human prostatic adenocarcinoma cells. Prostate 2007;67:1699-1717.

[102] Graler MH, Goetzl EJ. The immunosuppressant FTY720 down-regulates sphingosine 1-phosphate G-protein-coupled receptors. FASEB J 2004;18:551-553.

[103] Sabbadini RA. Targeting sphingosine-1-phosphate for cancer therapy. Br J Cancer 2006;95:1131-1135.

[104] Visentin B, Vekich JA, Sibbald BJ, Cavalli AL, Moreno KM, Matteo RG, Garland WA, Lu Y, Yu S, Hall HS, Kundra V, Mills GB, Sabbadini RA. Validation of an anti-sphingosine-1-phosphate antibody as a potential therapeutic in reducing growth, invasion, and angiogenesis in multiple tumor lineages. Cancer Cell 2006;9:225-238.

[105] Schwab SR, Pereira JP, Matloubian M, Xu Y, Huang Y, Cyster JG. Lymphocyte sequestration through S1P lyase inhibition and disruption of S1P gradients. Science 2005;309:1735-1739.

[106] Lo CG, Xu Y, Proia RL, Cyster JG. Cyclical modulation of sphingosine-1-phosphate receptor 1 surface expression during lymphocyte recirculation and relationship to lymphoid organ transit. J Exp Med 2005;201:291-301.

[107] Gardell SE, Dubin AE, Chun J. Emerging medicinal roles for lysophospholipid signaling. Trends Mol Med 2006;12:65-75.

[108] Huwiler A, Pfeilschifter J. New players on the center stage: sphingosine 1-phosphate and its receptors as drug targets. Biochem Pharmacol 2008;75:1893-1900.

[109] Mandala S, Hajdu R, Bergstrom J, Quackenbush E, Xie J, Milligan J, Thornton R, Shei GJ, Card D, Keohane C, Rosenbach M, Hale J, Lynch CL, Rupprecht K, Parsons W, Rosen H. Alteration of lymphocyte trafficking by sphingosine-1-phosphate receptor agonists. Science 2002;296:346-349.

[110] Rosen H, Alfonso C, Surh CD, McHeyzer-Williams MG. Rapid induction of medullary thymocyte phenotypic maturation and egress inhibition by nanomolar sphingosine 1-phosphate receptor agonist. Proc Natl Acad Sci U S A 2003;100:10907-10912.

[111] Zhang Z, Schluesener HJ. FTY720: a most promising immunosuppressant modulating immune cell functions. Mini Rev Med Chem 2007;7:845-850.

[112] Bagdanoff JT, Donoviel MS, Nouraldeen A, Tarver J, Fu Q, Carlsen M, Jessop TC, Zhang H, Hazelwood J, Nguyen H, Baugh SD, Gardyan M, Terranova KM, Barbosa J, Yan J, Bednarz M, Layek S, Courtney LF, Taylor J, Digeorge-Foushee AM, Gopinathan S, Bruce D, Smith T, Moran L, O'Neill E, Kramer J, Lai Z, Kimball SD, Liu Q, Sun W, Yu S, Swaffield J, Wilson A, Main A, Carson KG, Oravecz T, Augeri DJ. Inhibition of sphingosine-1-phosphate lyase for the treatment of autoimmune disorders. J Med Chem 2009;52:3941-3953.

[113] Bandhuvula P, Fyrst H, Saba JD. A rapid fluorescence assay for sphingosine-1-phosphate lyase enzyme activity. J Lipid Res 2007;48:2769-2778.

[114] Vogel P, Donoviel MS, Read R, Hansen GM, Hazlewood J, Anderson SJ, Sun W, Swaffield J, Oravecz T. Incomplete inhibition of sphingosine 1-phosphate lyase mod-

ulates immune system function yet prevents early lethality and non-lymphoid lesions. PLoS One 2009;4:e4112.

[115] Fleischmann R. Novel small-molecular therapeutics for rheumatoid arthritis. Curr Opin Rheumatol 2012;24:335-341.

[116] Gonzalez-Cabrera PJ, Hla T, Rosen H. Mapping pathways downstream of sphingosine 1-phosphate subtype 1 by differential chemical perturbation and proteomics. J Biol Chem 2007;282:7254-7264.

[117] Oo ML, Thangada S, Wu MT, Liu CH, Macdonald TL, Lynch KR, Lin CY, Hla T. Immunosuppressive and anti-angiogenic sphingosine 1-phosphate receptor-1 agonists induce ubiquitinylation and proteasomal degradation of the receptor. J Biol Chem 2007;282:9082-9089.

[118] Fukuhara S, Simmons S, Kawamura S, Inoue A, Orba Y, Tokudome T, Sunden Y, Arai Y, Moriwaki K, Ishida J, Uemura A, Kiyonari H, Abe T, Fukamizu A, Hirashima M, Sawa H, Aoki J, Ishii M, Mochizuki N. The sphingosine-1-phosphate transporter Spns2 expressed on endothelial cells regulates lymphocyte trafficking in mice. J Clin Invest 2012;122:1416-1426.

[119] Okamoto H, Takuwa N, Yokomizo T, Sugimoto N, Sakurada S, Shigematsu H, Takuwa Y. Inhibitory regulation of Rac activation, membrane ruffling, and cell migration by the G protein-coupled sphingosine-1-phosphate receptor EDG5 but not EDG1 or EDG3. Mol Cell Biol 2000;20:9247-9261.

[120] Pham TH, Okada T, Matloubian M, Lo CG, Cyster JG. S1P1 receptor signaling overrides retention mediated by G alpha i-coupled receptors to promote T cell egress. Immunity 2008;28:122-133.

[121] Sawicka E, Dubois G, Jarai G, Edwards M, Thomas M, Nicholls A, Albert R, Newson C, Brinkmann V, Walker C. The sphingosine 1-phosphate receptor agonist FTY720 differentially affects the sequestration of CD4+/CD25+ T-regulatory cells and enhances their functional activity. J Immunol 2005;175:7973-7980.

[122] LaMontagne K, Littlewood-Evans A, Schnell C, O'Reilly T, Wyder L, Sanchez T, Probst B, Butler J, Wood A, Liau G, Billy E, Theuer A, Hla T, Wood J. Antagonism of sphingosine-1-phosphate receptors by FTY720 inhibits angiogenesis and tumor vascularization. Cancer Res 2006;66:221-231.

[123] Schmid G, Guba M, Ischenko I, Papyan A, Joka M, Schrepfer S, Bruns CJ, Jauch KW, Heeschen C, Graeb C. The immunosuppressant FTY720 inhibits tumor angiogenesis via the sphingosine 1-phosphate receptor 1. J Cell Biochem 2007;101:259-270.

[124] Cinamon G, Matloubian M, Lesneski MJ, Xu Y, Low C, Lu T, Proia RL, Cyster JG. Sphingosine 1-phosphate receptor 1 promotes B cell localization in the splenic marginal zone. Nat Immunol 2004;5:713-720.

[125] Kahan BD. Frontiers in immunosuppression. Transplant Proc 2008;40:11-15.

[126] Kappos L, Antel J, Comi G, Montalban X, O'Connor P, Polman CH, Haas T, Korn AA, Karlsson G, Radue EW. Oral fingolimod (FTY720) for relapsing multiple sclerosis. N Engl J Med 2006;355:1124-1140.

[127] Cohen JA, Barkhof F, Comi G, Hartung HP, Khatri BO, Montalban X, Pelletier J, Capra R, Gallo P, Izquierdo G, Tiel-Wilck K, de Vera A, Jin J, Stites T, Wu S, Aradhye S, Kappos L. Oral fingolimod or intramuscular interferon for relapsing multiple sclerosis. N Engl J Med 2010;362:402-415.

[128] Kappos L, Radue EW, O'Connor P, Polman C, Hohlfeld R, Calabresi P, Selmaj K, Agoropoulou C, Leyk M, Zhang-Auberson L, Burtin P. A placebo-controlled trial of oral fingolimod in relapsing multiple sclerosis. N Engl J Med 2010;362:387-401.

[129] Martin R. Multiple sclerosis: closing in on an oral treatment. Nature 2010;464:360-362.

[130] Tsunemi S, Iwasaki T, Kitano S, Imado T, Miyazawa K, Sano H. Effects of the novel immunosuppressant FTY720 in a murine rheumatoid arthritis model. Clin Immunol 2010;136:197-204.

[131] Matsuura M, Imayoshi T, Chiba K, Okumoto T. Effect of FTY720, a novel immunosuppressant, on adjuvant-induced arthritis in rats. Inflamm Res 2000;49:404-410.

[132] Terato K, Hasty KA, Reife RA, Cremer MA, Kang AH, Stuart JM. Induction of arthritis with monoclonal antibodies to collagen. J Immunol 1992;148:2103-2108.

Chapter 2

New Therapeutic Targets for the Control of Inflammatory Arthritis: A Pivotal Role for Endothelins

Maria das Graças Muller de Oliveira Henriques

Additional information is available at the end of the chapter

http://dx.doi.org/10.5772/53738

1. Introduction

Rheumatoid arthritis (RA) is a complex, debilitating, chronic, systemic autoimmune disease characterised by immunological, inflammatory and mesenchymal tissue reactions in the synovium that are accompanied by polyarticular synovitis and ultimately lead to the progressive destruction of articular and periarticular structures [1,2]. A critical factor that contributes to joint damage is the excessive production of inflammatory mediators by resident and/or infiltrating inflammatory cells. Among the main mediators involved in the join damage process are free radicals, extracellular matrix–degrading enzymes, pro-inflammatory cytokines, including interleukin(IL)-6, IL-1 and tumour necrosis factor (TNF)-α, as well as chemokines, such as CXCL1, and lipid mediators, such as leukotriene (LT)B_4 [3,4,5].

Endothelins (ETs) are a family of naturally occurring peptides [6] with well-established growth-promoting, vasoactive, and nociceptive properties that affect the function of a number of tissues and systems [7]. ETs have pathophysiological roles in pulmonary hypertension, arterial hypertension, atherosclerosis, cerebral vasospasm and inflammatory processes [8,9,10,11].

Recently, new evidence has demonstrated that endogenous endothelins (ETs) also play a role in articular inflammation by regulating inflammatory pain, edema formation, leukocyte influx and the production of inflammatory mediators. The present chapter attempts to provide an overview of the evidence accumulated to date, which suggests that ETs play a pivotal role in articular inflammation, and the blockade of these endogenous peptides can represent a promising therapeutic tool for the treatment of RA and other articular inflammatory diseases. To address this issue in a comprehensive manner, however, it is important to briefly provide some fundamental aspects of endothelin biosynthesis and release as well as information about the receptors that they interact with and the modes of action of these peptides.

2. The endothelin system

The endothelin system comprises a family of three highly conserved vasoactive peptides, which bind to two endothelin receptors (endothelin receptor types A [ETA] and B [ETB]), with differing affinities that are determined by the N-terminal domain of the peptide. ET-1 has a higher affinity than ET-2, which, in turn, has a higher affinity than ET-3. In humans, the affinity of ET-1 for the ETA receptor is 1,000-fold higher than that of ET-3 [12] (Fig 1).

ET -1, the most prominent representative of the ET family, was first identified as a potent vasoconstrictor secreted by vascular endothelial cells [13]. Since the initial description of ET-1 [14], it has become evident that in addition to modulating vascular tone, ET peptides are also involved in numerous other pathophysiological processes and are produced not only by endothelial cells but by a wide variety of cells in virtually all organs [7] (Table 1).

Tissue	Cell type	Reference
Lung	Alveolar epithelium	[15-17]
Liver	Hepatocytes	[18]
	Kupffer cells	
Skin	fibroblast	[19, 20]
Synovia	synoviocytes	[21, 22]
Heart	myocytes	[23]

Table 1. Localization of ET system in different cells

Numerous lines of evidence indicate that ET-1 acts locally via both autocrine and paracrine mechanisms in physiological and pathological situations. Contribution of the ET system to disease progression can occur due to either an increase in tissue ET-1 production or an increase in the tissue expression of its receptors. ET-1 is upregulated by angiotensin II, vasopressin, thrombin, lipopolysaccharide, insulin, TGF-β, epithelial growth factor, and EGF-2 and is downregulated by nitric oxide, prostaglandin, and natriuretic hormone [24, 25].

The release of endothelins is regulated both at the gene expression level and at the peptide synthesis level. Preproendothelins are synthesized via the transcriptional activation of the preproendothelin gene, which is regulated by c-fos and c-jun, nuclear factor-1, AP-1 and GATA-2 [26, 27]. The translational product is a 203-amino acid peptide known as preproendothelin, which is cleaved at dibasic sites by furin-like endopeptidases to form big endothelins. These biologically inactive 37- to 41-amino acid intermediates [25] are cleaved at Trp21–Val 22 by a family of endothelin-converting enzymes (ECE) to produce mature ET-1 [28, 29] (Fig 1). Three isoforms of ECE have been reported [30]: ECE-1, ECE-2 and ECE-3. Four variants of ECE-1 have been reported in humans [31], ECE-1a ECE-1b, ECE-1c and ECE-1d, which are the result of alternative splicing of ECE-1 mRNA. Interestingly, chymase, the mast cell-derived serine protease, also hydrolyses big ET-1 [1–38] into the intermediate peptide ET-1 [1–31] which is then readily transformed to ET-1 by neutral endopeptidase 24-11 (NEP) in tissue homogenates [32]. Recently, the chymase-dependent production of ET-1 was proposed to play an important role in cardiovascular and pulmonary pathologies [7, 33].

The ETA and ETB receptors belong to the superfamily of G-protein–coupled receptors with seven transmembrane domains and are differentially expressed according to cell type [34, 35]. The ETA receptor is found predominantly in smooth muscle cells and cardiac muscles [36]. Both receptors, however, have a fairly widespread distribution across many cell types (Table 2)

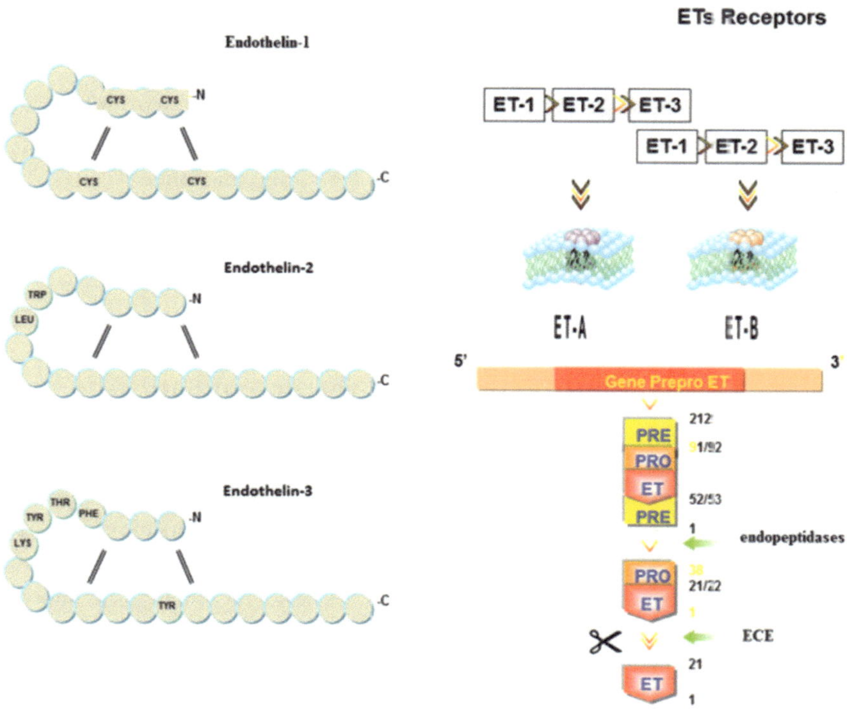

Figure 1. Endothelin structure, receptors and production

3. Endothelin signaling

The detailed mechanism by which ET induces intracellular responses remains unclear. ET receptor activation leads to diverse cellular responses through interaction with a chain of pathways that includes the G-protein-activated cell surface receptor, the coupling of G-proteins and the phospholipase (PLC) pathway as well as other G protein-activated effectors. In one of the canonical signalling pathways, ETA induced activation of phospholipase C leads to the formation of inositol triphosphate and diacylglycerol from phosphatidylinositol. Inositol

1,4,5-triphosphate (IP3] then diffuses to specific receptors on the endoplasmic reticulum and releases stored Ca2+ into the cytosol. This causes a rapid elevation in intracellular Ca2+, which, in turn, causes cellular contraction, followed by vasoconstriction [37-39].

Additionally, ET-1 is known to stimulate arachidonic acid production and prostaglandin release in rabbit iris [40], porcine coronary artery [41] and mouse paw [42]. This occurs as a result of the activation of phospholipase A2 and increased intracellular Ca2+ [43].

In addition to phospholipase activation and prostaglandin production, endothelin-1 also stimulates protein tyrosine kinases (PTK), such as FAK and RAS, in neoplastic cells [44]. The activation of PTKs results in the induction of the RAF/MEK/MAPK pathway, which subsequently stimulates the transcription of proto-oncogenes, such as c-FOS, c-MYC, c-JUN, and, in turn, activates cell growth and metastasis.

Nitric oxide (NO) is a versatile molecule with a multitude of functions, including the regulation of vascular tone, neuronal signalling and host defence [45]. In a classic ET-1 signalling pathway, ET-1 stimulates NO production in endothelial cells by activating endothelial cell NO synthase (eNOS) [46, 47] via PI3-K/Akt activation, which in turn, stimulates the phosphorylation of eNOS and subsequent NO production [47]. Interestingly, NO appears to antagonize ET-1 synthesis by inhibiting preproET-1 transcription [48].

4. Evidence for the involvement of ET-1 in rheumatoid arthritis

ET-1 has been demonstrated to participate in the pathogenesis of a number of diseases, such as sepsis, bronchial asthma and pulmonary hypertension [49]. In addition to their well-recognised vasoconstrictive properties, ETs play an important role in inflammatory reactions modulating hyperalgesia, edema formation [50-52] and cell migration [53, 54]. Considering their pro-inflammatory properties and the presence of ETs in the plasma and synovial fluid from RA patients, the participation of ETs in RA is strongly indicated. These findings will be described in the following sections.

5. Presence of endothelins in plasma and synovial fluid from human RA patients

High levels of ET-1 are detected in the synovial fluid of RA, osteoarthritis (OA), and gout patients. Plasma levels of ET-1 in patients with active RA exceed the values in patients with non-active RA. Moreover, ET-1 is secreted from macrophage-like synoviocytes, and the levels of ET-1-like immunoreactivity in synovial fluid are several times higher than those in plasma [21, 22, 55, 56]. In addition, specific 125I-labeled-ET-1-binding sites that are characteristic of the ETA receptor were localised to the media of the synovial blood vessels in sections of rheumatoid, osteoarthritic, and normal synovium, suggesting that endothelin may act locally to modulate synovial perfusion and exacerbate hypoxia in chronic arthritis.[Table 2].

Disease	Source	Number of patients	References
Gout	Serum	81	[58]
Rheumatoid Arthritis	Serum	20, 397, 23	[55, 59]
	Plasma	12	[60, 61]
	Synovial Fluid	20	[55-57]
Hypertrophic osteoarthropathy	Plasma	20	[62]

Table 2. Presence of ET-1 Serum, Pasma or Synovial Fluid from Patients

6. Evidences from *in vitro* studies

Exogenous ET-1 presents a remarkable variety of inflammatory properties, including the activation of resident and inflammatory cells and the stimulation of cytokine production [11, 63, 64], (table 3).

Accordingly, increased expression of the preproET-1 gene and significant amounts of endothelin-1 are produced by resident cells of the synovia, including endothelial cells of the synovial blood vessels [57], fibroblasts [65], articular chondrocytes [66-70], macrophage-like synoviocyte and fibroblast-like synoviocytes [21, 22].

ET-1 modulates the expression of adhesion molecules on endothelial cells and on fibroblast-like synovial cells [65], stimulates the production of fibronectin and collagen in synoviocytes [65, 71],), stimulates cytokine production on monocytes and macrophages [53, 72, 73], and regulates neutrophil adhesion and migration [9, 53, 74].

Cell Type	Effect
Endothelial cells	Production of reactive oxygen species, TNF-α, IL-1, IL-6, NO, PGE2 Expression of ICAM-1, VCAM-1, E-Selectin
Fibroblasts	Production of reactive oxygen species, proliferation, resistance to apoptosis
Macrophages	Production of TNF-α, IL-1, IL-6, IL-8, GMCSF, reactive oxygen species, Chemotaxis
Mast Cells	Degranulation, release of histamine, production of LTC_4
Neutrophils	Agregation, chemotaxis, release of PAF, elastase

Table 3. Effect of exogenous ET-1 on different cells types

In addition to its pro-inflammatory effects, ET-1 is mitogenic to articular chondrocytes [75] and activates these cells. ET-1 binds to the specific endothelin A or endothelin B receptors expressed on chondrocytes [76, 77] and triggers a cascade of intracellular events, including phospholipase C activation [75] and the phosphorylation of p38, Akt, p44/42, and SAP/JNK, in a sequential manner [78] thereby inducing an increase in intracellular calcium [75, 79] and prostaglandin production [66]. ET-1 causes the overproduction of nitric oxide (NO) and metalloproteinase (MMP)-1 and -13 in human osteoarthritic chondrocytes [80]. The production of these enzymes seems to occur through the activation of at least two kinases, p38 MAP kinase and PKA [78]. NO seems to be a key molecule that is produced in parallel with the ET-1-induced overproduction of MMPs

Additionally, ET-1 also increases collagenase activity and decreases protein levels of tissue inhibitor of metalloproteinases 1 (TIMP-1), leading to type II collagen breakdown [81]. The endothelin-1 receptors expressed in articular chondrocytes can be up-regulated by the growth factors PDGF, EGF, IGF-1 and TGFα, which are increased in the synovial fluid of RA patients [68, 77].

It is interesting to note the age-related differences in the production of ET-1 and the expression of receptors from chondrocytes. *In vitro* studies have shown that chondrocytes obtained from older donors produce more ET-1 and express more ET-1-specific receptors (as shown by binding assays) both under basal conditions and after challenge with IL-1β or TNF-α, possibly implicating ET-1 in age-related osteoarthritis [69].

Thus, blocking the effects of ET-1 may become a useful therapeutic approach aimed at stopping cartilage destruction in rheumatic conditions such as rheumatoid arthritis and OA

7. Evidence from *in vivo* studies

Active rheumatoid arthritis is characterised by a strong inflammatory reaction and hyperplasia of synovial tissue that is an unremitting and profoundly debilitating consequence of the disease and can lead to substantial loss of function and mobility. [82, 83]. In this regard, ETs are well documented as participating in a wide variety of inflammatory and/or pain-related processes (for summary see table 4).

Animal Model	Effect	References
Paw oedema	Edema	[52, 84, 85]
	Nociception	[86-90]
	Hyperalgesia	[42, 91, 92]
Mouse cheek model	Nociception	[55, 59, 93]
Pleurisy	Cell migration/ Cytokine production	[53, 73, 85, 94]
knee-joint inflammation	Hyperalgesia/edema	[95-100]
surgical osteoarthritis	nociception	[95]

Table 4. Endothelins in Vascular Permeability and Pain.

8. Effects of exogenous endothelins in vascular permeability and pain

ET-related peptides induce profound effects on the microvasculature *in vivo,* acting as powerful constrictors of arterioles and venules [101-103] and decreasing blood flow in rabbit and human skin [103, 104]. Exogenous ETs exhibit dual effects on vascular permeability that at first glance could be considered to be paradoxical.

Early reports demonstrated a marked inhibitory effect of ET-1 (when administered locally or intradermally) on vascular permeability. ET-1 inhibited plasma extravasation that was induced in rat or rabbit dorsal skin by several stimuli [105, 106]. ET-1 (0.5 pmol/site) also inhibited paw edema and pleural exudation induced by PAF in mice [107]. Notably, the studies that describe the anti-edematogenic effect of ETs have used the local or intradermic administration of low concentrations of ET-1 (between 0.01 pmol to 0.05 pmol). The mechanisms involved in this effect are not clear and may be a consequence of local vasoconstriction or may be explained by the differential effects of ETs on the smooth muscle of arterial and venous vasculature [108]. Nevertheless, the anti-edematogenic effect of exogenous ETs appears to be dependent both on concentration and on the vascular beds.

There are compelling data describing the edematogenic properties of exogenous ET-1. The vasoconstriction effect of ET-1 may actually be masking an edematogenic effect of the peptide because it was also found that ET-1 causes a flare reaction and oedema surrounding the ischaemic area in the human forearm [109, 110]. Accordingly, endothelin-1 (up to 10 pmol) is able to induce ETA receptor mediated oedema in the mouse hind paw [85, 87]. ET-1 markedly enhances extravasation of plasma proteins from the microvasculature in distal organs when administered intravenously [51, 111-113]. This effect is mediated indirectly via the release of PAF and TXA2 in response to ETA receptor activation [112, 114-116]. Endothelin-1 enhances neutrophil adhesion to human coronary artery endothelial cells via ETA receptors [54]. ET-1(1–30 pmol/cavity) or sarafotoxin S6c [0.1–30 pmol/cavity) also triggered edema formation and neutrophil accumulation within 6 h when injected in the synovial cavity [117].

The nociceptive properties of exogenous ET-1 are also well described. Human subjects report a deep burning pain and tenderness following ET-1 injection into the forearm [50, 109]. Recent results confirm that exogenous ET-1 is capable of evoking acute pain in humans. Spontaneous pain was found to develop rapidly after intradermal injection of ET-1 into the volar aspect of the forearm of healthy males at high concentrations (10^{-7} and 10^{-6} M). It decreasing gradually, ending 30 and 60 min after ET-1 administration, respectively [118].

Endothelin-1 triggers ETA receptor-mediated nociception, hyperalgesia and oedema in the mouse hind paw [87]. In mice, ET-1 also causes ETA receptor-mediated enhancement of capsaicin-induced nociception [86], potentiates formalin-induced nociception and paw edema [86, 119] and prostate cancer-induced pain [120].

Endothelin-1 also causes articular nociception as well as hyperalgesia to prostaglandin E2 in dogs [50] and carrageenan in rats [98] when injected into a naive knee-joint. Nociception induced by endothelin-1 in the naive articulation of the rat is mediated largely via ETA receptors [42, 99], whereas both ETA and ETB receptors underlie its action in the joint primed (pre-inflamed) with carrageenan. Interestingly, ET-1 peptide-induced hypernociception was not altered by the inhibition of neutrophil migration or ET(B) receptor antagonism but rather by ET(A) receptor antagonism. Furthermore, LPS-induced nociception in the carrageenan-primed joint of the rat is largely mediated by endothelin release and the activation of ETB receptors within the joint itself [98]. The pro-nociceptive role of ETB receptors was confirmed by the fact that when its highly selective agonist, sarafotoxin S6c [34], was injected 72 h after priming with carrageenan, pain was increased, indicating incapacitation. Surprisingly, sarafotoxin produced an anti-nociceptive effect when it was given 24 h before either the initial injection of carrageenan into the naive joint or restimulation of the primed joint with carrageenan, ET-1, or S6c [96]. ETB activation exerts an apparent prophylactic action, inhibiting the development of inflammatory (carrageenan-induced) pain. In addition, ETB receptor-operated mechanisms limit the priming effect of carrageenan to nociception evoked by subsequent inflammatory insult. These findings dramatically illustrate the dual pro- and anti-nociceptive roles of the ETB receptors under the same inflammatory conditions. These roles are dependent upon the order in which these stimulus occur.

9. Effects of endogenous endothelins in inflammatory process

Consistent with the observed pro-inflammatory effects of endothelins, the studies with ETA and ETB receptor antagonists have confirmed the role of endothelins in a wide range of inflammatory reactions.

ETA receptor antagonists inhibit allergic paw oedema in mice and plasma extravasation during endotoxin shock in rats [121]. The ETA receptor antagonist BQ-123 inhibits eosinophil migration and lymphocyte accumulation in allergic pleurisy. BQ-123 also inhibited interleukin-5 levels in the exudate and plasma, as well as intracellular staining of interleukin-4, interleukin-5, and interferon-gamma in CD4+ lymphocytes [73]. Endogenous endothelins also participate in delayed eosinophil and neutrophil recruitment in murine pleurisy. Mononuclear and eosinophil accumulation triggered by OVA were reduced by BQ-123 (150 pmol/cavity) or bosentan (by 68 and 43% inhibition of eosinophilia) but were unaffected BQ-788, the ETB receptor antagonist. BQ-123 and bosentan also inhibited LPS-induced increases in neutrophils (by 67 and 40%) and eosinophils (by 63 and 74%) at 24 h [53, 94] and abrogated the increase in tumour necrosis factor alpha, interleukin-6 and keratinocyte-derived chemokine/CXC chemokine ligand 1 4 h after LPS stimulation [74].

Endogenous endothelins contribute to ovalbumin elicited nociceptive responses in the hind paw of sensitised mice, which are mediated locally by IL-15-triggered ETA and ETB receptor mechanisms [42, 88, 122]. Interestingly, ET-1 peptide-induced hypernociception was not altered by the inhibition of neutrophil migration or ET(B) receptor antagonism but rather by ET(A) receptor antagonism. Furthermore, ET(A), but not ET(B), receptor antagonism inhibited antigen-induced PGE[2] production, whereas either the selective or combined blockade of ET(A) and/or ET(B) receptors reduced antigen challenge-induced hypernociception and neutrophil recruitment [122].

http://dx.doi.org/10.5772/53738

10. Protective effect of the dual ET receptor antagonist on RA in animal models

As indicated above, exogenous ET-1 exhibits well established inflammatory properties and elicits acute nociception. There is also compelling evidence that endogenous endothelins play a role in different aspects of the inflammatory reaction and hyperalgesia. However, the implication of endothelins in the inflammatory process during experimental rheumatoid arthritis was only recently addressed. Most of these studies used the selective ETA receptor antagonist BQ123, the selective ETB receptor antagonist BQ788, or the dual ET receptor antagonist bosentan, which is the prototype sentan-class drug and was first approved by the US Food and Drug Administration (FDA) for human use in pulmonary arterial hypertension [123, 124].

In the murine model of zymosan-induced arthritis, the intra-articular administration of selective ETA or ETB receptor antagonists (BQ-123 and BQ-788, respectively) markedly reduced knee joint edema formation and neutrophil influx into the synovial cavity 6 and 24 h after stimulation. Moreover, increased expression of pre-pro-ET-1 mRNA and the ETA and ETB receptors in knee joint synovial tissue was observed in parallel with the inflammatory process [117]. Likewise, the dual blockade of ETA/ETB with bosentan (10 mg/kg, i.v.) also reduced edema formation and neutrophil counts 6 h after zymosan stimulation. Pretreatment with BQ-123 or BQ-788 (i.a.; 15 pmol/cavity) also decreased zymosan-induced TNF production within 6 h, keratinocyte-derived chemokine/CXCL1 production within 24 h, and leukotriene B4 at both time points. These findings suggest that endogenous ETs contribute to knee joint inflammation, acting through ETA and ETB receptors to modulate edema formation, neutrophil recruitment, and the production of inflammatory mediators [117].

Daily oral administration of bosentan significantly attenuated knee joint swelling and inflammation to an extent that was comparable to dexamethasone in antigen-induced arthritis (AIA). In addition, bosentan reduced inflammatory mechanical hyperalgesia. Chronic bosentan administration also inhibited joint swelling and protected against inflammation and joint destruction during AIA flare-up reactions. Unlike in the zymosan-induced arthritis model, the use of the ETA-selective antagonist ambrisentan failed to promote any detectable anti-inflammatory or antinociceptive activity in the AIA study [125].

Moreover, the lipid anti-inflammatory mediator lipoxin A_4 was described as exerting anti-inflammatory effects on articular inflammation, inhibiting oedema and neutrophil influx and the levels of preproET-1 mRNA, KC/CXCL1, LTB_4 and TNF-α through a mechanism that involved the inhibition of ET-1 expression and its effects. Likewise, lipoxin A_4 treatment also inhibited ET-1-induced oedema formation and neutrophil influx into mouse knee joints [126].

The efficacy of the dual ET receptor antagonist bosentan was described in the collagen-induced arthritis (CIA) model, which is the animal model that best resembles human RA [127]. Oral treatment with bosentan (100 mg/kg) markedly ameliorated the clinical aspects of CIA (visual clinical score, paw swelling and hyperalgesia). Bosentan treatment also reduced joint damage, leukocyte infiltration and proinflammatory cytokine levels (IL-1β, TNF-α and IL-17) in the joint tissues. Bosentan treatment also inhibited the preproET mRNA expression that is elevated in the lymph nodes of arthritic mice. In this same article, Donate and co-workers [127] demonstrated that pre-pro-ET mRNA expression increased in PBMCs from rheumatoid arthritis (RA) patients but returned to basal levels in PBMCs from patients undergoing anti-TNF therapy. Further supporting the involvement of TNF-α in the upregulation of ET system genes, the authors showed that TNF-α increased the expression of pre-pro-ET-1, ETA and ETB in PBMCs from healthy donors and RA patients. TNF-α also increased the expression of IL-1β mRNA in PBMCs. Interestingly, the effect of TNF-α on the ET system genes was more prominent in cells from RA patients than in cells from healthy donors. However, this effect was not observed for IL-1β expression, suggesting a specific effect of TNF-α on the ET system.

11. Concluding remarks

Taken together, these data highlight the importance of ETs in the context of articular inflammation suggesting a central role for these peptides and represent innovative and promising therapeutic tools for the treatment of RA (Fig 2).

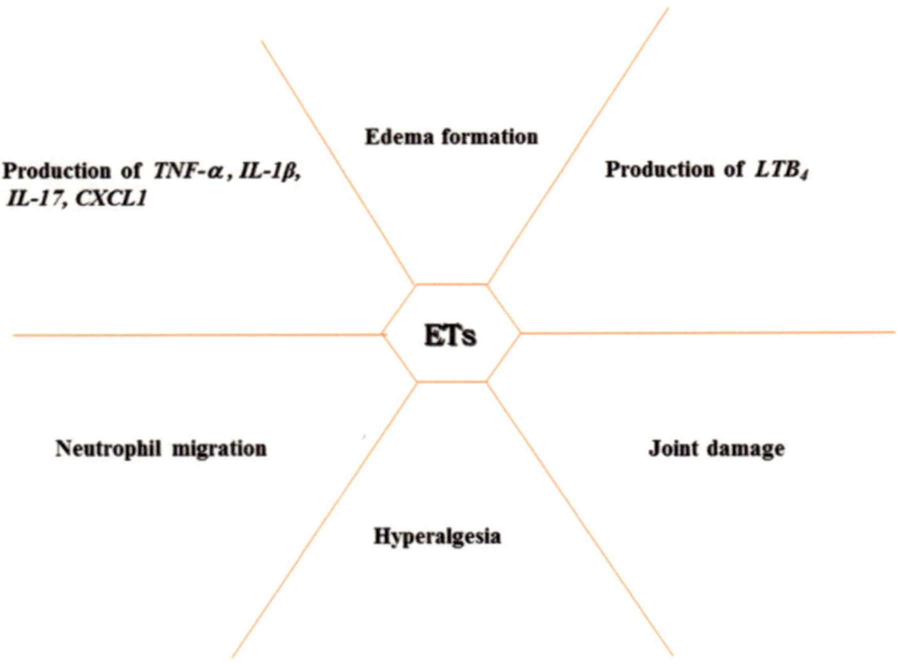

Figure 2. Role of endogenous endothelins in development of RA

Acknowledgements

The author wish to thank the support of CNPq; CAPES and FAPERJ.

Author details

Maria das Graças Muller de Oliveira Henriques*

Address all correspondence to: gracahenriques@fiocruz.br

Laboratory of Applied Pharmacology, Department of Pharmacolgy, Farmanguinhos, Oswaldo Cruz Foundation (FIOCRUZ), Brazil

References

[1] Arend WP. The innate immune system in rheumatoid arthritis. Arthritis Rheum. 2001 Oct;44(10):2224-34. PubMed PMID: 11665962. eng.

[2] Yamamura Y, Gupta R, Morita Y, He X, Pai R, Endres J, et al. Effector function of resting T cells: activation of synovial fibroblasts. J Immunol. 2001 Feb;166(4):2270-5. PubMed PMID: 11160281. eng.

[3] Maini RN, Taylor PC, Paleolog E, Charles P, Ballara S, Brennan FM, et al. Anti-tumour necrosis factor specific antibody (infliximab) treatment provides insights into the pathophysiology of rheumatoid arthritis. Ann Rheum Dis. 1999 Nov;58 Suppl 1:I56-60. PubMed PMID: 10577974. Pubmed Central PMCID: PMC1766574. eng.

[4] Feldmann M, Bondeson J, Brennan FM, Foxwell BM, Maini RN. The rationale for the current boom in anti-TNFalpha treatment. Is there an effective means to define therapeutic targets for drugs that provide all the benefits of anti-TNFalpha and minimise hazards? Ann Rheum Dis. 1999 Nov;58 Suppl 1:I27-31. PubMed PMID: 10577970. Pubmed Central PMCID: PMC1766587. eng.

[5] Lajas C, Abasolo L, Bellajdel B, Hernández-García C, Carmona L, Vargas E, et al. Costs and predictors of costs in rheumatoid arthritis: a prevalence-based study. Arthritis Rheum. 2003 Feb;49(1):64-70. PubMed PMID: 12579595. eng.

[6] Usuki S, Saitoh T, Sawamura T, Suzuki N, Shigemitsu S, Yanagisawa M, et al. Increased maternal plasma concentration of endothelin-1 during labor pain or on delivery and the existence of a large amount of endothelin-1 in amniotic fluid. Gynecol Endocrinol. 1990 Jun;4(2):85-97. PubMed PMID: 2204252. eng.

[7] Iglarz M, Clozel M. At the heart of tissue: endothelin system and end-organ damage. Clin Sci (Lond). 2010 Dec;119(11):453-63. PubMed PMID: 20712600. eng.

[8] Masaki T. Historical review: Endothelin. Trends Pharmacol Sci. 2004 Apr;25(4): 219-24. PubMed PMID: 15063086. eng.

[9] Dhaun N, Pollock DM, Goddard J, Webb DJ. Selective and mixed endothelin receptor antagonism in cardiovascular disease. Trends Pharmacol Sci. 2007 Nov;28(11):573-9. PubMed PMID: 17950470. eng.

[10] Khodorova A, Zou S, Ren K, Dubner R, Davar G, Strichartz G. Dual Roles for Endothelin-B Receptors in Modulating Adjuvant-Induced Inflammatory Hyperalgesia in Rats. Open Pain J. 2009;2:30-40. PubMed PMID: 20559459. Pubmed Central PMCID: PMC2886510. ENG.

[11] Rae, G.A. & Henriques, MG. Endothelins in inflammation Dekker M, editor. New York 1998. 163-202 p.

[12] Wagner OF, Christ G, Wojta J, Vierhapper H, Parzer S, Nowotny PJ, et al. Polar secretion of endothelin-1 by cultured endothelial cells. J Biol Chem. 1992 Aug;267(23): 16066-8. PubMed PMID: 1644793. eng.

[13] Hickey KA, Rubanyi G, Paul RJ, Highsmith RF. Characterization of a coronary vasoconstrictor produced by cultured endothelial cells. Am J Physiol. 1985 May;248(5 Pt 1):C550-6. PubMed PMID: 3993773. eng.

[14] Yanagisawa M, Kurihara H, Kimura S, Goto K, Masaki T. A novel peptide vasoconstrictor, endothelin, is produced by vascular endothelium and modulates smooth muscle Ca2+ channels. J Hypertens Suppl. 1988 Dec;6(4):S188-91. PubMed PMID: 2853725. eng.

[15] Markewitz BA, Kohan DE, Michael JR. Endothelin-1 synthesis, receptors, and signal transduction in alveolar epithelium: evidence for an autocrine role. Am J Physiol. 1995 Feb;268(2 Pt 1):L192-200. PubMed PMID: 7864140. eng.

[16] Sun G, De Angelis G, Nucci F, Ackerman V, Bellini A, Mattoli S. Functional analysis of the preproendothelin-1 gene promoter in pulmonary epithelial cells and monocytes. Biochem Biophys Res Commun. 1996 Apr;221(3):647-52. PubMed PMID: 8630015. eng.

[17] Odoux C, Crestani B, Lebrun G, Rolland C, Aubin P, Seta N, et al. Endothelin-1 secretion by alveolar macrophages in systemic sclerosis. Am J Respir Crit Care Med. 1997 Nov;156(5):1429-35. PubMed PMID: 9372656. eng.

[18] Gandhi CR, Harvey SA, Olson MS. Hepatic effects of endothelin: metabolism of (125I)endothelin-1 by liver-derived cells. Arch Biochem Biophys. 1993 Aug;305(1): 38-46. PubMed PMID: 8342954. eng.

[19] Kawaguchi Y, Suzuki K, Hara M, Hidaka T, Ishizuka T, Kawagoe M, et al. Increased endothelin-1 production in fibroblasts derived from patients with systemic sclerosis.

Ann Rheum Dis. 1994 Aug;53(8):506-10. PubMed PMID: 7944534. Pubmed Central PMCID: PMC1005389. eng.

[20] Brenner M, Degitz K, Besch R, Berking C. Differential expression of melanoma-associated growth factors in keratinocytes and fibroblasts by ultraviolet A and ultraviolet B radiation. Br J Dermatol. 2005 Oct;153(4):733-9. PubMed PMID: 16181453. eng.

[21] Yoshida H, Ohhara M, Ohsumi K. Production of endothelin-1 by cultured human synoviocytes. Clin Chim Acta. 1997 Mar;259(1-2):187-9. PubMed PMID: 9086307. eng.

[22] Yoshida H, Imafuku Y, Ohhara M, Miyata M, Kasukawa R, Ohsumi K, et al. Endothelin-1 production by human synoviocytes. Ann Clin Biochem. 1998 Mar;35 (Pt 2): 290-4. PubMed PMID: 9547903. eng.

[23] Amedeo Modesti P, Zecchi-Orlandini S, Vanni S, Polidori G, Bertolozzi I, Perna AM, et al. Release of preformed Ang II from myocytes mediates angiotensinogen and ET-1 gene overexpression in vivo via AT1 receptor. J Mol Cell Cardiol. 2002 Nov; 34(11):1491-500. PubMed PMID: 12431448. eng.

[24] Rubanyi GM, Polokoff MA. Endothelins: molecular biology, biochemistry, pharmacology, physiology, and pathophysiology. Pharmacol Rev. 1994 Sep;46(3):325-415. PubMed PMID: 7831383. eng.

[25] Kedzierski RM, Yanagisawa M. Endothelin system: the double-edged sword in health and disease. Annu Rev Pharmacol Toxicol. 2001;41:851-76. PubMed PMID: 11264479. eng.

[26] Inoue A, Yanagisawa M, Takuwa Y, Mitsui Y, Kobayashi M, Masaki T. The human preproendothelin-1 gene. Complete nucleotide sequence and regulation of expression. J Biol Chem. 1989 Sep;264(25):14954-9. PubMed PMID: 2670930. eng.

[27] Yanagisawa M, Inoue A, Takuwa Y, Mitsui Y, Kobayashi M, Masaki T. The human preproendothelin-1 gene: possible regulation by endothelial phosphoinositide turnover signaling. J Cardiovasc Pharmacol. 1989;13 Suppl 5:S13-7; discussion S8. PubMed PMID: 2473287. eng.

[28] Xu D, Emoto N, Giaid A, Slaughter C, Kaw S, deWit D, et al. ECE-1: a membrane-bound metalloprotease that catalyzes the proteolytic activation of big endothelin-1. Cell. 1994 Aug;78(3):473-85. PubMed PMID: 8062389. eng.

[29] McMahon EG, Palomo MA, Moore WM, McDonald JF, Stern MK. Phosphoramidon blocks the pressor activity of porcine big endothelin-1-(1-39) in vivo and conversion of big endothelin-1-(1-39) to endothelin-1-(1-21) in vitro. Proc Natl Acad Sci U S A. 1991 Feb;88(3):703-7. PubMed PMID: 1992461. Pubmed Central PMCID: PMC50881. eng.

[30] D'Orléans-Juste P, Plante M, Honoré JC, Carrier E, Labonté J. Synthesis and degradation of endothelin-1. Can J Physiol Pharmacol. 2003 Jun;81(6):503-10. PubMed PMID: 12839262. eng.

[31] Valdenaire O, Rohrbacher E, Mattei MG. Organization of the gene encoding the human endothelin-converting enzyme (ECE-1). J Biol Chem. 1995 Dec;270(50):29794-8. PubMed PMID: 8530372. eng.

[32] Hayasaki-Kajiwara Y, Naya N, Shimamura T, Iwasaki T, Nakajima M. Endothelin generating pathway through endothelin1-31 in human cultured bronchial smooth muscle cells. Br J Pharmacol. 1999 Jul;127(6):1415-21. PubMed PMID: 10455291. Pubmed Central PMCID: PMC1760661. eng.

[33] D'Orléans-Juste P, Houde M, Rae GA, Bkaily G, Carrier E, Simard E. Endothelin-1 (1-31): from chymase-dependent synthesis to cardiovascular pathologies. Vascul Pharmacol. 2008 2008 Aug-Sep;49(2-3):51-62. PubMed PMID: 18675382. eng.

[34] Arai H, Hori S, Aramori I, Ohkubo H, Nakanishi S. Cloning and expression of a cDNA encoding an endothelin receptor. Nature. 1990 1990 Dec 20-27;348(6303):730-2. PubMed PMID: 2175396. eng.

[35] Sakurai T, Yanagisawa M, Takuwa Y, Miyazaki H, Kimura S, Goto K, et al. Cloning of a cDNA encoding a non-isopeptide-selective subtype of the endothelin receptor. Nature. 1990 1990 Dec 20-27;348(6303):732-5. PubMed PMID: 2175397. eng.

[36] Huggins JP, Pelton JT, Miller RC. The structure and specificity of endothelin receptors: their importance in physiology and medicine. Pharmacol Ther. 1993;59(1): 55-123. PubMed PMID: 8259382. eng.

[37] Simonson MS, Dunn MJ. Cellular signaling by peptides of the endothelin gene family. FASEB J. 1990 Sep;4(12):2989-3000. PubMed PMID: 2168326. eng.

[38] Simonson MS, Osanai T, Dunn MJ. Endothelin isopeptides evoke Ca2+ signaling and oscillations of cytosolic free (Ca2+) in human mesangial cells. Biochim Biophys Acta. 1990 Oct;1055(1):63-8. PubMed PMID: 2171677. eng.

[39] Simonson MS, Dunn MJ. Endothelin. Pathways of transmembrane signaling. Hypertension. 1990 Feb;15(2 Suppl):I5-12. PubMed PMID: 2153630. eng.

[40] Abdel-Latif AA, Yousufzai SY, el-Mowafy AM, Ye Z. Prostaglandins mediate the stimulatory effects of endothelin-1 on cyclic adenosine monophosphate accumulation in ciliary smooth muscle isolated from bovine, cat, and other mammalian species. Invest Ophthalmol Vis Sci. 1996 Feb;37(2):328-38. PubMed PMID: 8603837. eng.

[41] Suzuki Y, Tanoi C, Shibuya M, Sugita K, Masuzawa-Ito K, Asano M. Different utilization of Ca2+ in the contractile action of endothelin-1 on cerebral, coronary and mesenteric arteries of the dog. Eur J Pharmacol. 1992 Sep;219(3):401-8. PubMed PMID: 1425968. eng.

[42] Verri W, Cunha T, Parada C, Wei X, Ferreira S, Liew F, et al. IL-15 mediates immune inflammatory hypernociception by triggering a sequential release of IFN-gamma, endothelin, and prostaglandin. Proceedings of the National Academy of Sciences of the

United States of America. 2006 JUN 20 2006;103(25):9721-5. PubMed PMID: WOS: 000238660400060. English.

[43] Suzuki S, Suzuki A, Kajikuri J, Itoh T. Endothelin-1-induced prostaglandin E2 production: modulation of contractile response to endothelin-1 in porcine coronary artery. Eur J Pharmacol. 1992 Jun;217(1):97-100. PubMed PMID: 1397025. eng.

[44] Nelson J, Bagnato A, Battistini B, Nisen P. The endothelin axis: emerging role in cancer. Nat Rev Cancer. 2003 Feb;3(2):110-6. PubMed PMID: 12563310. eng.

[45] Albrecht EW, Stegeman CA, Heeringa P, Henning RH, van Goor H. Protective role of endothelial nitric oxide synthase. J Pathol. 2003 Jan;199(1):8-17. PubMed PMID: 12474221. eng.

[46] Liu S, Premont RT, Kontos CD, Huang J, Rockey DC. Endothelin-1 activates endothelial cell nitric-oxide synthase via heterotrimeric G-protein betagamma subunit signaling to protein jinase B/Akt. J Biol Chem. 2003 Dec;278(50):49929-35. PubMed PMID: 14523027. eng.

[47] Herrera M, Hong NJ, Ortiz PA, Garvin JL. Endothelin-1 inhibits thick ascending limb transport via Akt-stimulated nitric oxide production. J Biol Chem. 2009 Jan;284(3): 1454-60. PubMed PMID: 19033447. Pubmed Central PMCID: PMC2615526. eng.

[48] Alonso D, Radomski MW. The nitric oxide-endothelin-1 connection. Heart Fail Rev. 2003 Jan;8(1):107-15. PubMed PMID: 12652164. eng.

[49] Shah R. Endothelins in health and disease. Eur J Intern Med. 2007 Jul;18(4):272-82. PubMed PMID: 17574100. eng.

[50] Ferreira SH, Romitelli M, de Nucci G. Endothelin-1 participation in overt and inflammatory pain. J Cardiovasc Pharmacol. 1989;13 Suppl 5:S220-2. PubMed PMID: 2473319. eng.

[51] Sirois MG, Filep JG, Rousseau A, Fournier A, Plante GE, Sirois P. Endothelin-1 enhances vascular permeability in conscious rats: role of thromboxane A2. Eur J Pharmacol. 1992 Apr;214(2-3):119-25. PubMed PMID: 1516634. eng.

[52] SAMPAIO A, RAE G, DORLEANSJUSTE P, HENRIQUES M. ET(A) RECEPTOR ANTAGONISTS INHIBIT ALLERGIC INFLAMMATION IN THE MOUSE. Journal of Cardiovascular Pharmacology. 1995 1995;26:S416-S8. PubMed PMID: WOS:A1995TH91200122. English.

[53] Sampaio A, Rae G, Henriques M. Participation of endogenous endothelins in delayed eosinophil and neutrophil recruitment in mouse pleurisy. Inflammation Research. 2000 APR 2000;49(4):170-6. PubMed PMID: WOS:000087042300006. English.

[54] Zouki C, Baron C, Fournier A, Filep JG. Endothelin-1 enhances neutrophil adhesion to human coronary artery endothelial cells: role of ET(A) receptors and platelet-acti-

vating factor. Br J Pharmacol. 1999 Jun;127(4):969-79. PubMed PMID: 10433505. Pubmed Central PMCID: PMC1566081. eng.

[55] Haq A, El-Ramahi K, Al-Dalaan A, Al-Sedairy ST. Serum and synovial fluid concentrations of endothelin-1 in patients with rheumatoid arthritis. J Med. 1999;30(1-2): 51-60. PubMed PMID: 10515240. eng.

[56] Miyasaka N, Hirata Y, Ando K, Sato K, Morita H, Shichiri M, et al. Increased production of endothelin-1 in patients with inflammatory arthritides. Arthritis Rheum. 1992 Apr;35(4):397-400. PubMed PMID: 1567488. eng.

[57] Wharton J, Rutherford RA, Walsh DA, Mapp PI, Knock GA, Blake DR, et al. Autoradiographic localization and analysis of endothelin-1 binding sites in human synovial tissue. Arthritis Rheum. 1992 Aug;35(8):894-9. PubMed PMID: 1642655. eng.

[58] Lebedeva MV, Stakhova TIu, Zaĭtseva LI, Selivanova OIu, Severova MM. (Antihypertensive therapy optimization and endothelial function in patients with gout and chronic urate tubulointerstitial nephritis). Ter Arkh. 2010;82(6):43-6. PubMed PMID: 20731110. rus.

[59] Panoulas VF, Douglas KM, Smith JP, Taffé P, Stavropoulos-Kalinoglou A, Toms TE, et al. Polymorphisms of the endothelin-1 gene associate with hypertension in patients with rheumatoid arthritis. Endothelium. 2008 2008 Jul-Aug;15(4):203-12. PubMed PMID: 18663623. eng.

[60] Pache M, Schwarz HA, Kaiser HJ, Wüest P, Klöti M, Dubler B, et al. Elevated plasma endothelin-1 levels and vascular dysregulation in patients with rheumatoid arthritis. Med Sci Monit. 2002 Sep;8(9):CR616-9. PubMed PMID: 12218941. eng.

[61] Ikonomidis I, Lekakis JP, Nikolaou M, Paraskevaidis I, Andreadou I, Kaplanoglou T, et al. Inhibition of interleukin-1 by anakinra improves vascular and left ventricular function in patients with rheumatoid arthritis. Circulation. 2008 May;117(20):2662-9. PubMed PMID: 18474811. eng.

[62] Silveri F, De Angelis R, Argentati F, Brecciaroli D, Muti S, Cervini C. Hypertrophic osteoarthropathy: endothelium and platelet function. Clin Rheumatol. 1996 Sep; 15(5):435-9. PubMed PMID: 8894355. eng.

[63] Fonseca C, Abraham D, Renzoni EA. Endothelin in pulmonary fibrosis. Am J Respir Cell Mol Biol. 2011 Jan;44(1):1-10. PubMed PMID: 20448055. eng.

[64] Khimji AK, Rockey DC. Endothelin--biology and disease. Cell Signal. 2010 Nov; 22(11):1615-25. PubMed PMID: 20466059. eng.

[65] Schwarting A, Schlaak J, Lotz J, Pfers I, Meyer zum Büschenfelde KH, Mayet WJ. Endothelin-1 modulates the expression of adhesion molecules on fibroblast-like synovial cells (FLS). Scand J Rheumatol. 1996;25(4):246-56. PubMed PMID: 8792802. eng.

[66] Khatib AM, Ribault D, Quintero M, Barbara A, Fiet J, Mitrovic DR. The mechanism of inhibition of endothelin-1-induced stimulation of DNA synthesis in rat articular

chondrocytes. Mol Cell Endocrinol. 1997 Sep;132(1-2):25-31. PubMed PMID: 9324043. eng.

[67] Appleton CT, McErlain DD, Henry JL, Holdsworth DW, Beier F. Molecular and histological analysis of a new rat model of experimental knee osteoarthritis. Ann N Y Acad Sci. 2007 Nov;1117:165-74. PubMed PMID: 17646269. eng.

[68] Usmani SE, Appleton CT, Beier F. Transforming growth factor-alpha induces endothelin receptor A expression in osteoarthritis. J Orthop Res. 2012 Sep;30(9):1391-7. PubMed PMID: 22407503. eng.

[69] Khatib AM, Lomri A, Mitrovic RD, Moldovan F. Articular chondrocyte aging and endothelin-1. Cytokine. 2007 Jan;37(1):6-13. PubMed PMID: 17382552. eng.

[70] Vallender TW, Lahn BT. Localized methylation in the key regulator gene endothelin-1 is associated with cell type-specific transcriptional silencing. FEBS Lett. 2006 Aug;580(18):4560-6. PubMed PMID: 16870175. eng.

[71] Gutierrez S, Palacios I, Egido J, Gómez-Garre D, Hernández P, González E, et al. Endothelin-1 induces loss of proteoglycans and enhances fibronectin and collagen production in cultured rabbit synovial cells. Eur J Pharmacol. 1996 Apr;302(1-3):191-7. PubMed PMID: 8791007. eng.

[72] Speciale L, Roda K, Saresella M, Taramelli D, Ferrante P. Different endothelins stimulate cytokine production by peritoneal macrophages and microglial cell line. Immunology. 1998 Jan;93(1):109-14. PubMed PMID: 9536126. Pubmed Central PMCID: PMC1364113. eng.

[73] Sampaio A, Rae G, Henriques M. Role of endothelins on lymphocyte accumulation in allergic pleurisy. Journal of Leukocyte Biology. 2000 FEB 2000;67(2):189-95. PubMed PMID: WOS:000086630800007. English.

[74] Sampaio A, Rae G, das Gracas M, Henriques M. Effects of endothelin ETA receptor antagonism on granulocyte and lymphocyte accumulation in LPS-induced inflammation. Journal of Leukocyte Biology. 2004 JUL 2004;76(1):210-6. PubMed PMID: WOS: 000222283400026. English.

[75] Stojilkovic SS, Vukicevic S, Luyten FP. Calcium signaling in endothelin- and platelet-derived growth factor-stimulated chondrocytes. J Bone Miner Res. 1994 May;9(5): 705-14. PubMed PMID: 8053400. eng.

[76] Khatib AM, Lomri A, Moldovan F, Soliman H, Fiet J, Mitrovic DR. Endothelin 1 receptors, signal transduction and effects on DNA and proteoglycan synthesis in rat articular chondrocytes. Cytokine. 1998 Sep;10(9):669-79. PubMed PMID: 9770328. eng.

[77] Messai H, Panasyuk A, Khatib A, Barbara A, Mitrovic DR. Endothelin-1 receptors on cultured rat articular chondrocytes: regulation by age, growth factors, and cytokines, and effect on cAMP production. Mech Ageing Dev. 2001 May;122(6):519-31. PubMed PMID: 11295169. eng.

[78] Manacu C, Martel-Pelletier J, Roy-Beaudry M, Pelletier J, Fernandes J, Shipkolye F, et al. Endothelin-1 in osteoarthritic chondrocytes triggers nitric oxide production and upregulates collagenase production. Arthritis Research & Therapy. 2005 2005;7(2):R324-R32. PubMed PMID: WOS:000227579900023. English.

[79] Kinoshita A, Tamura T, Aoki C, Nakanishi T, Sobue S, Suzuki F, et al. Demonstration of endothelin (ET) receptors on cultured rabbit chondrocytes and stimulation of DNA synthesis and calcium influx by ET-1 via its receptors. Cell Biol Int. 1995 Aug; 19(8):647-54. PubMed PMID: 7550073. eng.

[80] Khatib AM, Siegfried G, Messai H, Moldovan F, Mitrovic DR. Mechanism of inhibition of endothelin-1-stimulated proteoglycan and collagen synthesis in rat articular chondrocytes. Cytokine. 2002 Mar;17(5):254-61. PubMed PMID: 12027406. eng.

[81] Roy-Beaudry M, Martel-Pelletier J, Pelletier JP, M'Barek KN, Christgau S, Shipkolye F, et al. Endothelin 1 promotes osteoarthritic cartilage degradation via matrix metalloprotease 1 and matrix metalloprotease 13 induction. Arthritis Rheum. 2003 Oct; 48(10):2855-64. PubMed PMID: 14558091. eng.

[82] Firestein GS. Evolving concepts of rheumatoid arthritis. Nature. 2003 May;423(6937): 356-61. PubMed PMID: 12748655. eng.

[83] McDougall JJ. Arthritis and pain. Neurogenic origin of joint pain. Arthritis Res Ther. 2006;8(6):220. PubMed PMID: 17118212. Pubmed Central PMCID: PMC1794504. eng.

[84] Andrade D, Serra R, Svensjö E, Lima AP, Ramos ES, Fortes FS, et al. Trypanosoma cruzi invades host cells through the activation of endothelin and bradykinin receptors: a converging pathway leading to chagasic vasculopathy. Br J Pharmacol. 2012 Mar;165(5):1333-47. PubMed PMID: 21797847. Pubmed Central PMCID: PMC3372720. eng.

[85] Kassuya CA, Rogerio AP, Calixto JB. The role of ET(A) and ET(B) receptor antagonists in acute and allergic inflammation in mice. Peptides. 2008 Aug;29(8):1329-37. PubMed PMID: 18632188. eng.

[86] Piovezan AP, D'Orléans-Juste P, Tonussi CR, Rae GA. Effects of endothelin-1 on capsaicin-induced nociception in mice. Eur J Pharmacol. 1998 Jun;351(1):15-22. PubMed PMID: 9698200. eng.

[87] Piovezan AP, D'Orléans-Juste P, Souza GE, Rae GA. Endothelin-1-induced ET(A) receptor-mediated nociception, hyperalgesia and oedema in the mouse hind-paw: modulation by simultaneous ET(B) receptor activation. Br J Pharmacol. 2000 Mar; 129(5):961-8. PubMed PMID: 10696096. Pubmed Central PMCID: PMC1571931. eng.

[88] Piovezan A, D'Orleans-Juste P, Frighetto M, Souza G, Henriques M, Rae G. Endothelins contribute towards nociception induced by antigen in ovalbumin-sensitised mice. British Journal of Pharmacology. 2004 FEB 2004;141(4):755-63. PubMed PMID: WOS:000220379200024. English.

[89] Piovezan AP, D'Orléans-Juste P, Tonussi CR, Rae GA. Endothelins potentiate formalin-induced nociception and paw edema in mice. Can J Physiol Pharmacol. 1997 Jun; 75(6):596-600. PubMed PMID: 9276135. eng.

[90] Motta EM, Chichorro JG, D'Orléans-Juste P, Rae GA. Roles of endothelin ETA and ETB receptors in nociception and chemical, thermal and mechanical hyperalgesia induced by endothelin-1 in the rat hindpaw. Peptides. 2009 May;30(5):918-25. PubMed PMID: 19428770. eng.

[91] Verri W, Schivo I, Cunha T, Liew F, Ferreira S, Cunha F. Interleukin-18 induces mechanical hypernociception in rats via endothelin acting on ETB receptors in a morphine-sensitive manner. Journal of Pharmacology and Experimental Therapeutics. 2004 AUG 2004;310(2):710-7. PubMed PMID: WOS:000222728500035. English.

[92] Verri W, Cunha T, Parada C, Poole S, Liew F, Ferreira S, et al. Antigen-induced inflammatory mechanical hypernociception in mice is mediated by IL-18. Brain Behavior and Immunity. 2007 JUL 2007;21(5):535-43. PubMed PMID: WOS: 000247652200004. English.

[93] Gomes LO, Hara DB, Rae GA. Endothelin-1 induces itch and pain in the mouse cheek model. Life Sci. 2012 Mar. PubMed PMID: 22483687. ENG.

[94] Sampaio AL, Rae GA, Henriques MG. Effects of endothelin ETA receptor antagonism on granulocyte and lymphocyte accumulation in LPS-induced inflammation. J Leukoc Biol. 2004 Jul;76(1):210-6. PubMed PMID: 15107459. eng.

[95] Kaufman GN, Zaouter C, Valteau B, Sirois P, Moldovan F. Nociceptive tolerance is improved by bradykinin receptor B1 antagonism and joint morphology is protected by both endothelin type A and bradykinin receptor B1 antagonism in a surgical model of osteoarthritis. Arthritis Res Ther. 2011;13(3):R76. PubMed PMID: 21575197. Pubmed Central PMCID: PMC3218886. eng.

[96] Daher JB, Souza GE, D'Orléans-Juste P, Rae GA. Endothelin ETB receptors inhibit articular nociception and priming induced by carrageenan in the rat knee-joint. Eur J Pharmacol. 2004 Aug;496(1-3):77-85. PubMed PMID: 15288578. eng.

[97] Verri W, Cunha T, Magro D, Domingues A, Vieira S, Souza G, et al. Role of IL-18 in overt pain-like behaviour in mice. European Journal of Pharmacology. 2008 JUL 7 2008;588(2-3):207-12. PubMed PMID: WOS:000257187600010. English.

[98] De-Melo JD, Tonussi CR, D'Orléans-Juste P, Rae GA. Articular nociception induced by endothelin-1, carrageenan and LPS in naive and previously inflamed knee-joints in the rat: inhibition by endothelin receptor antagonists. Pain. 1998 Sep;77(3):261-9. PubMed PMID: 9808351. eng.

[99] De-Melo JD, Tonussi CR, D'Orléans-Juste P, Rae GA. Effects of endothelin-1 on inflammatory incapacitation of the rat knee joint. J Cardiovasc Pharmacol. 1998;31 Suppl 1:S518-20. PubMed PMID: 9595530. eng.

[100] Pinto LG, Cunha TM, Vieira SM, Lemos HP, Verri WA, Cunha FQ, et al. IL-17 mediates articular hypernociception in antigen-induced arthritis in mice. Pain. 2010 Feb; 148(2):247-56. PubMed PMID: 19969421. eng.

[101] Vemulapalli S, Chiu PJ, Griscti K, Brown A, Kurowski S, Sybertz EJ. Phosphoramidon does not inhibit endogenous endothelin-1 release stimulated by hemorrhage, cytokines and hypoxia in rats. Eur J Pharmacol. 1994 May;257(1-2):95-102. PubMed PMID: 8082712. eng.

[102] Morise Z, Ueda M, Aiura K, Endo M, Kitajima M. Pathophysiologic role of endothelin-1 in renal function in rats with endotoxin shock. Surgery. 1994 Feb;115(2):199-204. PubMed PMID: 8310408. eng.

[103] Nambi P, Pullen M, Slivjak MJ, Ohlstein EH, Storer B, Smith EF. Endotoxin-mediated changes in plasma endothelin concentrations, renal endothelin receptor and renal function. Pharmacology. 1994 Mar;48(3):147-56. PubMed PMID: 8153142. eng.

[104] Pernow J, Hemsén A, Hallén A, Lundberg JM. Release of endothelin-like immunoreactivity in relation to neuropeptide Y and catecholamines during endotoxin shock and asphyxia in the pig. Acta Physiol Scand. 1990 Nov;140(3):311-22. PubMed PMID: 2082700. eng.

[105] Lundberg JM, Ahlborg G, Hemsén A, Nisell H, Lunell NO, Pernow J, et al. Evidence for release of endothelin-1 in pigs and humans. J Cardiovasc Pharmacol. 1991;17 Suppl 7:S350-3. PubMed PMID: 1725378. eng.

[106] Myhre U, Pettersen JT, Risøe C, Giercksky KE. Endothelin-1 and endotoxemia. J Cardiovasc Pharmacol. 1993;22 Suppl 8:S291-4. PubMed PMID: 7509968. eng.

[107] Henriques M, Rae G, Cordeiro R, Williams T. Endothelin-1 Inhibits Paf-Induced paw edema and pleurisy in the mouse. British Journal of Pharmacology. 1992 JUL 1992;106(3):579-82. PubMed PMID: WOS:A1992JA35800015. English.

[108] D'Orléans-Juste P, Claing A, Regoli D, Sirois P, Plante GE. Endothelial and smooth muscle pharmacology of pre- and post-capillary microcirculation: correlation with plasma extravasation. Prostaglandins Leukot Essent Fatty Acids. 1996 Jan;54(1):31-7. PubMed PMID: 8992491. eng.

[109] Dahlöf B, Gustafsson D, Hedner T, Jern S, Hansson L. Regional haemodynamic effects of endothelin-1 in rat and man: unexpected adverse reaction. J Hypertens. 1990 Sep;8(9):811-7. PubMed PMID: 2172370. eng.

[110] Brain SD. The direct observation of arteriolar constriction induced by endothelin in vivo. Eur J Pharmacol. 1989 Feb;160(3):401-3. PubMed PMID: 2653847. eng.

[111] Filep JG, Sirois MG, Rousseau A, Fournier A, Sirois P. Effects of endothelin-1 on vascular permeability in the conscious rat: interactions with platelet-activating factor. Br J Pharmacol. 1991 Dec;104(4):797-804. PubMed PMID: 1667286. Pubmed Central PMCID: PMC1908850. eng.

[112] Filep JG, Fournier A, Földes-Filep E. Endothelin-1-induced myocardial ischaemia and oedema in the rat: involvement of the ETA receptor, platelet-activating factor and thromboxane A2. Br J Pharmacol. 1994 Jul;112(3):963-71. PubMed PMID: 7921626. Pubmed Central PMCID: PMC1910206. eng.

[113] Lopez-Belmonte J, Whittle BJ. Endothelin-1 induces neutrophil-independent vascular injury in the rat gastric microcirculation. Eur J Pharmacol. 1995 May;278(1):R7-9. PubMed PMID: 7664809. eng.

[114] Filep JG, Clozel M, Fournier A, Földes-Filep E. Characterization of receptors mediating vascular responses to endothelin-1 in the conscious rat. Br J Pharmacol. 1994 Nov;113(3):845-52. PubMed PMID: 7858876. Pubmed Central PMCID: PMC1510416. eng.

[115] Filep JG, Fournier A, Földes-Filep E. Acute pro-inflammatory actions of endothelin-1 in the guinea-pig lung: involvement of ETA and ETB receptors. Br J Pharmacol. 1995 May;115(2):227-36. PubMed PMID: 7670725. Pubmed Central PMCID: PMC1908312. eng.

[116] Kurose I, Miura S, Fukumura D, Tsuchiya M. Mechanisms of endothelin-induced macromolecular leakage in microvascular beds of rat mesentery. Eur J Pharmacol. 1993 Nov;250(1):85-94. PubMed PMID: 8119327. eng.

[117] Conte FeP, Barja-Fidalgo C, Verri WA, Cunha FQ, Rae GA, Penido C, et al. Endothelins modulate inflammatory reaction in zymosan-induced arthritis: participation of LTB4, TNF-alpha, and CXCL-1. J Leukoc Biol. 2008 Sep;84(3):652-60. PubMed PMID: 18515326. eng.

[118] Hans G, Deseure K, Robert D, De Hert S. Neurosensory changes in a human model of endothelin-1 induced pain: a behavioral study. Neurosci Lett. 2007 May;418(2): 117-21. PubMed PMID: 17403578. eng.

[119] Yuyama H, Koakutsu A, Fujiyasu N, Fujimori A, Sato S, Shibasaki K, et al. Inhibitory effects of a selective endothelin-A receptor antagonist YM598 on endothelin-1-induced potentiation of nociception in formalin-induced and prostate cancer-induced pain models in mice. J Cardiovasc Pharmacol. 2004 Nov;44 Suppl 1:S479-82. PubMed PMID: 15838353. eng.

[120] Yuyama H, Koakutsu A, Fujiyasu N, Tanahashi M, Fujimori A, Sato S, et al. Effects of selective endothelin ET(A) receptor antagonists on endothelin-1-induced potentiation of cancer pain. Eur J Pharmacol. 2004 May;492(2-3):177-82. PubMed PMID: 15178362. eng.

[121] Filep JG. Role for endogenous endothelin in the regulation of plasma volume and albumin escape during endotoxin shock in conscious rats. Br J Pharmacol. 2000 Mar; 129(5):975-83. PubMed PMID: 10696098. Pubmed Central PMCID: PMC1571901. eng.

[122] Verri W, Cunha T, Magro D, Guerrero A, Vieira S, Carregaro V, et al. Targeting endothelin ETA and ETB receptors inhibits antigen-induced neutrophil migration and

mechanical hypernociception in mice. Naunyn-Schmiedebergs Archives of Pharmacology. 2009 MAR 2009;379(3):271-9. PubMed PMID: WOS:000263062400007. English.

[123] Sitbon O, Badesch DB, Channick RN, Frost A, Robbins IM, Simonneau G, et al. Effects of the dual endothelin receptor antagonist bosentan in patients with pulmonary arterial hypertension: a 1-year follow-up study. Chest. 2003 Jul;124(1):247-54. PubMed PMID: 12853530. eng.

[124] Hiramoto Y, Shioyama W, Kuroda T, Masaki M, Sugiyama S, Okamoto K, et al. Effect of bosentan on plasma endothelin-1 concentration in patients with pulmonary arterial hypertension. Circ J. 2007 Mar;71(3):367-9. PubMed PMID: 17322637. eng.

[125] Imhof AK, Glück L, Gajda M, Bräuer R, Schaible HG, Schulz S. Potent anti-inflammatory and antinociceptive activity of the endothelin receptor antagonist bosentan in monoarthritic mice. Arthritis Res Ther. 2011;13(3):R97. PubMed PMID: 21689431. Pubmed Central PMCID: PMC3218912. eng.

[126] Conte F, Menezes-de-Lima O, Verri W, Cunha F, Penido C, Henriques M. Lipoxin A(4) attenuates zymosan-induced arthritis by modulating endothelin-1 and its effects. British Journal of Pharmacology. 2010 OCT 2010;161(4):911-24. PubMed PMID: WOS:000282179000015. English.

[127] Donate P, Cunha T, Verri W, Junta C, Lima F, Vieira S, et al. Bosentan, an endothelin receptor antagonist, ameliorates collagen-induced arthritis: the role of TNF-alpha in the induction of endothelin system genes. Inflammation Research. 2012 APR 2012;61(4):337-48. PubMed PMID: WOS:000301778300008. English.

Chapter 3

The Role of Micro-RNAs in Rheumatic Diseases: An Update

Giovanni Ciancio, Manuela Ferracin, Massimo Negrini and Marcello Govoni

Additional information is available at the end of the chapter

http://dx.doi.org/10.5772/54273

1. Introduction

MicroRNAs (miRNAs) are small non-coding RNAs of approximately 22 nucleotides in length, whose main function is to modulate the expression of multiple target genes at the post-transcriptional level through messenger-RNA (mRNA) degradation or repression of translation [1-3]. More than 30% of all human genes are regulated by miRNAs, with each miRNA controlling multiple mRNA targets, and each mRNA targeted by various miRNAs [2]. These intriguing molecules has been first described in 1993 in *Caenorhabditis elegans* [4] and first demonstrated in humans in 2001 [5]. Since then, several miRNAs have been identified and more than 2.042 miRNAs have been described in humans to date (miRBase release 19, at http:// www.mirbase.org/).

MiRNA play a crucial role in modulating a large range of biologic functions from developmental timing to organogenesis [6,7]. They have a key role in cellular differentiation, homeostasis, apoptosis and anti-viral defence [1,8]. More recently, it has become evident that miRNAs play a crucial role in the development of immune cells and in regulating the immune response [9-11].

Altered expression of miRNAs profiles has been initially related to the development of cancer and subsequently to various non-malignant diseases such as cardiovascular disorders, lung diseases, schizophrenia, Alzheimer disease, neuro psychiatric disorders, viral infections, primary biliary cirrhosis and chronic inflammatory and autoimmune diseases [12-17]

In the last two decades, increasing evidences have linked miRNA abnormal expression with pathogenic mechanisms of cancer, and a lot of causes that led to their dysregulation have been discovered [18]. Many miRNAs have been associated with cancer development [19,20], metastatic capability [21] and resistance to anti-cancer drugs [22]. In this field, they are also considered as new potential diagnostic and prognostic biomarkers [20, 23]. Furthermore the application of miRNAs as a candidate molecular target for anticancer therapeutics seems very promising [18,24].

More recently, some studies have highlighted the role of miRNAs in the development of several rheumatic diseases [25-33]and this argument today represents an emerging and exciting field of research. This is not surprising since miRNAs altered expression may lead either to persistent inflammation or to impaired tolerance against self-antigens, thus promoting the development of both autoimmune and inflammatory chronic diseases [11, 34].

In this article we summarize the new acquisitions about the growing importance of miRNAs in rheumatic diseases as pathogenetic factors, potential biomarkers and possible new therapeutic targets. We also focus on new developments about the possible role of miRNA in the pathogenesis of psoriatic arthritis (PsA) on the basis of our recent experimental results.

2. MiRNAs in rheumatic diseases

2.1. Connective tissue disorders

2.1.1. Systemic lupus erythematosus

Systemic lupus erithematosus (SLE) is an autoimmune systemic disease of unknown etiology characterized by abnormal autoantibody production, inflammatory involvement of various organ systems including skin, mucous membranes, joints, serous membranes, kidney, brain, lung and heart and significant morbidity and mortality [35].A number of studies carried out so far, have demonstrated that miRNA have an important role in SLE pathogenesis and can be predictive of disease activity and severity, helpful as biomarkers and useful for development of new therapeutic strategies [36-42].

In the study of Dai et al. [36], peripheral blood mononuclear cell (PBMC) miRNA profiles of 23 patients with SLE, 10 healthy controls and 10 patients with idiopathic thrombocytopenic purpura (ITP) were analyzed. In comparison with healthy controls, miRNA microarray analysis identified 19 miRNA differentially expressed in ITP (14 down-regulated and 5 up-regulated) and 16 miRNAs differentially expressed in SLE (7 *down-regulated*: miR-196a, miR-17-5p, miR-409-3p,HMP-PREDICTED-miR141, miR-383, HMP-PREDICTED-miR112 and miR-184; and 9 *up-regulated*: HMP-PREDICTED-miR189, HMP-PREDICTED-miR-61, HMP-PREDICTED-miR78, miR-21,miR-142-3p, miR-342, miR-299-3p,miR-198 and mmu-miR-298). Interestingly, from the comparison between the two pathologic groups,13 miRNAs resulted dysregulated both in SLE and ITP, 6 downregulated in ITP only, and finally 3 dysregulated in SLE only: miR-184 (underexpressed) and miR198 and miR21 (overexpressed) [36]. Furthermore, 8 miRNA (miR-494, miR-188, miR-501, mmu-miR-298, HMP-PREDICTED-miR61, HMP-PREDICTED-miR78, miR-296 and miR-299-3p) were downregulated in SLE patients with more active disease (SLE Disease Activity Index score

[SLEDAI] ≥15) in comparison with patients with inactive disease (SLEDAI ≤12), which led to hypothesized that these 8 miRNA could be involved in SLE progress, recrudescence and organ injure [36]. The same group examined miRNA expression in renal biopsy of patients with WHO Class II lupus nephritis (LN), showing 66 dysregulated miRNA (36 up- and 30 down-regulated) in comparison with healthy controls [37].

Te et al. investigated PBMCs miRNA expression profile of LN patients (African American and European American) in comparison with unaffected controls and found 5 miRNA differentially expressed in LN: 4 up-regulated (miR-371–5P, miR-423–5P, miR-638 and miR-663) and 1 down-regulated (miR-1224–3P) [43]. In particular, miR-371-5P, miR-423-5P and miR-1224-3P were reported for the first time to be associated with lupus nephritis [43].

In a study performed by using the TaqMan miRNA assay, Tang et al. showed in SLE PBMCs 42 miRNAs differentially expressed in comparison with healthy controls, with 7 miRNA being more than six-fold down-regulated in SLE: miR-31, miR-95, miR-99a, miR-130b, miR-10a, miR-134, and miR-146a [40]. Notably, underexpression of miR-146a negatively correlated with clinical disease activity and with interferon (IFN) scores in SLE patients. Moreover, inhibition of endogenous miR-146a in PBMCs through transfection with synthetic miRNA-146a hairpin inhibitor increased the induction of type I IFN, which is known to have a role in the pathogenesis of SLE. These findings highlighted that underexpression of miR-146a could have an important role in the pathogenesis of SLE, thus providing potential novel strategies for therapeutic intervention [40].

Consistent with these results, Wang et al. showed that in SLE patients serum miR-146a and miR-155 levels were lower, and the urinary level of miR-146a was higher in comparison with healthy controls [44]. Moreover, estimated glomerular filtration rate (eGFR) correlated with both serum miR-146a and miR-155, and serum miR-146a inversely correlated with proteinuria and the SLE Disease Activity Index, which suggested that both miR-146a and miR-155 participated in the pathophysiology of SLE and might be used as biomarkers of SLE [44]. The same authors recently confirmed that urinary levels of miR-146a and miR-155 in patients with SLE were significantly higher than that in healthy controls [45]. In another study they also evidenced that the serum levels of miR-200a, miR-200b, miR-200c, miR-429, miR-205 and miR-192, and urinary levels of miR-200a, miR-200c, miR-141, miR-429 and miR-192 of SLE patients were lower than those of controls,with SLEDAI index that inversely correlated with serum miR-200a [46]. Hai-yan et al. confirmed in their study the lower expression of miR-146a in PBMCs of SLE patients compared to healthy controls [47].

In comparison with healthy controls, miR-21 and miR-148a [48] and miR-126 [42] resulted up-regulated in SLE CD4+ T cells and promoted cell hypomethylation by repressing DNA methyltransferase 1 (DNMT1) expression, which led to hypothsized that they contribute to T cell autoreactivity in SLE.

Compared with controls, miR-21 has been also found upregulated in SLE CD4+ T lymphocytes by Stagakis et al. [39]. MiR21 strongly correlated with SLE disease activity and investigation of putative gene-targets showed that it suppressed PDCD4, thus regulating aberrant T cell responses in human SLE.

Most recently, Ding et al. demonstrated that miR-142-3p/5p were significantly down-regulated in SLE CD4+ T cells compared with healthy controls and that their reduced expression caused T cell activity and B cell hyperstimulation[49]. Lu et al. showed a different intra-renal expression of miR-638, miR-198 and miR-146a between LN patients and normal controls [38]. In particular, miR-638 had lower glomerular expression and higher tubulointerstitial expression; miR-198 resulted up-regulated in both glomerulus and in tubulointerstitium; and miR-146a was overexpressed in glomerulus. Interestingly, tubulointerstitial miR-638 expression significantly correlated with clinical disease severity (estimated GFR/histological activity index and proteinuria/disease activity score, respectively), while glomerular miR-146a expressions were correlated with estimated GFR and histological activity index [38].

Main miRNA dysregulated in SLE are shown in Tab.1.

Up-regulated	Down-regulated
-miR198 and miR21 (PBMC)[36]	-miR-184 (PBMC) [36]
-miR-371–5P,miR-423–5P, miR-638 and miR-663 (PBMC)[43]	-miR-1224–3P (PBMC) [43]
-miR-21 and miR-148a (CD4+ T cells)[48]	- miR-31, miR-95, miR-99a, miR-130b, miR-10a, miR-134, and miR-146a (PBMC) [40]
-miR-21 (CD4+ T cells) [39]	-miR-146a and miR-155 (serum) [44]
-miR-126(CD4+ T cells)[42]	-miR-142-3p/5p (CD4+ T cells) [49]
-miR-638, miR-198 and miR-146a (intra-renal) [38]	-miR-638 (intra-renal) [38]
	-miR-146a (urine)[44]

Abbreviations: PBMC, peripheral blood mononuclear cells

Table 1. Main microRNA dysregulated in SLE

2.1.2. Sjögren Syndrome (SS)

SS is an inflammatory autoimmune disease primarily affecting the exocrine glands and characterized by the presence of typical autoantibodies such as anti-Ro (SSA) and anti-La (SSB), keratoconjunctivitis sicca, xerostomia, pulmonary involvement, nonerosive polyarthritis and increased risk of lymphoid malignancy [50]. The relatively easy access to the target tissue (salivary glands and saliva) makes Sjogren's syndrome appealing to study microRNAs [41]. Michael et al. demonstrated a prominent difference between miRNAs profile in saliva obtained from patients with SS and healthy donors [51]. Alevizos et al. showed a different miRNA expression profile in glands of SS in comparison with controls. Moreover, in half of the patients with a focus score of 12, the miR-17-92 cluster resulted downregulated [52].

Lu et al. showed that miR-574 and miR-768-3p resulted overexpressed in the SS salivary glands, while miRNA-146a was increased in PBMCs and salivary glands [53]. Interestingly, the overexpression of miR146a was confirmed in PBMC of patients with SS [54, 55] as well as in PBMCs and in the salivary glands of a SS mouse model [54]. These results are promising for the development of future diagnostic and prognostic biomarkers in SS.

Main miRNA dysregulated in SS are shown in Tab.2.

Up-regulated	Down-regulated
-miR-574 and miR-768-3p (salivary glands) [53] -miR-146a (PBMCs and salivary glands) [53] -miR-146a (PBMCs) [54, 55]	miR-17-92 (salivary glands) [52]

Abbreviations: PBMC, peripheral blood mononuclear cells

Table 2. Main microRNA dysregulated in SS

2.1.3. Systemic Sclerosis (SSc)

SSc is a generalized connective tissue disease affecting skin and internal organs and characterized by abnormal extracellular collagen accumulation. It is tipically associated with specific autoantibodies (anticentromere and anti-topoisomerase Scl-70) [56].

Recently, Maurer et al. found that miR-29a was strongly down-regulated in SSc fibroblasts and skin sections as compared with the healthy controls and, similarly to human SSc, the expression of miR-29a was reduced in the bleomycin model of skin fibrosis [57]. Interestingly, overexpression in SSc fibroblasts decreased, and knockdown in normal fibroblasts increased the levels of messenger RNA for type I and type III collagen, which highlighted the role of miR-29a as post-transcriptional regulators of pro-fibrotic genes [57].These results appear very intriguing and reveal that miR29 could be considered a potential therapeutic target in SSc [57, 58]. In comparison with the normal skin tissues, Zhu et al. identified some miRNAs aberrantly expressed in limited cutaneous scleroderma and diffuse cutaneous scleroderma skin tissues, such as miR-21 (up-regulated) and miR-145 and miR-29b (down-regulated) both in the skin tissues and fibroblasto [59].

Main miRNA dysregulated in SSc are shown in Tab.3.

Up-regulated	Down-regulated
-miR-21 (SSc skin tissues and fibroblasts)[59]	-miR-29a (SSc fibroblasts) [57] -miR-145 and miR-29b (SSc skin tissues and fibroblasts) [59]

Table 3. Main microRNA dysregulated in SSc

2.2. Osteoarthritis (OA)

OA is the most common age related disorder whose main features are the damage of the articular cartilage, the increased activity in the subchondral bone and osteophyte formation. A moderate synovitis may appear especially in advanced cases [60]. In comparison with normal cartilage, Iliopoulos et al. evidenced 16 miRNAs differentially expressed in OA cartilage [61].

Out of these, miR-22 resulted up-regulated and contributed to decreased expression of aggrecan and increased levels of IL-1b and MMP-13 in chondrocytes, while miR-140 was found down-regulated and its under-expression was related to the development of age-related OA-like changes [61]. In the cartilage of late-stage OA, Jones et al. described several differentially expressed miRNAs, out of these miR-146a resulted down-regulated, miR-9 and miR-98 up-regulated [62]. Interestingly, functional analysis revealed that miR-9 and miR-98 reduced the IL-1β-induced production of TNFα in primary chondrocytes, while miR-9 also inhibited MMP-13 secretion in vitro, a scenario which led to hypothesized their protective role in OA [62]. MiR-27a was also found down-regulated in OA chondrocytes and its underexpression indirectly inhibited MMP-13 and IGFBP-5 (insulin-like growth factor binding protein) [63]. A protective role on OA cartilage and in modulating pain symptoms has been hypothesized for miR-146A [64]. Most recently, overexpression of miR-146a, miR-155, miR-181a and miR-223 was demonstrated in PBMCs of OA patients in comparison with healthy controls, with miR-146a and miR-223 significantly higher in the early stages of OA than at later stages [65].

However, although several OA-associated miRNA have been reported to date, their potential role in OA needs to be further elucidated and their targets need to be discovered in the future.

Main miRNA dysregulated in OA are shown in Tab.4

Up-regulated	Down-regulated
-miR-22 (OA cartilage) [61]	-miR-140 (OA cartilage) [61]
-miR-9 and MiR-98 (OA cartilage) [62]	-miR-146a (OA cartilage) [62]
-miR-146a, miR-155, miR-181a (OA PBMCs) [65]	-miR-27a (OA chondrocytes) [63]

Abbreviations: PBMC, peripheral blood mononuclear cells

Table 4. Main microRNA dysregulated in OA

2.3. Rheumatoid arthritis

Rheumatoid arthritis (RA) is a chronic inflammatory joint disorder that is characterized by immune-driven inflammation of synovial membrane which results in erosion, joint destruction and disability. Extra-articular symptoms, such as serositis, nodules and vasculitis are common and usually associated to a more severe disease. The etiology of rheumatoid arthritis (RA) is still unknown, and many uncertainties regarding its pathogenetic mechanisms persist yet [66].

Many recent studies have demonstrated that different miRNAs are significantly dysregulated in RA tissues.

2.3.1. Synovium

In comparison with healthy controls and/or OA patients, some miRNA have been found up-(miR-155, miR-203 and miR-146a) or down-(miR124a and miR-34a*) regulated in RA synovial tissue and/or synovial fluid [67-74].

MiR-155 has emerged as one of the most attractive and thoroughly studied miRNA in RA. It was found significantly up-regulated in RA-synovial fibroblasts (RA-SFs) [74], in the lining layer CD68+ macrophages [68] and in synovial fluid CD14+ cells [68, 74] of the RA synovial compartment.

Since overexpression of miR-155 in RA-SFs was shown to decrease the levels of matrix metalloproteinase 3 (MMP-3) and 1 (MMP-1) *in vitro*, it was initially hypothesized a protective role of miR-155 by modulating destructive properties of RA-synovial fibroblasts (RA-SFs) [74]. However, *in vivo* data have shown an opposite role for miR-155 in the development of arthritis [68, 75]. Up-regulation of miR-155 in synovial fluid CD14+ cells increased the expression of TNF-α, IL-1β, IL-6, and IL-8 and downregulated the expression of the miR-155 target SHIP-1 (Src homology 2-containing inositol phosphatase-1), an inhibitor of inflammation [68], and miR-155-deficient mice are resistant to collagen-induced arthritis [75].These data, together with the observation that specific inhibition of miR-155 in RA synovial macrophages reduced TNF-alpha production led to ascribe to miR-155 a role in excessive proinflammatory activation of myeloid cells in RA and to suggest that miR-155 may represent an intriguing therapeutic target [68]. Interestingly, Worm et al. first reported on miR-155 silencing in vivo in a mouse inflammation model [76], which further underlines the potentiality of miR-155 antagonists as novel therapeutics for treatment of chronic inflammatory diseases

MiR-203, was found significantly up-regulated in RA-SFs in comparison with OA-SFs [73]. It resulted in higher release of MMP-1 and secretion of IL-6 via the NF-kappa B pathway, which led to hypothesize a role in activating RA-SFs and triggering inflammation [73]. However, the direct targets of miR-203 in RA-SFs still need to be highlighted [73].

Mir-146a resulted greatly expressed in RA synovial tissue when compared with OA and it has been demonstrated in CD3+ T cells, IL-17 producing T cells, CD68+ cells, in some B lymphocytes [70, 72, 74] and in RA-SF, where its expression resulted induced by several pro-inflammatory mediators such as TNF-alpha and IL-1beta [70, 74]. However, its role in synovial tissue has yet to be elucidate.

MiR-124a was found significantly lower in RA-SFs in comparison with OA [69]. Its down-regulation appears to play an important role in the pathogenesis of RA by mediating the enhancement of both cyclin-dependent kinase 2 (CDK-2), involved in the cell cycle regulation, and monocyte chemoattractant protein 1 (MCP-1),which are able to attract into the synovial tissue inflammatory cells, memory T lymphocytes and natural killer cells [67, 69]. These intriguing findings have suggested that miR-124a could also have a therapeutic potential [67, 69].

Finally miR-34a* was found significantly down-regulated in RA-SFs in comparison with OA as a result of higher DNA methylation, which would contribute to the RA-SFs resistance to apoptosis, a typical feature of these RA cells [71]

2.3.2. *Blood*

MiR-146a was found overexpressed in PBMC obtained from RA patients, expecially those with early RA and with high disease activity, compared with healthy and disease control individuals [72, 77]. Other studies confirmed miR-146a overexpression in PBMC [78], in CD4+

T lymphocytes from peripheral blood [79] and in plasma [80] of RA patients. The observation that miR-146a was able to silence in PBMC the expression of interleukin-1 receptor-associated kinase 1 (IRAK1) and TNF receptor associated factor 6 (TRAF6), members of the TLR4 signaling cascade [81], led to hypothesized that miR-146a could act as a negative regulator of inflammation, as supported by other recent studies [77, 82, 83]. However, in the study of Pauley et al. PBMC expression of IRAK-1 and TRAF6 was no different between RA patients and healthy controls, as expected [77], which led to hypothesized that was a defect in regulation of these molecules by miR-146a that promoted inflammation, with an extensive and prolonged TNF-alpha production [77].

Consistent with the data on synovial compartment, miR-155 has been found increased in PBMC from RA patients compared with healthy controls and upregulated during the differentiation of IL-17 producing cells [72, 77]. Conversely, concentrations of miR-155 and other examined miRNA (miR-16, miR-132, miR-146a and miR-223) resulted not differently expressed between RA and OA patients in plasma, although plasma levels of miR-155,miR-16, miR-146a and miR-223 inversely correlated with clinical indices, such as tender joint count and 28-joint Disease Activity Score (DAS 28).

Recently, Fulci et al showed a clear up-regulation of miR-223 and a significant downregulation of miR-142, miR-28 and miR-30e in T-lymphocytes from peripheral blood from RA patients in comparison with healthy controls [84]. The same group confirmed the overexpression of miR-223 in T-lymphocytes of early rheumatoid arthritis patients [85] which led the authors to speculate that this aberrant over-expression could contribute to the pathogenesis of the disease.

Other miRNAs resulted disregulated in RA, such as miR-16, miR-132, miR-26a, and miR-150 which resulted up-regulated in PBMC from patients with RA compared with healthy controls. [72, 77]. Of these, miR-16 and miR-150 correlated with disease activity [72, 77], whereas miR-26 and miR-150 resulted upregulated in IL-17 producing T cells [72].

Main miRNA dysregulated in RA are shown in Tab.5

Up-regulated	Down-regulated
-miR-155 (synovium) [68, 74]	-miR-124a (synovium) [69]
-miR-155 (PBMC) [72, 77]	-miR-34a* (synovium) [71]
-miR-203 (synovium) [73]	
-miR-146a (synovium) [70, 72, 74]	
-miR-146a (PBMC/ CD4+ T lymphocytes/plasma) [72, 77-80]	
-miR-223 (blood T-lymphocytes [84, 85]	
- miR-16, miR-132, miR-26a, and miR-150 (PBMC) [72, 77]	

Abbreviations: PBMC, peripheral blood mononuclear cells

Table 5. Main microRNA dysregulated in RA

2.4. Psoriatic arthritis

Psoriatic arthritis (PsA) is a chronic inflammatory disease that develops in ~ 20% of individuals with psoriasis [86]. PSA pathogenesis is not yet fully understood and lymphocytes, in particular CD8+ T cells, appear to play an important role in the pathogenesis of both psoriasis and PsA [87, 88]. In addition, several pro-inflammatory cytochines seem to be involved, including TNF-α, IL-1, IL-6 and IL-12 [89-91]. While several studies have shown an altered expression of miRNAs in psoriasis, to date – at the best of our knowledge - no studies have been performed about the miRNA expression profile in PsA. On this background, we evaluated a comprehensive global miRNA expression profile in PBMCs of patients with PsA in comparison with healthy controls, with the main purpose to characterise the miRNA signature in PsA (*Clin Drug Investig, in press*). Below, the results of the principal studies on psoriasis and the main results of our study on PsA are summarized.

2.4.1. Psoriasis

Several miRNA have been found disregulated in psoriatic skin when compared with healthy skin, such as miR-203,miR-146a, miR-99a and miR-21 (up-regulated) or miR 125b (down- regulated).

Up-regulation of miR-203 correlated with the underexpression of SOCS-3 (suppressor of cytokine signalling 3) which is implicated in inflammatory response and keratinocyte functions [92]. Recently, Primo et al. confirmed the up-regulation of miR-203 in psoriatic lesions, with TNF-alpha and IL24 as its direct targets [93]. The over-expressed miR-146a was related to the TNF-α signalling control in the skin [94]. Up-regulation of miR-99a was correlated with a slow keratinocyte proliferation and induction of their differentiation through regulation of IGF-1R [95]. Elevated levels of miR-21 in psoriatic skin have been found by Meisgen et al. [96]. The authors evidenced that overexpression of this miRNA was related to apoptosis suppression in activated T cells, which contributed to T cell-derived psoriatic skin inflammation [96].

Downregulation of miR-125b has been associated with high TNF-α production [94] and with the modulation of keratinocyte differentiation and proliferation by targeting FGFR2 (fibroblast growth factor receptor 2) [97].

Other miRNA have been found dysregulated in psoriasis. Zibbert et al. identified 42 upregulated miRNAs and 5 downregulated miRNAs in psoriasis skin compared with healthy skin [98]. Out of these, up-regulated miR-21, miR-205, miR-221 and miR-222 were found to have potential mRNA targets in psoriatic skin such as PDCD4, TPM1, P57, C-KIT, RTN4, SHIP2, TIMP3, RECK and NFIB, which were likely to be involved in cellular growth, proliferation, apoptosis and degradation of the extracellular matrix [98].

Down-regulation of miR-424 in the skin [99] and up-regulation of miR-1266 in the serum [100] of PsA patients have also been demonstrated. Underexpression of miR-124 was related to increased levels of MEK1 or cyclin E1 proteins, thus to enhanced keratinocyte proliferation [99]. Overexpression of miR-1266 in the PsA serum was quite unexpected being this miRNA a putative regulator of IL-17A, a key cytokine in PsA pathogenesis, so the authors hypothesized that miR-1266 could be involved in the pathogenesis of psoriasis by regulating other target molecules [100].

Main miRNA dysregulated in psoriasis are shown in Tab.6.

Up-regulated	Down-regulated
-miR-203 (psoriatic skin) [92, 93]	-miR 125b (psoriatic skin) [92]
-miR-146a (psoriatic skin) [92]	-miR-424 (psoriatic skin) [99]
-miR-99a (psoriatic skin) [95]	
-miR-21 (psoriatic skin) [96]	
-miR-21, miR-205, miR-221 and miR-222 (psoriatic skin)[98]	
-miR-1266 (serum) [100]	

Table 6. Main microRNA dysregulated in Psoriasis

2.4.2. Psoriatic arthritis

In our recent study (*Clin Drug Investig, in press*), we evaluated global miRNA expression profile in PBMCs of 13 patients with early active and untreated PsA. In comparison with healthy controls, the PBMC of PsA group revealed the presence of 9 up-modulated and 7 down-regulated miRNAs. Within the group of up-regulated, miR-21, miR-34a and miR-125a appeared of particular interest considering the extent of their modulation and their emerging role in inflammatory processes (*Clin Drug Investig, in press*) (Tab.7). Instead, all down-regulated miRNAs belonged to two large adjacent miRNA clusters located on chromosome 14, which makes this chromosome worthy of further investigation in the field of psoriasis and PsA genetic susceptibility (*Clin Drug investig, in press*). Quantitative RT-PCR (RT-qPCR) analysis for specific miRNA (miR-21, miR-34a, miR-125a), performed in the entire series of 13 PsA patients plus 5 additional PsA patients and in healthy controls, confirmed the up-regulation of these three miRNA (unpublished data). (Figure 1A-C). Moreover, based on its emerging role in immunity control and the proved involvement in other autoimmune diseases [40, 77, 81, 101, 102] we also evaluated by RT-qPCR miR-146a levels in the entire group of 18 PsA patients. Also in this case, real time results were in agreement with microarray and did not show significant differences between patients and controls (unpublished data) (Figure 1D). The demonstration of a miRNA signature in PsA could be a novel starting point for understanding pathogenic mechanisms of this disease. Moreover, altered miRNAs expression in patients with active disease makes them attractive as potential biomarkers of disease.

Up-regulated	Down-regulated
MiR-21, miR-34a and miR-125a (PBMC) (Ciancio et al., Clin Drug Investig,*in press*)	
Abbreviations: PBMC, peripheral blood mononuclear cells	

Table 7. Main microRNA dysregulated in PsA

http://dx.doi.org/10.5772/54273

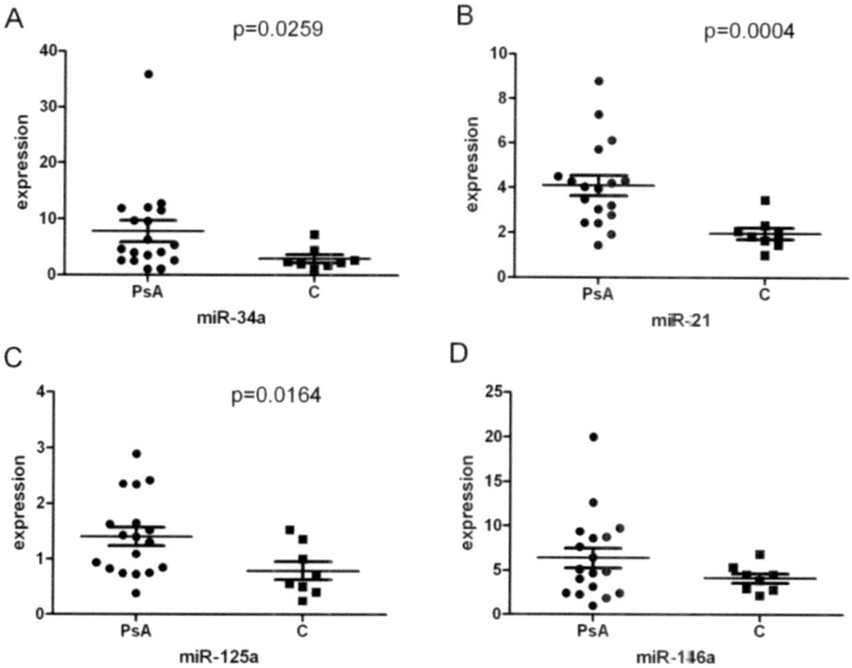

Figure 1. Validation of miR-34a (A), miR-21 (B), miR-125a (C) and miR-146a (D) levels by quantitative RT-PCR. MiRNAs expression in 18 PsA patients and 8 controls was quantified using RT-qPCR. Each expression data was normalized on endogenous U6 RNA level by 2-ΔCt method. Each sample was analyzed in triplicate. Data are displayed using vertical scatter plot (GraphPad v.5), bars represent means ± SEM. Two-tailed t-test was used to determine the p-values.

3. Conclusions

MiRNA are fine regulators of gene expression at the post-trascriptional level and it is today known that they partecipate in the regulation of almost every aspect of cell physiology, including the development of immune cells and the regulation of the immune response.

MiRNA altered expression has been related to the development of several chronic inflammatory and autoimmune diseases such as systemic lupus erithematosus, rheumatoid arthritis, Sjogren syndrome, systemic sclerosis, psoriasis and psoriatic arthritis. Osteoarthritis, the most common age related disorder, seems also to be related to an altered expression of miRNAs. Besides their crucial role in the pathogenesis of rheumatic diseases, miRNAs can also be predictive of disease activity and severity, helpful as biomarkers and useful for development of new therapeutic strategies. However, this exciting field of research is still at an early stage and larger studies are still desirable to define the specific roles that individual miRNAs may play in rheumatic diseases.

Author details

Giovanni Ciancio[1*], Manuela Ferracin[2], Massimo Negrini[2] and Marcello Govoni[1]

*Address all correspondence to: g.ciancio@ospfe.it

1 Rheumatology Unit, Department of Clinical and Experimental Medicine, University of Ferrara and Azienda Ospedaliera-Universitaria Sant'Anna, Ferrara, Italy

2 Department of Experimental and Diagnostic Medicine and Laboratory for Technologies of Advanced Therapies (LTTA), University of Ferrara, Italy

References

[1] Ambros V. The functions of animal microRNAs. Nature 2004;431(7006):350-5.

[2] Guo H, Ingolia NT, Weissman JS, Bartel DP. Mammalian microRNAs predominantly act to decrease target mRNA levels. Nature 2010;466(7308):835-40.

[3] Lagos-Quintana M, Rauhut R, Lendeckel W, Tuschl T. Identification of novel genes coding for small expressed RNAs. Science 2001;294(5543):853-8.

[4] Lee RC, Feinbaum RL, Ambros V. The C. elegans heterochronic gene lin-4 encodes small RNAs with antisense complementarity to lin-14. Cell 1993;75(5):843-54.

[5] Hutvagner G, McLachlan J, Pasquinelli AE, Balint E, Tuschl T, Zamore PD. A cellular function for the RNA-interference enzyme Dicer in the maturation of the let-7 small temporal RNA. Science 2001;293(5531):834-8.

[6] Ambros V. MicroRNA pathways in flies and worms: growth, death, fat, stress, and timing. Cell 2003;113(6):673-6.

[7] Bartel DP. MicroRNAs: genomics, biogenesis, mechanism, and function. Cell 2004;116(2):281-97.

[8] Krek A, Grun D, Poy MN, et al. Combinatorial microRNA target predictions. Nat Genet 2005;37(5):495-500.

[9] Baltimore D, Boldin MP, O'Connell RM, Rao DS, Taganov KD. MicroRNAs: new regulators of immune cell development and function. Nat Immunol 2008;9(8):839-45.

[10] Lodish HF, Zhou B, Liu G, Chen CZ. Micromanagement of the immune system by microRNAs. Nat Rev Immunol 2008;8(2):120-30.

[11] Lu LF, Liston A. MicroRNA in the immune system, microRNA as an immune system. Immunology 2009;127(3):291-8.

[12] Houzet L, Yeung ML, de Lame V, Desai D, Smith SM, Jeang KT. MicroRNA profile changes in human immunodeficiency virus type 1 (HIV-1) seropositive individuals. Retrovirology 2008;5:118.

[13] Jiang Q, Wang Y, Hao Y, et al. miR2Disease: a manually curated database for microRNA deregulation in human disease. Nucleic Acids Res 2009;37(Database issue):D98-104.

[14] Niwa R, Zhou F, Li C, Slack FJ. The expression of the Alzheimer's amyloid precursor protein-like gene is regulated by developmental timing microRNAs and their targets in Caenorhabditis elegans. Dev Biol 2008;315(2):418-25.

[15] Padgett KA, Lan RY, Leung PC, et al. Primary biliary cirrhosis is associated with altered hepatic microRNA expression. J Autoimmun 2009;32(3-4):246-53.

[16] Sarasin-Filipowicz M, Krol J, Markiewicz I, Heim MH, Filipowicz W. Decreased levels of microRNA miR-122 in individuals with hepatitis C responding poorly to interferon therapy. Nat Med 2009;15(1):31-3.

[17] Zhu Y, Kalbfleisch T, Brennan MD, Li Y. A MicroRNA gene is hosted in an intron of a schizophrenia-susceptibility gene. Schizophr Res 2009;109(1-3) 86-9.

[18] Schoof CR, Botelho EL, Izzotti A, Vasques Ldos R. MicroRNAs in cancer treatment and prognosis. Am J Cancer Res 2012;2(4):414-33.

[19] Galasso M, Sandhu SK, Volinia S. MicroRNA expression signatures in solid malignancies. Cancer J 2012;18(3):238-43.

[20] Lu J, Getz G, Miska EA, et al. MicroRNA expression profiles classify human cancers. Nature 2005;435(7043):834-8.

[21] Lopez-Camarillo C, Marchat LA, Arechaga-Ocampo E, et al. MetastamiRs: Non-Coding MicroRNAs Driving Cancer Invasion and Metastasis. Int J Mol Sci 2012;13(2):1347-79.

[22] Rodrigues AS, Dinis J, Gromicho M, Martins C, Laires A, Rueff J. Genomics and cancer drug resistance. Curr Pharm Biotechnol 2012;13(5):651-73.

[23] Calin GA, Ferracin M, Cimmino A, et al. A MicroRNA signature associated with prognosis and progression in chronic lymphocytic leukemia. N Engl J Med 2005;353(17):1793-801.

[24] Rutnam ZJ, Yang BB. The involvement of microRNAs in malignant transformation. Histol Histopathol 2012;27(10):1263-70.

[25] Baxter D, McInnes IB, Kurowska-Stolarska M. Novel regulatory mechanisms in inflammatory arthritis: a role for microRNA. Immunol Cell Biol 2012;90(3):288-92.

[26] Ceribelli A, Nahid MA, Satoh M, Chan EK. MicroRNAs in rheumatoid arthritis. FEBS Lett 2011;585(23):3667-74.

[27] Ceribelli A, Yao B, Dominguez-Gutierrez PR, Nahid MA, Satoh M, Chan EK. MicroRNAs in systemic rheumatic diseases. Arthritis Res Ther 2011;13(4):229.

[28] Duroux-Richard I, Jorgensen C, Apparailly F. What do microRNAs mean for rheumatoid arthritis? Arthritis Rheum 2012;64(1):11-20.

[29] Duroux-Richard I, Presumey J, Courties G, et al. MicroRNAs as new player in rheumatoid arthritis. Joint Bone Spine 2011;78(1):17-22.

[30] Furer V, Greenberg JD, Attur M, Abramson SB, Pillinger MH. The role of microRNA in rheumatoid arthritis and other autoimmune diseases. Clin Immunol 2010;136(1):1-15.

[31] Nakasa T, Nagata Y, Yamasaki K, Ochi M. A mini-review: microRNA in arthritis. Physiol Genomics 2011;43(10):566-70.

[32] Tili E, Michaille JJ, Costinean S, Croce CM. MicroRNAs, the immune system and rheumatic disease. Nat Clin Pract Rheumatol 2008;4(10):534-41.

[33] Wittmann J, Jack HM. microRNAs in rheumatoid arthritis: midget RNAs with a giant impact. Ann Rheum Dis 2011;70 Suppl 1:i92-6.

[34] Sonkoly E, Pivarcsi A. Advances in microRNAs: implications for immunity and inflammatory diseases. J Cell Mol Med 2009;13(1):24-38.

[35] Boumpas DT, Austin HA, 3rd, Fessler BJ, Balow JE, Klippel JH, Lockshin MD. Systemic lupus erythematosus: emerging concepts. Part 1: Renal, neuropsychiatric, cardiovascular, pulmonary, and hematologic disease. Ann Intern Med 1995;122(12):940-50.

[36] Dai Y, Huang YS, Tang M, et al. Microarray analysis of microRNA expression in peripheral blood cells of systemic lupus erythematosus patients. Lupus 2007;16(12):939-46.

[37] Dai Y, Sui W, Lan H, Yan Q, Huang H, Huang Y. Comprehensive analysis of microRNA expression patterns in renal biopsies of lupus nephritis patients. Rheumatol Int 2009;29(7):749-54.

[38] Lu J, Kwan BC, Lai FM, et al. Glomerular and tubulointerstitial miR-638, miR-198 and miR-146a expression in lupus nephritis. Nephrology (Carlton) 2012;17(4):346-51.

[39] Stagakis E, Bertsias G, Verginis P, et al. Identification of novel microRNA signatures linked to human lupus disease activity and pathogenesis: miR-21 regulates aberrant T cell responses through regulation of PDCD4 expression. Ann Rheum Dis 2011;70(8):1496-506.

[40] Tang Y, Luo X, Cui H, et al. MicroRNA-146A contributes to abnormal activation of the type I interferon pathway in human lupus by targeting the key signaling proteins. Arthritis Rheum 2009;60(4):1065-75.

[41] Alevizos I, Illei GG. MicroRNAs as biomarkers in rheumatic diseases. Nat Rev Rheumatol 2010;6(7):391-8.

[42] Zhao S, Wang Y, Liang Y, et al. MicroRNA-126 regulates DNA methylation in CD4+ T cells and contributes to systemic lupus erythematosus by targeting DNA methyltransferase 1. Arthritis Rheum 2011;63(5):1376-86.

[43] Te JL, Dozmorov IM, Guthridge JM, et al. Identification of unique microRNA signature associated with lupus nephritis. PLoS One 2010;5(5):e10344.

[44] Wang G, Tam LS, Li EK, et al. Serum and urinary cell-free MiR-146a and MiR-155 in patients with systemic lupus erythematosus. J Rheumatol 2010;37(12):2516-22.

[45] Wang G, Tam LS, Kwan BC, et al. Expression of miR-146a and miR-155 in the urinary sediment of systemic lupus erythematosus. Clin Rheumatol 2012;31(3):435-40.

[46] Wang G, Tam LS, Li EK, et al. Serum and urinary free microRNA level in patients with systemic lupus erythematosus. Lupus 2011;20(5):493-500.

[47] Hai-yan W, Yang L, Mei-hong C, Hui Z. Expression of MicroRNA-146a in peripheral blood mononuclear cells in patients with systemic lupus Erythematosus. Zhongguo Yi Xue Ke Xue Yuan Xue Bao 2011;33(2):185-8.

[48] Pan W, Zhu S, Yuan M, et al. MicroRNA-21 and microRNA-148a contribute to DNA hypomethylation in lupus CD4+ T cells by directly and indirectly targeting DNA methyltransferase 1. J Immunol 2010;184(12):6773-81.

[49] Ding S, Liang Y, Zhao M, et al. Decreased microRNA-142-3p/5p expression causes CD4+ T cell activation and B cell hyperstimulation in systemic lupus erythematosus. Arthritis Rheum 2012;64(9):2953-63.

[50] Moutsopoulos HM. Sjogren's syndrome: autoimmune epithelitis. Clin Immunol Immunopathol 1994;72(2):162-5.

[51] Michael A, Bajracharya SD, Yuen PS, et al. Exosomes from human saliva as a source of microRNA biomarkers. Oral Dis 2010;16(1):34-8.

[52] Alevizos I, Illei GG. MicroRNAs in Sjogren's syndrome as a prototypic autoimmune disease. Autoimmun Rev 2010;9(9):618-21.

[53] Lu Q, Renaudineau Y, Cha S, et al. Epigenetics in autoimmune disorders: highlights of the 10th Sjogren's syndrome symposium. Autoimmun Rev 2010;9(9):627-30.

[54] Pauley KM, Stewart CM, Gauna AE, et al. Altered miR-146a expression in Sjogren's syndrome and its functional role in innate immunity. Eur J Immunol 2011;41(7):2029-39.

[55] Zilahi E, Tarr T, Papp G, Griger Z, Sipka S, Zeher M. Increased microRNA-146a/b, TRAF6 gene and decreased IRAK1 gene expressions in the peripheral mononuclear cells of patients with Sjogren's syndrome. Immunol Lett 2012;141(2):165-8.

[56] LeRoy EC, Black C, Fleischmajer R, et al. Scleroderma (systemic sclerosis): classification, subsets and pathogenesis. J Rheumatol 1988;15(2):202-5.

[57] Maurer B, Stanczyk J, Jungel A, et al. MicroRNA-29, a key regulator of collagen expression in systemic sclerosis. Arthritis Rheum 2010;62(6):1733-43.

[58] Peng WJ, Tao JH, Mei B, et al. MicroRNA-29: a potential therapeutic target for systemic sclerosis. Expert Opin Ther Targets 2012;16(9):875-9.

[59] Zhu H, Li Y, Qu S, et al. MicroRNA expression abnormalities in limited cutaneous scleroderma and diffuse cutaneous scleroderma. J Clin Immunol 2012;32(3):514-22.

[60] Felson DT. The course of osteoarthritis and factors that affect it. Rheum Dis Clin North Am 1993;19(3):607-15.

[61] Iliopoulos D, Malizos KN, Oikonomou P, Tsezou A. Integrative microRNA and proteomic approaches identify novel osteoarthritis genes and their collaborative metabolic and inflammatory networks. PLoS One 2008;3(11):e3740.

[62] Jones SW, Watkins G, Le Good N, et al. The identification of differentially expressed microRNA in osteoarthritic tissue that modulate the production of TNF-alpha and MMP13. Osteoarthritis Cartilage 2009;17(4):464-72.

[63] Tardif G, Hum D, Pelletier JP, Duval N, Martel-Pelletier J. Regulation of the IGFBP-5 and MMP-13 genes by the microRNAs miR-140 and miR-27a in human osteoarthritic chondrocytes. BMC Musculoskelet Disord 2009;10:148.

[64] Li X, Gibson G, Kim JS, et al. MicroRNA-146a is linked to pain-related pathophysiology of osteoarthritis. Gene 2011;480(1-2):34-41.

[65] Okuhara A, Nakasa T, Shibuya H, et al. Changes in microRNA expression in peripheral mononuclear cells according to the progression of osteoarthritis. Mod Rheumatol 2012;22(3):446-57.

[66] Klareskog L, Catrina AI, Paget S. Rheumatoid arthritis. Lancet 2009;373(9664):659-72.

[67] Kawano S, Nakamachi Y. miR-124a as a key regulator of proliferation and MCP-1 secretion in synoviocytes from patients with rheumatoid arthritis. Ann Rheum Dis 2011;70 Suppl 1:i88-91.

[68] Kurowska-Stolarska M, Alivernini S, Ballantine LE, et al. MicroRNA-155 as a proinflammatory regulator in clinical and experimental arthritis. Proc Natl Acad Sci U S A 2011;108(27):11193-8.

[69] Nakamachi Y, Kawano S, Takenokuchi M, et al. MicroRNA-124a is a key regulator of proliferation and monocyte chemoattractant protein 1 secretion in fibroblast-like synoviocytes from patients with rheumatoid arthritis. Arthritis Rheum 2009;60(5): 1294-304.

[70] Nakasa T, Miyaki S, Okubo A, et al. Expression of microRNA-146 in rheumatoid arthritis synovial tissue. Arthritis Rheum 2008;58(5):1284-92.

[71] Niederer F, Trenkmann M, Ospelt C, et al. Down-regulation of microRNA-34a* in rheumatoid arthritis synovial fibroblasts promotes apoptosis resistance. Arthritis Rheum 2012;64(6):1771-9.

[72] Niimoto T, Nakasa T, Ishikawa M, et al. MicroRNA-146a expresses in interleukin-17 producing T cells in rheumatoid arthritis patients. BMC Musculoskelet Disord 2010;11:209.

[73] Stanczyk J, Ospelt C, Karouzakis E, et al. Altered expression of microRNA-203 in rheumatoid arthritis synovial fibroblasts and its role in fibroblast activation. Arthritis Rheum 2011;63(2):373-81.

[74] Stanczyk J, Pedrioli DM, Brentano F, et al. Altered expression of MicroRNA in synovial fibroblasts and synovial tissue in rheumatoid arthritis. Arthritis Rheum 2008;58(4):1001-9.

[75] Bluml S, Bonelli M, Niederreiter B, et al. Essential role of microRNA-155 in the pathogenesis of autoimmune arthritis in mice. Arthritis Rheum 2011;63(5):1281-8.

[76] Worm J, Stenvang J, Petri A, et al. Silencing of microRNA-155 in mice during acute inflammatory response leads to derepression of c/ebp Beta and down-regulation of G-CSF. Nucleic Acids Res 2009;37(17):5784-92.

[77] Pauley KM, Satoh M, Chan AL, Bubb MR, Reeves WH, Chan EK. Upregulated miR-146a expression in peripheral blood mononuclear cells from rheumatoid arthritis patients. Arthritis Res Ther 2008;10(4):R101.

[78] Feng ZT, Li J, Ren J, Lv Z. [Expression of miR-146a and miR-16 in peripheral blood mononuclear cells of patients with rheumatoid arthritis and their correlation to the disease activity]. Nan Fang Yi Ke Da Xue Xue Bao 2011;31(2):320-3.

[79] Li J, Wan Y, Guo Q, et al. Altered microRNA expression profile with miR-146a upregulation in CD4+ T cells from patients with rheumatoid arthritis. Arthritis Res Ther 2010;12(3):R81.

[80] Murata K, Yoshitomi H, Tanida S, et al. Plasma and synovial fluid microRNAs as potential biomarkers of rheumatoid arthritis and osteoarthritis. Arthritis Res Ther 2010;12(3):R86.

[81] Taganov KD, Boldin MP, Chang KJ, Baltimore D. NF-kappaB-dependent induction of microRNA miR-146, an inhibitor targeted to signaling proteins of innate immune responses. Proc Natl Acad Sci U S A 2006;103(33):12481-6.

[82] Nakasa T, Shibuya H, Nagata Y, Niimoto T, Ochi M. The inhibitory effect of microRNA-146a expression on bone destruction in collagen-induced arthritis. Arthritis Rheum 2011;63(6):1582-90.

[83] Yamasaki K, Nakasa T, Miyaki S, et al. Expression of MicroRNA-146a in osteoarthritis cartilage. Arthritis Rheum 2009;60(4):1035-41.

[84] Fulci V, Scappucci G, Sebastiani GD, et al. miR-223 is overexpressed in T-lymphocytes of patients affected by rheumatoid arthritis. Hum Immunol 2010;71(2):206-11.

[85] Sebastiani GD, Fulci V, Niccolini S, et al. Over-expression of miR-223 in T-lymphocytes of early rheumatoid arthritis patients. Clin Exp Rheumatol 2011;29(6):1058-9.

[86] Szodoray P, Alex P, Chappell-Woodward CM, et al. Circulating cytokines in Norwegian patients with psoriatic arthritis determined by a multiplex cytokine array system. Rheumatology (Oxford) 2007;46(3):417-25.

[87] Costello P, Bresnihan B, O'Farrelly C, FitzGerald O. Predominance of CD8+ T lymphocytes in psoriatic arthritis. J Rheumatol 1999;26(5):1117-24.

[88] Fitzgerald O, Winchester R. Psoriatic arthritis: from pathogenesis to therapy. Arthritis Res Ther 2009;11(1):214.

[89] Partsch G, Steiner G, Leeb BF, Dunky A, Broll H, Smolen JS. Highly increased levels of tumor necrosis factor-alpha and other proinflammatory cytokines in psoriatic arthritis synovial fluid. J Rheumatol 1997;24(3):518-23.

[90] Alenius GM, Eriksson C, Rantapaa Dahlqvist S. Interleukin-6 and soluble interleukin-2 receptor alpha-markers of inflammation in patients with psoriatic arthritis? Clin Exp Rheumatol 2009;27(1):120-3.

[91] Mortel MR, Emer J. Prospective new biologic therapies for psoriasis and psoriatic arthritis. J Drugs Dermatol 2010;9(8):947-58.

[92] Sonkoly E, Wei T, Janson PC, et al. MicroRNAs: novel regulators involved in the pathogenesis of psoriasis? PLoS One 2007;2(7):e610.

[93] Primo MN, Bak RO, Schibler B, Mikkelsen JG. Regulation of pro-inflammatory cytokines TNFalpha and IL24 by microRNA-203 in primary keratinocytes. Cytokine 2012.

[94] Sonkoly E, Stahle M, Pivarcsi A. MicroRNAs: novel regulators in skin inflammation. Clin Exp Dermatol 2008;33(3):312-5.

[95] Lerman G, Avivi C, Mardoukh C, et al. MiRNA expression in psoriatic skin: reciprocal regulation of hsa-miR-99a and IGF-1R. PLoS One 2011;6(6):e20916.

[96] Meisgen F, Xu N, Wei T, et al. MiR-21 is up-regulated in psoriasis and suppresses T cell apoptosis. Exp Dermatol 2012;21(4):312-4.

[97] Xu N, Brodin P, Wei T, et al. MiR-125b, a microRNA downregulated in psoriasis, modulates keratinocyte proliferation by targeting FGFR2. J Invest Dermatol 2011;131(7):1521-9.

[98] Zibert JR, Lovendorf MB, Litman T, Olsen J, Kaczkowski B, Skov L. MicroRNAs and potential target interactions in psoriasis. J Dermatol Sci 2010;58(3):177-85.

[99] Ichihara A, Jinnin M, Yamane K, et al. microRNA-mediated keratinocyte hyperproliferation in psoriasis vulgaris. Br J Dermatol 2011;165(5):1003-10.

[100] Ichihara A, Jinnin M, Oyama R, et al. Increased serum levels of miR-1266 in patients with psoriasis vulgaris. Eur J Dermatol 2012;22(1):68-71.

[101] Chan EK, Satoh M, Pauley KM. Contrast in aberrant microRNA expression in systemic lupus erythematosus and rheumatoid arthritis: is microRNA-146 all we need? Arthritis Rheum 2009;60(4):912-5.

[102] Tsitsiou E, Lindsay MA. microRNAs and the immune response. Curr Opin Pharmacol 2009;9(4):514-20.

Chapter 4

Catecholestrogens in Rheumatoid Arthritis (RA): Hidden Role

Wahid Ali Khan and Mohd. Wajid Ali Khan

Additional information is available at the end of the chapter

http://dx.doi.org/10.5772/51794

1. Introduction

Sex hormones are implicated in immune response, with estrogens acting as enhancers [10]. Estrogens not only have anti-inflammatory but also pro-inflammatory roles depending upon different influencing factors [66]. Metabolism of estrogen within the body is a complex and important subject. Estrone and estradiol are biochemically interconvertable and yield the same family of estrogen metabolites. The metabolism of estrogen takes place primarily in the liver through Phase I (hydroxylation) and Phase II (methylation, glucuronidation, and sulfation) pathways with ultimate excretion in the urine and feces [26].

Cytochrome P-450 enzymes mediate the hydroxylation of estradiol and estrone, which is the major Phase I metabolic pathway for endogenous estrogens. Several extrahepatic target tissues or cultured cells from target tissue express estrogen-hydroxylating enzymes activities [28]. Each cytochrome P-450 favors the hydroxylation of specific carbons, altogether, these enzymes can hydroxylate virtually all carbons in the molecule, with the exception of the inaccessible carbons. Different functional groups produced by the action of P-450 at the specific sites of steroid nucleus markedly effects the biological properties of different estrogen metabolites. For example, different hydroxylation reaction give estrogenic or carcinogenic metabolites. Functionally, the important reactions catalyzed by cytochrome P-450 are at carbon number 2, 4 and 16.

In this chapter, we venture into the area of the ambiguous relationship between catecholestrogens (CEs) and rheumatoid arthritis (RA). This analysis is focused in a part on the possible role of CEs in the pathogenesis of RA and on exploring the mechanism behind the generation of autoantibodies taken consideration the role of CEs. It also explains a unique hypothesis, which showed that CEs formed in various tissues undergo oxidative metabolism (enzymatic or non-enzymatic) to produce reactive oxygen species (ROS), which could modified DNA and alter it immunogenicity. This would lead to the induction and elevated levels of RA autoantibodies. In addition, chapter further explain the role of CEs in antigen-driven induction of RA autoantibodies that may unfold various aspects of RA.

2. Catecholestrogens (CEs)

Catecholestrogens (CEs) are biological active metabolites of estrogen which are synthesized by estrogen 2- and 4- hydroxylase in the liver, brain and other organ [29]. They are produced by the actions of genes encoded by CYP1A1, CYP1A2 and CYP1B1, which is an estrogen 4-hydroxylase (Figure 1).

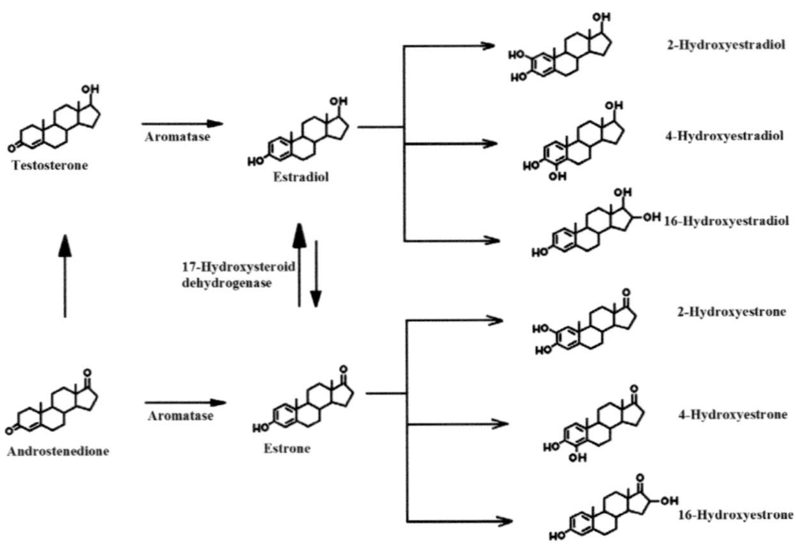

Figure 1. Pathway of estrogen metabolism including estradiol, estrone and various estrogen metabolites (including CEs).

CEs also yield potent genotoxic molecules implicated in carcinogenesis. 4-Hydroxyestrone/estradiol was found to be carcinogenic in the male Syrian golden hamster kidney tumor model, whereas 2-hydroxylated metabolites were without activity [46]. 4-Hydroxyestrogen can be oxidized to quinone intermediates that react with purine base of DNA, resulting in depurinating adduct that generates highly mutagenic apurinic sites. Quinones derived from 2-hydroxyestrogens produced stable DNA adducts and are presumed to be less genotoxic [67]. As described elsewhere, estrogen may be oxidized by hepatic cytochrome P-450 enzymes to hydroxyl CEs and further oxidized to the semiquinone and quinone form [1]. The quinone formed from oxidation of 4-hydroxyestrogen has half-life of 12 minutes as compared with the short life of 2-hydroxyestrogen ($t_{1/2}$ = 47 s) [30]. Estrone and estradiol are oxidized to lesser amount to 2-hydroxycatechols by CYP3A4 in liver and by CYP1A in extrahepatic tissues or to 4-hydroxycatechols by CYP1B1 in extrahepatic sites, with the 2-hydroxycatechol being formed to a larger extent. Catechol-o-methyl transferases (COMTs) inactivated 2- and 4-hydroxycatechols to their respective methyl derivatives [69]. COMT, a phase II enzyme, catalyses the transfer of methyl group from S-adenosyl methionine to hydroxyl groups of a number of catechol substrates, including the catecholestrogens. CEs under normal condition are o-methylated by COMT to form 2- and 4-o-methylethers, which are excreted in the urine [56]. Small amount of CEs may also be converted by peroxidase-catalysed reactions to semiquinones or quinones that are capable of forming DNA adducts or generating ROS via redox cycling that could oxidize DNA bases [69]. Estrogen metabolites have indirect and direct genotoxicity. Hydroxylation is an important elimination step for estrogen to generate CEs. Microsomal estradiol hydroxylation in human breast cancer showed significantly higher 4-hydroxy:2-hydroxyestradiol ratio in tumor tissue than in adjacent normal breast tissue [48], but the breast cancer tissue samples contained fourfold higher levels of 4-hydroxyestradiol (4-OHE_2) than in normal tissue from benign breast biopsies [57].

It has been observed that intra-tissue concentration of estrogens, hydroxyestrogens (16 α-hydroxyestrone, 2-hydroxyestrone, 2-hydroxyestradiol, 4-hydroxyestrone, and 4-hydroxyestradiol) and methoxyestrogens (2-methoxyestrone, 2-methoxyestradiol, 4-methoxyestrone, and 4-methoxyestradiol) in normal and malignant breast showed the highest concentration of 4-hydroxyestradiol in malignant tissue [4]. The concentration, as evaluated by combined high performance liquid chromatograpy (HPLC) and gas chromatograpy-mass spectrometry (GC-MS) was found to be more than twice as high as that of any other compound. CEs have been measured in rat brain and various endocrine tissues by sensitive radioenzymatic assay. The concentration of these CEs in the hypothalamus and pituitary are at least ten times higher than parent estrogen. CEs have potent endocrine effect i.e. they have an important role in neuroendocrine regulation [54].

In addition, brain is capable of 2-hydroxylation and consequently forms CEs from estrone and estradiol. Increased availability of estrogen and estradiol for binding and hypothalamic sites would facilitate formation of CEs. 2-Hydroxylated and 4-hydroxylated estrogen exerts biologic responses on the cyclic secretion of leutenising hormone (LH) perhaps even on follicle stimulating hormone (FSH) and prolactin. Catecholestradiol competes with estradiol for estrogen binding sites in the anterior pituitary gland and hypothalamus and dopamine binding sites on anterior pituitary membranes [41].

Mitogenicity associated with estrogen receptor (ER)-mediated cellular events was believed to be the mechanism by which estrogens contributed to carcinogenesis [59]. The role of CEs as genotoxic chemical procarcinogenesis, independent of ER mediation, has been well recognized [70]. Although oxidative metabolism of estrogen to CEs is generally thought to terminate the estrogenic signal, but CEs retain some binding affinity to the ER. Exposure of MCF-7 cells with 2- and 4-hydroxyestradiol increased the rate of cell proliferation and the expression of estrogen-inducible gene such as progesterone receptor (PR) gene and pS2. Compare to estradiol, 2- and 4-hydroxyestradiol increased proliferation rate, level of PR protein as well as pS2 mRNA expression to certain fold [62].

As describe previously, estrogens are metabolized via two pathways i.e. formation of CEs and to lesser extent, 16 α-hydroxylation. The catechols are formed as 2- and 4-hydroxylated estrogen. These two CEs can be inactivated by the enzyme COMT through o-methylation [69]. Other possible mechanism of inactivation includes conjugation of CEs by glucouronidation and sulphation. High concentration of 4-hydroxylated metabolites caused insufficient production of methyl, glucouronide or sulphate conjugate which in turn results in CE toxicity in cell and consequently competitive catalytic oxidation to semiquinone (CE-SQ) and quinone (CE-Q). CE-SQ and CE-Q may conjugate with glutathione (GSH), catalyse by S-transferase. CE-Q may also react with DNA to form stable and de-purinating adduct if this inactivating process is incomplete [47].

3. CEs and DNA

Endogenous estrogens can become carcinogenic via formation of catecholestrogen quinones, which react with DNA to form specific estrogen-DNA adducts. The mutations resulting from these adducts can cause cell transformation and initiation of breast cancer [58]. The 4-hydroxyestrogen generates free radicals from reductive-oxidative cycling with the corresponding CE-SQ/CE-Q forms, thus causing DNA damage extensively. In comparison to 4-hydroxyestrogen, 2-hydroxyestrogen is not carcinogenic and has potent inhibitory effect on the growth of tumor cells and on angiogenesis [17]. The DNA adducts generated by 2-hydroxyestrogen and 4-hydroxyestrogen can form stable modifications that remain in the DNA unless they are removed by repair. On the other hand, the modification bases can be released from DNA by destabilization of the glycosydic bond and result in the formation of depurinated or depyrimidinated sites [7].

Earlier studies from our lab showed that CE modified DNA brings about single and double strand breaks, hyperchromicity, damage at the restriction sites and modification of different bases (Table 1) [40, 36, 37, 38]. It has been observed that CE caused more damage to the DNA in presence of copper in comparison to nitric oxide (NO) as the extent of base modification was greatest for thymine followed by guanine, adenine and cytosine [40]. We proposed that CE and NO formed in different tissue may react with each other to produce CE-Q.

The quinone/semiquinone redox system produces superoxide ions (O_2^-) which can react with NO to form peroxynitrite, which could cause DNA damage [38]. Quenching studies of DNA modified with CEs in presence of C(II) showed that catalase and bathocuproine strongly (~ 80 %) inhibited the modification by CEs plus Cu(II) indicating the involvement of H_2O_2 and Cu(I) during the modification [36, 37]. These results demonstrate that CEs lead to the production of potent ROS, capable of causing DNA damage, thus playing important role not only in carcinogenesis [36] but also in systemic lupus erythematosus (SLE) [40, 37, 39] and RA [38].

Parameter	Native DNA	CE-modified DNA
Hyperchromicity	—	32.2
Absorbance ratio (A_{260}/A_{280})	1.86	1.52
Melting temperature (T_m) °C	88	80.5
S1 nuclease action	No digestion	Digestion
	Restriction enzymes	
PvuI (CGAT↓CG)	Digestion	No digestion
PvuII (CAG↓CTG)	Digestion	No digestion
SspI (AAT↓ATT)	Digestion	Digestion
	Circular dichroism (mdeg) Wavelength (nm)	
+274	0.77	0.52
–246	–1.3	–7.60
–210	–0.85	–0.58
Scavengers		*inhibition of modification*
Catalase	—	82
Sodium azide	—	21
Bathocuproine	—	80
Ascorbic acid	—	35
	Base modification	
Adenine	—	16.9%
Guanine	—	45.5%
Cytosine	—	12.6%
Thymine	—	47.1%

Table 1. Characterization of Native and CE-modified DNA under identical experimental conditions. (Adapted from [36]).

Over the last 2 decades, only two studies have been reported that explain the presence of CE adducts in human breast tissue. First study involves the analysis of CE adducts in the DNA from malignant breast tumor. DNA sample showed the presence of deoxyguanosine adducts of 4-hydroxyestradiol and 4-hydroxyestrone in almost every samples [21]. Other study showed the presence of CE quinone-derived DNA adduct in two breast samples that were collected from one women with and one woman without breast cancer [51]. The catechol quinone-derived adducts identified were 4-hydroxyestradiol-1-N3-adenosine, 4-hydroxyestrone-1-N3-adenosine and 4-hydroxyestradiol-1-N7-guanine. Animal experimentation involves the injection of 4-hydroxyestradiol (or estradiol-3,4-quinone) into the mammary glands of female ACI rats which resulted in the formation of the depurinating adducts, 4-

hydroxyestradiol-1-N3-adenosine and 4-hydroxyestradiol-1-N7-guanine. [47]. In addition to these adducts, 4-hydroxyestradiol-GSH conjugates was also detected. Another study demonstrates the presence of 4-hydroxy catecholestrogen conjugates with GSH or its hydrolytic product (cysteine and N-acetylcysteine) both in tumors and hyperplastic mammary tissues in ERKO/Wnt-1 mice [18]. Estradiol-3,4-quinone reacted rapidly to form 4-hydroxyestradiol-1-N3-adenosine adducts that are considered to be as depurinating adducts.

It has been shown that CEs can induce DNA lesions not only in plasmid DNA [40, 36, 37, 38] but also in calf thymus DNA [49]. In short, quinone intermediates produced by oxidation of the CE 4-hydroxyestradiol or 4-hydroxyestrone may react with purine bases of DNA to form depurinating adducts that generate highly mutagenic apurinic sites. In contrast, quinone of 2-hydroxylated estrogen produce less harmful and stable DNA adducts [7]. The CE metabolites may also produced potentially mutagenic oxygen radicals by metabolic redox cycling that can also caused DNA damage. The abasic sites resulting from the spontaneous depurination-depyrimidination of the modified bases and the aldehydic base and sugar lesions resulting from the oxidative damage to deoxyribose moieties in the DNA molecules [49], disturb the structural integrity of DNA and destabilize the double helix. This would alter it property and render DNA immunogenic.

4. CEs and Immune Response

Despite a large number of reports that may explain the role of estrogen (or estradiol) in modulation of immune response [10, 66], the role of CEs in the immune response is lacking. It has been observed that the conversion from 2-hydroxysetrogens to 4-hydroxyestrogen might be an additional pro-inflammatory signal because these endogenous metabolites can be oxidized to 3,4-quinone, which lead to depurination and mutation [49]. The 3,4-semiquinone and quinone produce ROS, which stimulate inflammation, whereas methylation and sulfation are detoxification pathways, which involve the release of detoxying agents in the urine [56]. Other pro-inflammatory role of 4- hydroxyestrogen can be explain by the fact that 4-hydroxyestradiol undergoes 2-electron oxidation to quinone via semiquinone and during this process, ROS can be generated to cause DNA damage and cell death [8]. A similar effect was observed in our studies that explained extensive DNA damage and base modification [40, 36, 37, 38, 39]. In contrast to the pro-oxidant activities of 4-hydroxyestradiol, 2-hydroxyestradiol is a antioxidant that show no carcinogenic activities and has potent inhibitory effect on the growth of tumor cells and on angiogenesis [17]. Thus, 4-hydroxyestradiol in comparison to 2-hydroxyestradiol induce carcinogenesis and have pro-inflammatory effects [20]. But now, we are unaware of the fact that whether pro-inflammatory mediators induce a shift from 2-hydroxyestrogen to 4- and 16-hydroxylated estrogens. From all these studies there is a clear evidence that 2-methoxyestradiol is a pro-apoptotic and cytostatic endogenous compound, which can inhibit not only angiogenesis [17] but also inflammation in animal models. In contrast, 4-hydroxylated estrogens might exert pro-inflammatory roles by inducing ROS and DNA damage. Just like conversion from 2-hydroxyestrogens to 4-hydroxyestrogens, a shift to 16 α-hydroxylated forms of estrogen can be an important pro-inflammatory and pro-proliferative signal [66].

The direct role of CEs in mediating immune response can be explain in our studies that demonstrate the production of antibodies to CE-modified plasmid DNA [40, 36, 37, 39, 38]. As reported earlier, CE-modified DNA (CE-DNA) was found to be highly immunogenic (> 1:12800) in animal model [36]. These antibodies were effectively used as probe for detecting oxidative lesions in human genomic DNA as well as for the estimation of 8-hydroxy-2′-deoxyguanosine (8-OHG) level in the urine of cancer patients [36] and RA patients [38]. Antibodies evaluated from competition ELISA showed strong specificity for the CE-DNA (immunogen) causing about 92 % inhibition in anibody binding at 20 μg/ml of the immunogen (competitor) concentration. Fifty percent inhibition was observed at 3.5 μg/ml of the immunogen. In addition, these antibodies showed a very high degree of binding toward 8-OHG that may explain the role of ROS in mediating various immune responses including inflammation. CE-modified form of different bases (adenine, guanine, cytosine, thymine), human and calf thymus DNA, ROS-DNA, poly nucleotides (dT, dA, dC, dG, dA-dT) were also recognized by these antibodies. Another evidence that explain the role of CEs in mediating immune responses comes from our previous study that showed that CE-DNA was not only recognized highly by cancer autoantibodies [36] but also by anti-DNA autoantibodies in SLE [40, 37] and RA [38]. Results from all these studies demonstrate that CEs somehow produce some antigenic stimulus that may contribute to the generation of antibodies which may directly or indirectly affect the immune system.

Dual pro-inflammatory and anti-inflammatory role of estrogens has been described earlier [66], which depend on the immune stimulus, subsequent antigen-specific immune response, the cell types involved during different disease phase, the specific microenvironment, timing of estrogen administration in relation to the disease course, the concentration of estrogen, the variability in expression of estrogen receptor depending on the microenvironment and the cell type and intracellular metabolism of estrogen leading to important biologically active metabolites (CEs) with quite different anti- and pro-inflammatory function. In addition, one of the striking property of estrogen is its ability to differentiate T and B cells, increase immunoglobulin production and increase immune complex-mediated disease such as SLE [9]. It has been found that women, who are diagnosed with breast cancer, have significantly elevated anti-HMdU autoantibodies [23]. This study is in agreement with our previous finding that explains the presence of circulating antibodies against CE-modified DNA in cancer patients [36]. The modified DNA presents unique epitopes which may be one of the factors for autoantibody induction in cancer. The presence of high levels of these antibodies proves to be the pro-oxidant conditions that have led to the oxidation of bases in genomic DNA and have stimulate an immune response. Since native DNA is a known weak immunogen, it appear that DNA damage by CE render it immunogenic leading to the induction of cancer autoantibodies. It has been suggested that the oxidative DNA damage and the immunologic responses it evokes (autoantibodies) start occurring not only in the carcinogenic process [36] but also in various autoimmune diseases [40, 36, 37, 39, 38] Estrogen also modulate the function of PMNs (poly morphonuclear leukocytes, neutrophils, granulocytes), which in turn cause the production of ROS on their stimulation. ROS generated by PMNs cause DNA modification as well as oxidation of protein and lipid peroxidation. It is interesting to note that 2-hydroxylated estrogens works as powerful inhibitors of PMNs activity, which shows one of the protective property of the 2-hydroxylated CEs. Therefore, estrogens (and estrogen metabolites like CEs) affect immunological responses and in turn, their activities are affected by the immunological products. In addition, estrogen in physiological concentration serves to enhance immune response by inducing the production of various types of cytokines and interleukins.

5. CEs and Cytokines

The sex hormones are likely to directly modulate the function of cells involved in the immune response [42]. The pro- and anti-inflammatory effects of estrogen and their metabolites (CEs) on secretion of pro-inflammatory cytokines have been a matter of debate for two or three decades. In fact, at physiological dose, estradiol induce IL-1α, a cytokine that can initiate a cascade of other cytokines, chemotactic and growth factors [12]. It is interesting to note that estradiol also inhibits IL-1α-induced IL-6 production. Therefore, estradiol not only results in increased human epithelial cell proliferation (a process important in tumor growth) but also inhibits the activity of natural killer cells, thus allowing tumor growth [52].

Estrogen and their metabolites (such as CEs) stabilized or increased cytokine secretion whereas testosterone inhibited this secretion [32]. This study explains that down stream estrogen, 2-hydroxyestradiol (2-OHE$_2$), 4-OHE$_2$ and 16-hydroxyestradiol (16-OHE$_2$) did not stimulate TNF secretion. However, the combination of 16-OHE$_2$ and 2-OHE$_2$ or 4-OHE$_2$ markedly stimulated TNF secretion that was observed in presence of cortisol. Therefore, at physiological concentration, estradiol and a combination of downstream estrogens (like 2-OHE$_2$, 4-OHE$_2$ and 16-OHE$_2$) increased (or stabilized) immune stimuli-induced TNF secretion. In addition, estradiol also caused the production of IL-6, IL-2, IFNγ, IL-4 and IL-10, caused by the pro-inflammatory influence of applied immune stimuli [32]. The study of Janele et al, 2006.] demonstrates that ratio of 16-hydroxylated estrogen in relation to 2-/4-hydroxylated estrogen is important for TNF secretion. It has been found that the ratio of 10:1 of 16-OHE$_2$ in relation to 2-/4- hydroxylated estrogen markedly stimulated TNF secretion in presence of cortisol (Figure 2).

In addition, in absence of cortisol, the combination of 16-hydroxylated and 2-hydroxylated estrogens even strongly inhibited TNF secretion. During chronic inflammatic conditions, administration of therapeutic estrogens increased 16-hydroxylated estrogens. In addition, during chronic inflammation in the situation of rheumatic diseases (example RA) the balance is switch to estrogen and particularly to 16-hydroxylated estrogen. In conclusion, one should assume that therapeutic administration of estrogen would enhance 16-OHE$_2$ over 2-/4-hydroxylated estrogens, which would support secretion of pro-inflammatory cytokines.

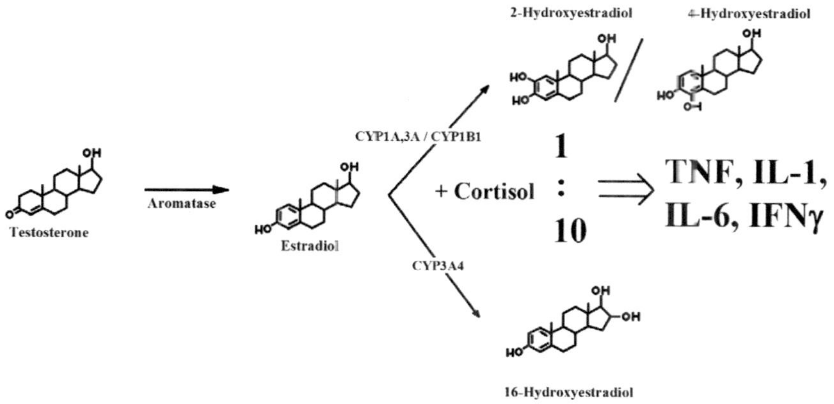

Figure 2. Effect of estrogen and their catechol metabolites (CEs) on the secretion of pro-inflammatory cytokines in RA.

It has been observed that estradiol increased IgG and IgM production by peripheral blood mononuclear cells (PBMC) in patients of SLE. This led to elevated levels of polyclonal IgG (including IgG anti-dsDNA) by enhancing B-cell activity by way of IL-10 [33]. It should be important to check these results in the presence of 16 α-hydroxyestrone (16-OHE$_1$) and the naturally occurring 2-hydroxylated CE. Previous study shown that decrease activity in SLE patients correlated negatively with urinary concentration of 2-hydroxylated estrogens [68]. Interestingly, estradiol increase IL-10 production by monocytes and exogenous IL-10 further enhances estradiol-induced increase in antibody production by B cells. Therefore, in SLE patients, estradiol increases IL-10 production by patient's monocytes and exogenous IL-10 acts additively with estradiol to increase antibody production of B cells. It is hypothesized that estradiol-estradiol receptor complexes may enhance the transcription of IL-10 genes by binding to estrogen-responsive elements or by binding to some transcription factor that directly bind those elements [24].

High doses of estrogen (1500-2000 pg/ml) administration to non-overiectomized mice ameliorated disease systems and significantly decreased the percentage of TNF α or IFNγ producing CNS antigen-specific T Cells in both the CNS and spleen [31]. However, similar studies in mice lacking IFNγ, IL-4 and IL-10 genes provide evidence that these cytokines may not be necessary for estradiol-mediated improvement of disease severity, discrediting the notion that an estrogen-induced shift towards Th 2 cytokine involved [31]. Estrogen also stimulates secretion of IL-4, -5, -6 and -10 by T_H 2 lymphocytes. These cytokines are potent stimulators of B-cell proliferation, maturation into plasma cells and synthesis of antibody. Interleukins 4, 5, 6 and 10 are expressed in greater amount in an estrogen-dominant hormonal milieu [53]. SLE patients have increased level of IL-6 and IL-10, product of T_H2 lymphocytes and macrophages, which can be directly correlated with clinical disease severity [53]. Patients with lupus also have an inherent defect in interferon gamma production. Under normal condition, increased estrogen leads to an increase interferon gamma concentration but in SLE patients, the estrogen-associated increase in interferon gamma secretion is absent

[53]. In addition, interesting changes of serum estrogens that correlated with cytokine variation have been found during pregnancy in SLE patients [19]. The local effect of sex hormones in autoimmune rheumatoid disease (RA) seem to consist mainly of altered cell proliferation (i.e. estrogen enhance) and cytokine production.

6. Reminding the concept of rheumatoid arthritis (RA)

Rheumatoid arthritis (RA) is an autoimmune disease whose aetiology and progression are multifactorial, including a range of immune, neuroendocrine and psychosocial variable [14]. How these variable interact with one another and how they ultimately influence the disease process in RA is only partially know. A growing body of evidence showed that the stress system and its interaction with the immune system, play a vital role in RA [14]. RA is more prevalent among women than men and 80 % of the total cases occurring between the age of 35 and 50 [34]. The primary presenting symptoms are pain, stiffness and swelling of the joints resulting in impaired physical function. Synovial inflammation underlines the cardinal manifestations of this disease, which include pain, swelling and tenderness followed by cartilage destruction, bone erosion and subsequent joint deformities. In RA, joint involvement is typically symmetric, a characteristic usually not found in other forms of arthritis [50]. Early theories on the pathogenesis of RA focused on autoantibodies and immune complexes, T cell-mediated antigen-specific responses, T cell-independent cytokine network and aggressive tumor-like behavior of synovium have also been implicated [22]. Recently the contribution of autoantibodies in RA has come in the front line and specific therapeutic interventions can be designed to suppress synovial inflammation and join destruction in RA [22].

RFs have been the hallmark autoantibody found in RA [71]. Autoantibodies to the major cartilaginous collagen have been found in the sera of some RA patients. In addition, cross-reactive natural autoantibodies (IgM) have been described in the sera of RA patients [25]. These antibodies are predominantly directed against histone moieties or against double-stranded DNA. Anti-ds DNA has also been reported following treatment of RA with IFNγ. Beside that, autoantibodies have been found in the sera of RA patients that showed preferentially high binding of CE-modified DNA [38]. In addition, the antibodies have been shown to represent a alternative immunochemical probe to detect oxidative lesions in DNA (genomic) as well as for the estimation of 8-OHdG level in different body fluid of RA patients [38], which may be used as marker in the diagnosis of the disease. Many autoantibody system that could participate in inflammatory joint disease are now recognized in RA, including rheumatoid factor, type II collagen, immunoglobulin heavy gene binding protein, heat shock proteins and hn RNP-33 [64]. Anti-collagen antibody and rheumatoid factor are produced by rheumatoid synovial B cells. The ability of ubiquitous antigen (glucose-6-phosphoisomerase) to induce synovial inflammation is probably related to their adherence to the cartilage surfaces. The presentation of immobilized antigen-antibody complexes on cartilage provides an exceptionally good substrate for complement fixation, similar to rheumatoid factor embedded in rheumatoid cartilage.

Macrophage-derived cytokines (like tumor necrosis factor alpha, TNF α) know to play an important role in the induction and perpetuation of the chronic inflammatory processes in rheumatoid joints as well as in the systemic manifestation of this disease [27]. Over production of this cytokines in the joints of RA patients triggers increase in synoviocyte proliferation and a cascade of secondary mediators involved in the recruitment of inflammatory cells and in the process of joint destruction [3]. It has been found that increase inflammatory markers are responsible for disease progression and joint destruction in early RA. Infect the rate of cartilage and joint destruction is correlated with plasma elevation in inflammatory acute phase reactants (C-reactive protein and vascular endothelial growth factor) and in the synovial concentration of matrix metalloproteinase, matrix digesting enzymes directly responsible for joint damage [2].

In recent years the treatment of RA has undergone somewhat of a revolution, with a strong consensus emerging in favor of early, aggressive therapy [63]. There is growing evidence that early treatment of the disease has a beneficial impact on treatment outcome. The goal to be achieved in managing RA are to explain the underline mechanism behind the generation of antibodies to cartilaginous collagen as well as other oxidative stress condition generated in the synovial fluid, which may be used as marker in the early diagnosis of the disease.

7. Role of CEs in the aetiopathogenesis of RA

Estrogen and their CE metabolites know to play an important role in autoimmune rheumatic diseases [38, 68, 15]. A role for estrogen in the pathogenesis of RA has been review for the last few years [66, 70, 38, 12, 32, 68, 15] but the exact patho-aetiology remains elusive. The evidences concerning the possibility of CEs in the development of RA are very limited and preliminary. It has been observed that the ratio of 16-OHE$_1$/4-OHE$_2$ in synovial fluid (SF) of RA was found to be significantly higher than control [6]. In addition, SF level of 4-OHE$_2$ was significantly increased in RA patients compared to controls [5]. Interestingly, urinary concentration of 2-hydroxylated estrogen were 10 times lower in patients with RA than in healthy individuals but the ratio of 16-OHE$_1$/2-hydroxylated was 20 times in RA patients as compared to control [68]. These finding suggests that the magnitude of conversion to the mitogenic 16-OHE$_1$ is extremely upregulated in RA which most likely contributes to the maintenance of the disease. Furthermore, peripheral estrogen hydroxylation was found to be increased in both men and women with SLE and estrogenic metabolites were reported to increase B cell differentiation and activate T cells [44].

Both RA and SLE are associated with an altered sex hormone balance characterized by lower amount of immunosuppressive androgens and higher amount of immune enhancing estrogens [15]. Increased estrogen to androgen ratios have been observed in RA patient's SF because of increased aromatase expression by inflammatory macrophages infiltrating synovial tissue [5]. Increased estrogen concentration in RA SF from patients of both sex likely results from the pro-inflammatory cytokines TNFα, IL-1β and IL-6, which accelerate the metabolic conversion of estrogen from androgen by inducing the synovial tissue aromatase (Figure 3). As a result, increased estrogen level might exert activating effects on synovial cell proliferation including macrophages and fibroblast [35]. Interestingly, renal excretion studies showed that the enhanced estrogen metabolism observed in both RA and SLE patients resulted in elevation of pro-inflammatory metabolites derived from estrone or estradiol such as 16-OHE_1, which exert mitogenic effects and may induce proliferation of synovial fibroblast [68, 13]. In addition, RA SF showed reduced amounts of anti-inflammatory estrogens metabolites such as 2-hydroxyestrogen that inhibits the growth promoting effects of estrogen. In contrast, 16-OHE_1 metabolites considered as enhancer of cell proliferation. In RA synovial tissue, biological effects of estrogen metabolites as a consequence of altered peripheral sex hormone synthesis mainly results in stimulation of cell proliferation and cytokine production [11].

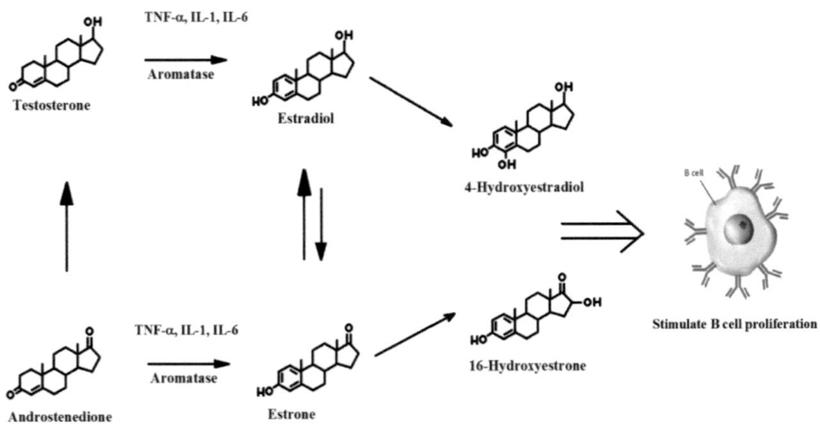

Figure 3. Immune modulation by estrogen and their metabolites in the synovial tissue of RA patients.

It has been observed that RA synovial cells mainly produce the cell pro-proliferation 16-$OHE_{1,}$ which in addition to 16-OHE_2, is the downstream estrogen metabolites that interferes with monocyte proliferation. In addition, urinary concentration and total urinary loss of 2-hydroxyestrogen was found to be 10 times higher in healthy subjects compared to RA [11]. Peripheral metabolic conversion of androgens to potent metabolites of estrogen that promote immune cell proliferation and activation may have role in the female predisposition to autoimmunity.

Estrogen represent a risk factor for the development of autoimmunity and therefore, their therapeutic use must be avoided in patients with active immune-mediated diseases specially RA [16]. In addition to estrogen, various CE metabolites know to increase the risk for the development of RA disease. The increased estrogen concentration has been observed in RA SF, where the hydroxylated forms make the major concentration in particular 16-OHE_1 and 4-OHE_2 whereas, the 2-OHE_1 was found to be similar to the controls [6, 5]. As describe early, 16-OHE_1 is a mitogenic and proliferative endogenous hormone which is responsible for the proliferation of synovial fibroblast [13]. 16-OHE$_1$ is formed from upstream estrone and estradiol, which show biological responses by covalent linkage to the receptor [61]. The other conversion product of estrone and estradiol are the 2-hydroxylated estrogens such as 2-OHE$_2$ and 2-OHE$_1$, which would classified as CE. In comparison to 16 hydroxylated estrogens, the 2-hydroxylated forms of estrogen inhibit growth-promoting effects of estradiol [61]. In one of the previous study, it has been observed that urinary levels of 2-hydroxylated estrogens were found 10 times lower in RA patients in comparison to normal subjects, whereas the ratio 16-OHE$_1$/2-hydroxyestrogens was found to be 20 times higher in RA patients than in healthy controls [68]. Decreased loss of 2-hydroxylated estrogen in relation to the mitogenic 16-OHE$_1$ might provide important stimulus to support proliferative state of the synovial cells in RA. Therefore, concentrated-related conversion to pro- and anti-inflammatory down stream metabolites of estrogen might support dual role of estrogen (pro- or anti-inflammatory) [13].

Estrogen at physiological concentration serves to enhance immune responses that may act as important driving force for human humoral immunity [65]. Estradiol increase IL-10 production by monocytes and exogenous IL-10 further enhance estradiol-induced increase in antibody production by B cells. In addition, estradiol enhances IgG and IgM production by PBMC, which leads to elevated levels of polyclonal IgG, including IgG anti-DNA in PBMC of SLE patients by enhancing B cell activity via interleukin 10 [33]. These studies are in agreement with our previous studies that describe the role of CEs in the etiopathogenesis of SLE, cancer and RA [40, 36, 37, 38, 39]. To have a better insight into the possible role of CEs in the aetiopathogenesis of RA, we have demonstrated that CE-modified DNA was highly recognized not only by SLE IgG [40, 37, 39] and cancer IgG [36] but also by RA IgG [38], pointing out the possible participation of modified DNA in the pathogenesis of various autoimmune diseases including RA, as it has been reported that CE-modified DNA bases cause DNA strand breakage and adduct formation in vivo and in vitro [7]. CE-modified DNA showed preferentially high binding with RA sera when compare with nDNA ($p < 0.001$). These studies clearly indicate that the modified DNA is an effective inhibitor showing substantial difference in the recognition of CE-modified DNA over the native form [38]. The results also demonstrate the pro-oxidant condition which is generated due to the oxidative metabolism of estrogen [40, 36]. Non-enzymatic oxidation of CE in the presence of NO [40] or Cu(II) [37] cause DNA modification and enhanced binding of these modified antigens to RA autoantibodies. To further confirm the role of CEs in RA, we evaluated the binding of autoantibodies by quantitive precipitin titration. The apparent association constant clearly indicates better recognition of CE-modified DNA over native by RA autoantibodies. The enhanced recognition of CE-modified DNA by RA IgG indicates possible participation of modified DNA in RA pathogenesis. The spontaneous production of autoantibodies in RA might arise as a consequence of antigenic change in DNA. Therefore, it could be possible that CE-modified bases of DNA might be one of the contributing factors towards the production of autoantibodies. However, the pro-inflammatory role of estrogen cannot be ruled out [65]. It might be possible that estrogen caused T and B cell differentiation and increase immunoglobulin production. These autoantibodies might be strongly bound with CE-modified DNA than native polymer. Further more, DNA isolated from sera and SF of different

RA patients caused appreciable inhibition in the activity of anti-CE-modified DNA antibodies clearly showing the presence of oxidatively altered epitopes on the isolated DNA molecules, which could be directly correlated to estrogen/radical mediated oxidative stress [38]. These studies show that hydroxylated estrogens (specially CEs) might have a role in the aetiopathogenesis of RA and other autoimmune diseases.

Various CE metabolites (4-OHE$_2$, 4-OHE$_1$, 2-OHE$_2$, 2-OHE$_1$) known to secret various cytokines from human peripheral blood leukocytes in presence of cortisol [32]. It has been demonstrated that the ratio of 16-hydroxylated estrogen in relation to 2-/4-hydroxylated estrogen is important for TNF secretion. The study showed that the ratio of 10:1 of 16-OHE$_2$ in relation to 2-/4-hydroxylated estrogens stimulate TNF secretion in the presence of cortisol otherwise this effect was not observed in absence of this hormone. Furthermore, absence of cortisol strongly inhibited TNF secretion if the combination of 16-OHE$_1$ and 2-hydroxylated estrogens were used in this experiment [32]. In addition, it has been demonstrated that estrogens are able to enhance secretion of matrix metalloproteinase and IL-1β-induced IL-6 secretion from human fibroblast-like synoviocytes in RA [35]. However, with respect to serum levels of estrogen in RA patients, they are not changed which is in strict contrast to androgen levels [13]. High estrogen concentration has been found in particular in SF of RA patients. The presence in the RA SF of an altered sex hormone balance resulting in lower immunosuppressive androgen and higher immunoenhancing estrogens might determine a favourable condition for the development of the immune-mediated RA synovitis. The appropriated explanation for high concentration of estrogen (and their CE metabolites) can be originated from the study that showed that the inflammatory cytokines (TNF-α, IL-1, IL-6) are particularly increased in RA synovitis and stimulate aromatase activity in peripheral tissues [55]. Therefore, enzyme complex is responsible for the peripheral conversion of androgen to estrogen (estrone and estradiol). In addition, a significant correlation was found between the aromatase activity and IL-6 production and aromatase has also been found significantly in synoviocytes [45]. Therefore, the increased aromatase activity induced by locally produced inflammatory cytokines (TNF-α, IL-1, IL-6) might explain the altered balance resulting in lower androgens and higher estrogen in RA SF as well as their effects on synovial cells [15, 6]. In conclusion, an increase in 16-hydroxyestrogen relative to the sum of all 2- and 4-hydroxylated estrogens (CE) must be viewed as a pro-inflammatory signal, which is particularly evident in RA patients.

Elevated serum concentration of 16-OHE$_1$ have been described in patients with SLE [43], indicating that abnormal pattern of estradiol metabolism may lead to increased estrogenic activity. Interestingly, similar phenomenon was observed in the synovial fluid of RA patients, where 16-OHE$_1$/4-OHE$_2$ was found to be significantly higher compared with control fluid [6, 5]. 4-Hydroxylated estrogens were found to be mitogenic and thus have pro-inflammatory effect [66, 68]. Importantly, all 2- and 4-hydroxylated estrogen demonstrated TNF-inhibitory effect, which was not observed with 16 α-hydroxylated estrogen. Thus the observed preference of 16 α-hydroxylated over 2-/4-hydroxylated estrogens must be considered an important pro-inflammatory signal, which occur particularly in RA patients. This study also describes methylation of hydroxylated estrogen metabolites (CEs) in addition to hydroxylation of estrone and estradiol. Catechol-o-methyl transferase, the only enzymes responsible for the methylation of CEs, was also present in primary synovial cells, although it doesn't show any preference with either estrone or estradiol-hydroxylated substrate. Similar to the 2- and 4-hydroxylated forms of estrogen, the 2- and 4-methoxy form inhibited TNF secretion from RA and osteoarthritis (OA) synovial cells [60]. These studies show that hydroxylated estrogen (especially CEs) might have a role in the aetiopathogenesis of RA and other autoimmune diseases.

7. Conclusion

Remarkable progress have been made in understanding the role of estrogen in the etiology of RA but the role of CEs in RA is lacking. Catechol metabolites known to play an important role in RA but the exact patho-aetiology remain elusive. The evidence concerning the possibility of CEs in the development of RA is very limited and preliminary. It has been observed that oxidative reactions, often catalyzed by isoforms of the cytochrome P-450, can result in the formation of CEs from parent estrogen and subsequently, semiquinones and quinones derived from CEs, are capable of forming either stable or depurinating DNA adducts. Oxidation of CEs also leads to high amount of ROS that can generate extensive DNA damage. This would probably alter its immunogenicity leading to the induction and elevated levels of RA autoantibodies (Figure 4). Therefore, it is possible that the CE-modified bases of DNA might be one of the contributing factors towards production of SLE autoantibodies. In addition, estrogen not only induces DNA damage but also modulate immune response and immune mediated disease. Estrogen was found to increase IgG and IgM from PBMC, which let to elevated level of polyclonal IgG including IgG anti-ds DNA by enhancing B cell activity via IL-10. These autoantibodies could be strongly bound to DNA and serve as an immunological marker for the diagnosis of diseases. Estrogen is thought to play both pro- and anti-inflammatory role in chronic inflammatory diseases that were found to be related to low and high concentration. Increased estrogen to androgen ratio have been observed in RA patients SF, perhaps due to increase aromatase expression by inflammatory macrophages infiltrating synovial tissues. The discovery of high concentration in SF from RA patients of both sexes can also be explain by the fact that inflammatory cytokines (i.e. TNFα, IL-1, IL-6) are increased in RA cynovitis and can markedly stimulate aromatase activity in peripheral tissue. But renal excretion studies showed that enhanced estrogen metabolism observed in RA resulted in elevation of pro-inflammatory metabolites derived from estrone and estradiol such as 16-OHE$_1$ (or 4-OHE$_2$, 4-OHE$_1$) which exert mitogenic effect on different synovial fibroblast. In contrast, RA SF have reduced amount of anti-inflammatory estrogen metabolites such as 2-hydroxyestrogen that inhibit the growth-promoting effect of estradiol. An unwanted shift from 2- to 4-hydroxyestrogen might be an additional pro-inflammatory signal because these 4-hydroxylated metabolites can be converted to 3,4-quinone, which lead to depurination and mutation in DNA. In conclusion, an increase in 16-OHE$_1$ relative to the sum of all 2- and 4-hydroxylated estrogens must be considered as pro-inflammatory signal which is particularly evident in RA [60].

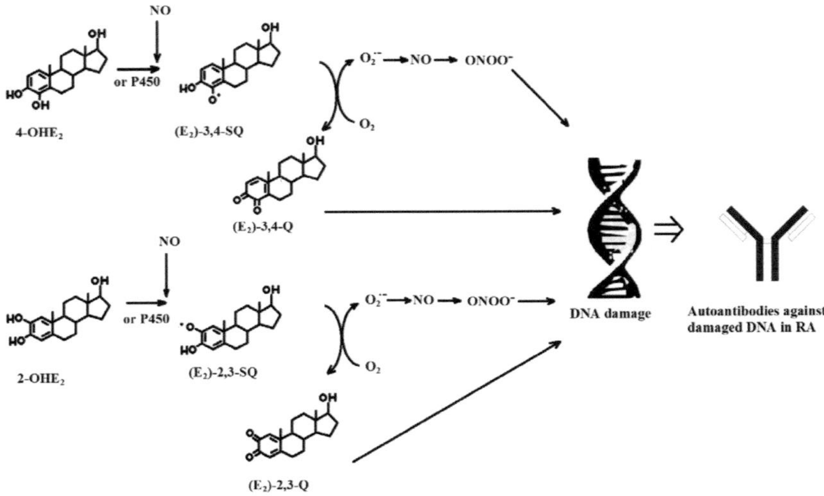

Figure 4. The proposed mechanism for the production autoantibodies in RA. 4-OHE_2 (4-hydroxyestradiol), 2-OHE_2 (2-hydroxyestradiol), (E_2)-3,4-SQ (Estradiol-3,4-semiquinone), (E_2)-2,3-SQ (Estradiol-2,3-semiquinone), (E_2)-3,4-Q (Estradiol-3,4-quinone), (E_2)-3,4-Q (Estradiol-2,3-quinone).

In light of these data, the review literature leads to the conclusion that CEs (and other metabolites) might have a role in the pathogenesis of RA. Based on the preliminary report, it appears that the production of antibodies in RA involves the generation of IgG against CE-modified DNA through oxidative induced DNA damage. Results imply that oxidative damage to DNA alter it immunogenicity leading to the induction and elevated levels of RA antibodies. RA is a chronic, systemic, inflammatory condition that is characterized by increased production of inflammatory cytokines as well as alteration in estrogen metabolites (CEs). Only by understanding the complex interaction between various estrogen metabolites and mechanism of autoantibodies production, we will able to generate therapeutic interventions that can be designed to suppress synovial inflammation in RA.

Acknowledgements

Authors like to thank Prof. Farhatullah for his valuable contribution to the editing of this manuscript.

Author details

Wahid Ali Khan[1*] and Mohd. Wajid Ali Khan[2]

*Address all correspondence to: wahidalikhan@rediffmail.com

1 Department of Clinical Biochemistry, College of Medicine, King Khalid University , Kingdom of Saudi Arabia

2 Institute of Infection and Immunity, School of Medicine, Cardiff University, United Kingdom

References

[1] Belous, A. R., Hachey, D. L., Dawling, S., Roodi, N., & Parl, F. F. (2007). Cytochrome p450 1B1-mediated estrogen metabolism results in estrogen-deoxyribonucleoside adduct formation. *Cancer Res*, 67, 812-817.

[2] Burrage, P. S., Mix, K. S., & Brinckerhoff, C. E. (2006). Matrix metalloproteinases: role in arthritis. *Front Biosci*, 1, 529-543.

[3] Camussi, G., & Lupia, E. (1998). The future role of anti-tumors necrosis factors (TNF) products in the treatment of rheumatoid arthritis. *Drugs*, 55, 613-620.

[4] Castagnetta, L. M. A., Granata, O. M., Traina, A., Ravazzolo, B., Amoroso, M., Miele, M., Bellavia, V., Agostara, B., & Carruba, G. (2002). Tissue content of hydroxyestrogens in relation to survival of breast cancer patients. *Clin Cancer Res*, 8, 3146-3155.

[5] Castnegnetta, L., Carruba, G., Granata, O. M., Stefano, R., Miele, M., Schmidt, M., Cutolo, M., & Straub, R. H. (2003). Increase estrogen formation and estrogen to androgen ratio in the SF of patients with rheumatoid arthritis. *J Rheumatoid*, 30, 2597-2605.

[6] Castnegnetta, L., Cutolo, M., Granata, O., Falco, M., Bellavia, V., & Carruba, G. (1999). Endocrine end points in rheumatoid arthritis. *Ann NY Acad Sci*, 876, 180-192.

[7] Cavalieri, E., Frenkel, K., Liehr, J. G., Rogan, E., & Roy, D. (2000). Estrogens as endogenous genotoxic agents-DNA adducts and mutations. *J Natl Cancer Inst Monogr*, 27, 75-93.

[8] Chen, Z. H., Na, H. K., Hurh, Y. J., & Surh, Y. J. (2005). Hydroxyestradiol induces oxidative stress and apoptosis in human mammary epithelial cells: possible protection by NF-κB and ERK/MAPK. Toxicol Appl Pharmacol , 208, 46-56.

[9] Cooke, M. S., Mistry, N., Wood, C., Herbert, K. E., & Lunec, J. (1997). Immunogenicity of DNA damaged by reactive oxygen species-implications for anti-DNA antibodies in lupus. *Free Radic Biol Med*, 22, 151-9.

[10] Cutolo, M., Capellino, S., Sulli, A., Serioli, B., Secchi, M. E., Villaggio, B., & Straub, R. H. (2006). Estrogens and autoimmune diseases. *Ann N Y Acad Sci*, 1089, 538-547.

[11] Cutolo, M., & Straub, H. (2012). Estrogen metabolism and autoimmunity. *Autoimmun Rev*, 11, 460-464.

[12] Cutolo, M., Sulli, A., Seriolo, B., Accardo, S., & Masi, A. T. (1995). Estrogen, the immune responses and autoimmunity. *Clin Exp Rheumatol*, 13, 217-226.

[13] Cutolo, M., Villaggio, B., Seriolo, B., Montagna, P., Capellino, S., Straub, R. H., & Sulli, A. (2004). Synovial fluid estrogen in rheumatoid arthritis. *Autoimmune Rev*, 3, 193-198.

[14] Cutolo, M. (1998). The role of the hypothalamus-pituitary-adrenocortical and-gonadal axis in rheumatoid arthritis. *Clin Exp Rheumatol*, 16, 3-6.

[15] Cutolo, M. (2004). Estrogen metabolites: increasing evidence for their role in rheumatoid arthritis and systemic lupus erythematosus. *J Rheumatol*, 31, 419-421.

[16] Cutolo, M. (2010). Hormone therapy in rheumatoid diseases. *Curr Opin Rheumatol*, 22, 257-263.

[17] Deng, H. W., & Shen, H. (2002). Current topics in human genetics: studies in complex diseases. In: Long JR. Genes in estrogen Metabolism Pathway and Breast Cancer, Long JR, World Scientific Publishing. 759-780.

[18] Devanesan, P., Santen, R. J., Bocchinfuso, W. P., Korach, K. S., Rogan, E. G., & Cavalieri, E. (2001). Catecholestrogen metabolites and conjugates in mammary tumors and hyperplastic tissue from estrogen receptor-α knock-out (ERKO)/Wnt-1 mice: Implications for initiation of mammary tumors. *Carcinogenesis*, 22, 1573-1576.

[19] Doria, A., Ghirardello, A., Iaccarino, L., Zampieri, S., Punzi, L., Tarricone, E., Ruffatti, A., Sulli, A., Sarzi-Puttini, P. C., Gambari, P. F., & Cutolo, M. (2004). Pregnancy cytokines and disease activity in systemic lupus erythematosus. *Arthritis Rheum*, 51, 989-995.

[20] Dubey, R. K., & Jackson, E. K. (2001). Cardiovascular protective effect of 17 β-estradiol metabolites. *J Appl Physio*, 91, 1868-1883.

[21] Embrechts, J., Lemiere, F., Van Dongen, W., Esmans, E. L., Buytaert, P., Van Marck, E., Kockx, M., & Makar, A. (2003). Detection of estrogen DNA-adducts in human breast tumor tissue and healthy tissue by combined nano LC-nano ES tandem mass spectroscopy. *J Am Soc Mass Spectrom*, 14, 482-491.

[22] Firestein, G. S. (2003). Evolving concepts of rheumatoid arthritis. *Nature*, 423, 356-361.

[23] Frenkel, K., Karkoszka, J., Glassman, T., Dublin, N., Toniolo, P., Taioli, E., Mooney, L. A., & Kato, I. (1998). Serum autoantibodies recognizing 5-hydroxymethyl-2′-deoxyuridine, an oxidized DNA base, as biomarkers of cancer risk in women. *Cancer Epidemiol Biomarkers Prev*, 7, 49-57.

[24] Gaub, M., Bellard, M., Sheuer, I., Chambon, P., & Sassone-Carsip, . (1990). Activation of the ovalbumin gene by the estrogen receptor involves the Fos-Jun complex. *Cell*, 63, 1267-1276.

[25] George, J., & Shoenfeld, Y. (1996). Natural autoantibodies. In: Autoantibodies, Peter JB, Shoenfeld Y, editors, Elsevier Scientifi, Amsterdam. 539.

[26] Granner, D. K. (1996). Hormones of the adrenal cortex. *In: Harper's Biochemistry, 24th edn, Murray RK, Granner DK, Mayes PA, Rodwell VW, Appleton & Lange, Stanford.*, 547-591.

[27] Grossman, J., & Brahn, M. (1997). Rheumatoid arthritis: current clinical and research directions. *J Womens Health*, 6, 627-638.

[28] Hammond, D. K., Zhu, B. T., Wang, M. Y., Ricci, M. J., & Liehr, J. G. (1997). Cytochrome p450 metabolism of estradiol in hamster liver and kidney. *Toxicol Appl Pharmacol*, 145, 54-60.

[29] Hoffman, A. R., Paul, S. M., & Axelrod, J. (1980). The enzymatic formation of catecholestrogen from 2 methoxyestrogens by rat liver microsomes. *Endocrinol*, 107, 1192-1197.

[30] Inversion, S. L., Shen, L., Anlor, N., & Bolton, J. L. (1996). Bioactivation of estrone and its catechol metabolites to quinoid-glutathione conjugates in rat liver microsomes. *Chem Res Toxicol*, 9, 492-499.

[31] Ito, A., Bebo, B. F., Jr, Mateguk, A., Zamora, A., Silverman, M., Fyfe-Johnson, A. ., & Offer, H. (2001). Estrogen treatment down-regulates TNF-alpha production and reduces the severity of experimental autoimmune encephalomyelitis in cytokine knockout mice. *J. Immunol*, 167, 542-552.

[32] Janele, D., Lang, T., Capellino, S., Cutolo, M., Dasilva, J. A. P., & Straub, R. H. (2006). Effect of testosterone, 17 β-estradiol and down stream estrogen on cytokine secretion from leukocytes in the presence and absence of cortisol. *Ann N Y Acad Sci*, 1069, 168-182.

[33] Kanda, N., Tsuchida, T., & Tamaki, K. (1999). Estrogen enhancement of anti-double-stranded DNA antibody and immunoglobin G production in peripheral blood mononuclear cells from patients with systemic lupus erythematosus. *Arthritis Rheum*, 42, 328-337.

[34] Kavanaugh, A., & Lipsky, P. E. (1996). Rheumatoid arthritis. *In: Chemical immunology: principles and practice, Rich RR, Schwartz BD, Fleisher TA, Shearer WT, Strober W, Mosby-Year Book, ST Louis, MO.*, 1093.

[35] Khalkhali-Ellis, Z., Seftor, E. A., Nieva, D. R., Handa, R. J., Price, R. H., Price, R H., Jr, Kirschmann, D. A., Baragi, V. M., Sharma, R. V., Bhalla, R. C., Moore, T. L., & Hendrix, M. J. (2000). Estrogen and progesterone regulation of human fibroblast-like synoviocyte function in vitro: implication in rheumatoid arthritis. *J Rheumatol*, 27, 1622-1631.

[36] Khan, W. A., Alam, K., & Moinuddin, . (2007). Catechol-estrogen modified DNA: a better antigen for cancer autoantibody. *Arch Biochem Biophys*, 465, 293-300.

[37] Khan, W. A., Habib, S., Khan, M. W. A., Alam, K., & Moinuddin. (2008). Enhanced binding of circulating SLE autoantibodies to catecholestrogen-copper-modified DNA. *Mol Cell Biochem*, 315, 143-150.

[38] Khan, W. A., & Moinuddin, Assiri. A. S. (2011). Immunochemical studies on catecholestrogen modified plasmid: possible role in rheumatoid arthritis. *J Clin Immunol*, 31, 22-29.

[39] Khan, W. A., Moinuddin, Khan. M. W. A., & Chabbra, H. S. (2009). Catecholestrogen: possible role in systemic lupus erythematosus. *Rheumatol (Oxford)*, 48, 1345-1351.

[40] Khan, W. A., & Moinuddin, . (2006). Binding characteristics of SLE anti-DNA autoantibodies to catecholestrogen-modified DNA. *Scand J Immunol*, 64, 677-683.

[41] Knobil, E., & Neil, J. D. (2006). Knobil and Neill's physiology of reproduction. 3rd Ed.Gulf Professional Publishing, , 2352-2376.

[42] Komi, J., & Lassila, O. (2000). Nonsteroidal anti-estrogens inhibit the functional differentiation of human monocyte-derived dendritic cells. *Blood*, 95, 2875-2882.

[43] Lahita, R. G., Bradlow, H. L., Kunkel, H. G., & Fishman, J. (1979). Alteration of estrogen metabolism in systemic lupus erythematosus. *Arthritis Rheum*, 22, 1195-1198.

[44] Lahita, R. G. (1996). The connective tissue diseases and the over all influence of gender. *Int J Fertil Menopausal Stud*, 41, 156-160.

[45] Le Bail, J., Liagre, B., Vergne, P., Bartin, P., Beneytout, J., & Habrioux, G. (2001). Aromatase in synovial cells from postmenopausal women. *Steroids*, 66, 749-753.

[46] Li, J. J., & Li, S. A. (1987). Estrogen carcinogenesis in Syrian hamster tissue: role of metabolism. *Fed Proc*, 46, 1858-1863.

[47] Li, K. M., Todovic, R., Devansen, P., Higginbotham, S., Kofeler, H., Ramanathan, R., Gross, M. L., Rogan, E. G., & Cavalieri, E. (2004). Metabolism and DNA binding studies of 4-hydroxyestradiol and estradiol-3,4-quinone invitro and in female ACI rat mammary gland invivo. Carciongenesis , 25, 289-297.

[48] Liehr, J. G., & Racci, M. J. (1996). 4-Hydroxylation of estrogens as marker of human mammary tumors. *Proc Natl Acad Sci USA*, 93, 3294-3296.

[49] Lin, P. H., Nakamura, J., Yamaguchi, S., Asakura, S., & Swenberg, J. A. (2003). Aldehydic DNA lesions induced by catecholestrogens in calf thymus DNA. *Carcinogenesis*, 24, 1133-1141.

[50] Majithia, V., & Geracia, S. A. (2007). Rheumatid arthritis: diagnosis and management. *Am J Med*, 120, 936-939.

[51] Markushin, Y., Zhong, W., Cavalieri, E. L., Rogan, E. G., Small, G. J., Yeung, E. S., & Jankowiak, R. (2003). Spectral characterization of catechol estrogen quinone (CEQ)-derived DNA- adducts and their identification in human breast tissue extract. *Chem Res Toxicol*, 16, 1107-1117.

[52] Mor, G., Wei, Y., Santen, R. J., Gutierrez, L., Eliza, M., Lev, B., Harada, N., Wang, J., Lysiak, J., Diano, S., & Naftolin, F. (1998). Macrophages, estrogen and the microenvironment of breast cancer. *J Steroid Biochem Mol Biol*, 67, 403-411.

[53] Parhan, P. (2000). The Immune System. *Elsevier Science Inc, New York, NY.*

[54] Paul, S. M., & Axelrod, J. (1977). Catecholestrogens: presence in brain and endocrine tissues. *Science*, 197, 657-659.

[55] Purohit, A., Ghilchic, M. W., & Duncan, L. (1995). Aromatase activity and interleukin-6 production by normal and malignant breast tissues. *J Clin Endocrinol Metab*, 80, 3052-3058.

[56] Roftogianis, R., Creveling, C., Weinshilboum, R., & Weisz, J. (2000). Estrogen metabolism by conjugation. *J Natl Cancer Inst Monogr*, 27, 113-124.

[57] Rogan, E. G., Badawi, A. F., Devanesan, P. D., Meza, J. L., Edney, J. A., West, W. W., Higginbotham, S. M., & Cavalieri, E. L. (2003). Relative imbalances in estrogen metabolism and conjugation in breast tissues of women with carcinoma: Potential biomarkers of susceptibility to cancer. *Carcinogenesis*, 24, 697-702.

[58] Saeed, M., Rogan, E., Fernandez, S. V., Sheriff, F., Russo, J., & Cavalieri, E. (2007). Formation of depurinating N3 Adenine and N7 Guanine adducts by MCF-10 F cells cultured in the presence of 4-hydroxyestradiol. *Int J Cancer*, 120, 1821-1824.

[59] Safe, S. H. (1998). Interactions between hormones and chemicals in breast cancer. *Annu Rev Pharmacol Toxicol*, 38, 121-158.

[60] Schmidt, M., Hartung, R., Capellino, S., Cutolo, M., Pfeifer-Leeg, A., & Straub, R. H. (2009). Estrone/17 β-estradiol conversion to and tumor necrosis factor inhibition by, estrogen metabolites in synovial cells of patients with rheumatoid arthritis and patients with osteoarthritis. *Arthritis Rheum*, 60, 2913-2922.

[61] Schneider, J., Huh, M. M., Bradlow, H. L., & Fishman, J. (1984) Antiestrogen action of 2-hydroxyestrone of MCF-7 human breast cancer cells. *J Biol Chem*, 259, 4840-4845.

[62] Schutze, N., Vollmer, G., & Knuppen, R. (1994). Catecholestrogens are agonists of estrogen receptor dependent gene expression in MCF-7 cells. *J Steroid Biochem Mol Biol*, 48, 453-461.

[63] Scott, D. L., & Kingsley, G. H. (2006). Tumor necrosis factor inhibitors for rheumatoid arthritis. *N Engl J Med*, 355, 704-712.

[64] Steiner, G., & Smolen, J. (2002). Autoantibodies in rheumatoid arthritis and clinical significance. Arthritis Res , 4, S 1-S5.

[65] Straub, R., & Cutolo, M. (2001). Impact of the hypothalamic pituitary-adrenal/gonadal oxes and the peripheral nervous system in rheumatoid arthritis: a systemic pathogenic view point. *Arthritis Rheum*, 44, 493-507.

[66] Straub, R. H. (2007). The complex role of estrogens in inflammation. *Endocr Rev*, 28, 521-574.

[67] Strauss, J. F., & Barbieri, R. L. (2009). *In: Yen and Jaffe's reproductive endocrinology: physiology, pathophysiology and clinical management.* 6th *Ed, Elsevier Health Science.*, 98.

[68] Weidler, C., Harle, P., Schedel, J., Schmidt, M., Scholmuich, J., & Straub, R. H. (2004). Patients with rheumatoid arthritis and systemic lupus erythematosus have increased renal excretion of mitogenic estrogens in relation to endogenous antiestrogens. *J Rheumatol*, 31, 489-494.

[69] Yue, W., Santen, R. J., Wang, J. P., Li, Y., Verderame, M. F., Bocchinfuso, W. P., Korach, K. S., Devanesan, P., Todorovic, R., Rogan, E. G., & Cavalieri, E. L. (2003). Genotoxic metabolites of estradiol in breast: potential mechanism of estradiol induced carcinogenesis. *J Steroid Biochem Mol Biol*, 86, 477-486.

[70] Zhu, B. T., & Conney, A. H. (1998). Functional role of estrogen metabolism in target cells: review and perspectives. *Carcinogenesis*, 19, 1-27.

[71] Zutshi, D. W., Reading, C. A., Epstein, W. V., Anseel, B. M., & Holborow, E. J. (1969). FII haemagglutination test for serum antigammaglobulin factors in arthritis sero-positive and sero-negative by other tests. *Ann Rheum Dis*, 28, 289-299.

Section 2

Clinical Science

Chapter 5

Treatment of Rheumatoid Arthritis with Biological Agents

Hiroaki Matsuno

Additional information is available at the end of the chapter

http://dx.doi.org/10.5772/53321

1. Introduction

Cytokines and Rheumatoid Arthritis

The term "cytokine" is coined from the combination of "cyto", a prefix which means cell, and "kine", which denotes movement.

Cytokines all have the following features:

1. They are low-molecular-weight glycoproteins that are not hormones.
2. They have an effect at very small concentrations.
3. Different cytokines can have the same function (redundancy).

For example, both tumor necrosis factor (TNF) and interleukin-6 (IL-6) have synovial proliferation activity and destroy articular cartilage and bone.

4. One cytokine can act on various organs at the same time (pleiotropy).

For example, TNF causes synovial proliferation, destroys articular cartilage, and promotes fever.

5. Each cytokine has a specific receptor and acts by binding to that receptor.

Inflammatory cytokines play a central role in rheumatoid arthritis. In the treatment of rheumatoid arthritis with biological agents, the effects of cytokines are suppressed by blocking the cytokine from binding to its specific receptor (Figure 1).

With respect to these cytokines, antibodies and antibody fusion proteins that inhibit the action of IL-1, IL-6, and TNF have already been commercialized, and development of an IL-17 inhibitor is underway (Figure 2,Table 1).

Antibodies for the treatment of rheumatoid arthritis can be divided into three groups: chimeric antibodies, humanized antibodies, and human antibodies. Experimental monoclonal antibodies are usually produced by immunizing a mouse with an antigen, and therefore, the antibody is 100% mouse antibody. When such an antibody is used as a therapeutic agent in humans, it causes a strong anaphylactic reaction. In an effort to reduce as far as possible the content of heterologous proteins, various chimeric antibodies, humanized antibodies, and human antibodies have been developed for the treatment of rheumatoid arthritis.

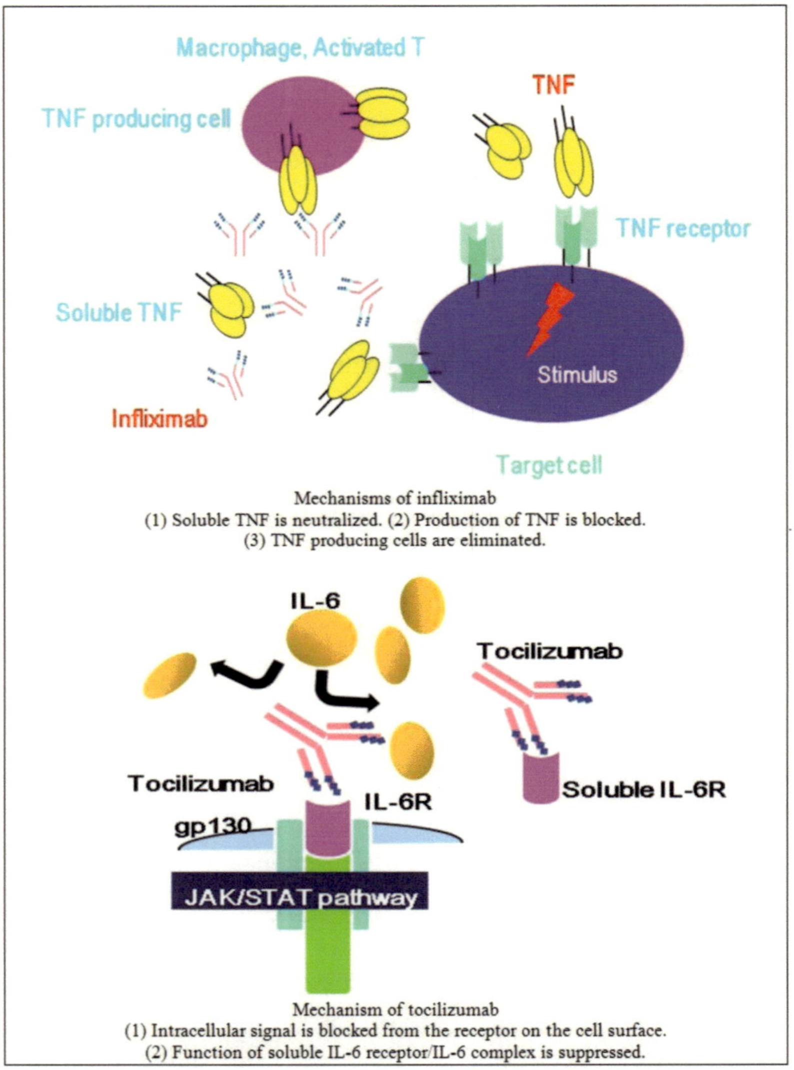

Figure 1. Mechanisms of infliximab and tocilizumab

http://dx.doi.org/10.5772/53321

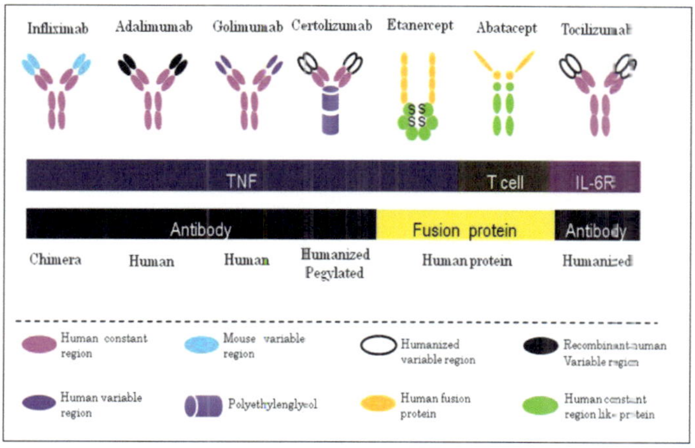

Figure 2. Types of biological agents developed for the treatment of rheumatoid arthritis.

A chimeric antibody is produced first as a mouse monoclonal antibody by immunizing a mouse with an antigen. Then the antigen binding site is preserved as it is, while the Fc site is artificially replaced with one of human origin such as IgG1 or IgG4. In chimeric antibodies, since about 25% mouse protein remains, anaphylactic reactions still occur about 10% of the time when they are administered. There are also reports of treatment with antibody preparations being impaired when antibodies to the chimeric antibody are produced.

A humanized antibody is produced first as a mouse monoclonal antibody, then only the variable parts of the antigen binding site on the heavy chain and light chain of the antibody are left as mouse protein, and the rest is replaced with human protein Since protein which codes the CDR1, CDR2, and CDR3 regions accounts for about 10% of the total, there is still a small chance of anaphylactic reaction with multiple administrations, though less than that with chimeric antibodies.

Human antibodies are fully human antibodies produced by the phage display method. A typical example is adalimumab. This antibody is produced as follows: An antibody light chain and antibody heavy chain, each with a strong affinity for TNF-α, are selected, and then the two are bound together. Therefore, while it is a fully human protein, it is not an antibody that is physiologically produced in humans. Consequently, it is reported that antibodies against the antibody are detected in 40% of cases or more, reducing the function of the antibody preparation. Combined use of an immunosuppressant to prevent antibody production is recommended.

Another fully humanized antibody on the market is golimumab. This antibody is produced by a method different from that of adalimumab. First, a humanized transgenic mouse is produced, the mouse is immunized with TNF, and the antibodies produced are purified and commercialized. This method has made it possible to produce an antibody which is closer to human than adalimumab.

Target	TNF-				
Product name	Remicade	Enbrel	Humira	Simponi	Cimzia
Non-proprietary name	Infliximab	Etanercept	Adalimumab	Golimumab	Certolizumab pegol
Indications	rheumatoid arthritis, uveitis, Behcet's disease, plaque psoriasis, pustular psoriasis, arthropathic psoriasis, erythrodermic psoriasis, Crohn's disease, ulcerative colitis	rheumatoid arthritis, poly juvenile idiopathic arthritis.	rheumatoid arthritis, poly juvenile idiopathic arthritis, plaque psoriasis, arthropathic psoriasis, ankylosing spondylitis, Crohn's disease	rheumatoid arthritis	rheumatoid arthritis, Crohn's disease
Administration method	Drip infusion	Subcutaneous injection	Subcutaneous injection	Subcutaneous injection	Subcutaneous injection
Administration interval	At wk 0, wk 2, wk 6, then every 8 wks	Every 1–2 wks	Every 2 wks	Every 4 wks	Every 4 wks
Structure	Chimeric antibody	TNFR–IgG1 fusion protein	Human antibody	Human antibody	Pegylated humanized antibody
Representative clinical study	ATTRACT[1] ASPIRE[2]	ERA[3] TEMPO[4]	PREMIER[5] DE019[6]	GO-FORWARD[7] AFTER[8]	GO-FAST4WARD[9] RAPID2[10]

Target	IL-1Rreceptor	IL-6Receptor	CD80/86	CD20
Product name	Kineret	Actemra (RoActemra)	Orencia	Rituxan (MabThera)
Non-proprietary name	Anakinra	Tocilizumab	Abatacept	Rituximab
Indications	rheumatoid arthritis	rheumatoid arthritis, poly juvenile idiopathic arthritis, systemic juvenile idiopathic arthritis, Castleman's disease	rheumatoid arthritis	rheumatoid arthritis, non-Hodgkin's lymphoma
Administration method	Subcutaneous injection	Drip infusion	Drip infusion	Drip infusion
Administration interval	Every 1 or 2 days	Every 4 wks	Every 4 wks	Day 1 and 15, then every 24 wks
Structure	IL-1 receptor antagonist	Humanized antibody	CTLA-4–IgG1 fusion protein	Chimeric antibody

	recombinant protein			
Representative clinical study	[11, 12]	SAMURAI[13] OPTION[14]	AIM[15] ATTAIN[16]	REFLEX[17] SERENE[18]

Table 1. Characteristics of various biological agents

2. Types of Cytokine Inhibitors (Biological Agents) and their effects on Rheumatoid Arthritis

Cytokine inhibitors used in the treatment of rheumatoid arthritis are inhibitors of IL-1 (anakinra), TNF (infliximab, etanercept, adalimumab, golimumab, and certolizumab pegol), and IL-6 (tocilizumab). In addition, biological agents other than cytokine inhibitors used in the treatment of rheumatoid arthritis include abatacept, which inhibits the action of T-cell co-stimulatory molecules CD80 and CD86, and rituximab, which targets CD20.

These drugs each have a stronger effect than methotrexate(MTX), which is considered to be most effective taken orally, and each has strong action to suppress bone and joint destruction (Figure 3, Figure. 4) [19].

Treatment with any biological agent is more effective than MTX monotherapy, and each suppresses bone and joint destruction.

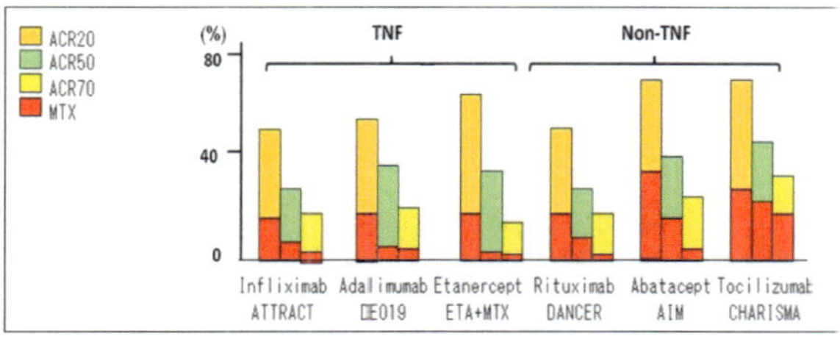

Figure 3. Improvement of clinical symptoms with biological agents

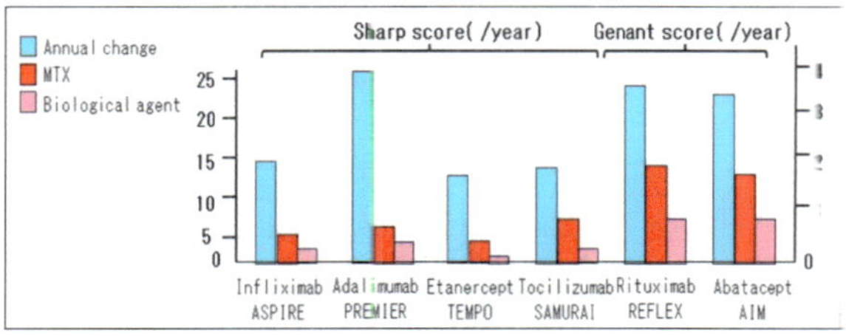

Figure 4. Suppression of joint destruction with biological agents

3. Recommendations for the Use of Biological Agents

Opinion is divided on which biological agent should be used to start with when active rheumatoid arthritis is diagnosed. Among typical rankings for the use of biological agents, there is the 2012 recommendation of the American College of Rheumatology (Figure 5) [20].

According to this recommendation, in the United States the first biological agent (1st Bio) recommended for treatment of early rheumatoid arthritis with disease duration of less than 6 months is a TNF inhibitor. For treatment of established RA with disease duration of 6 months or more, a TNF inhibitor and abatacept or rituximab are recommended as the 1st Bio.

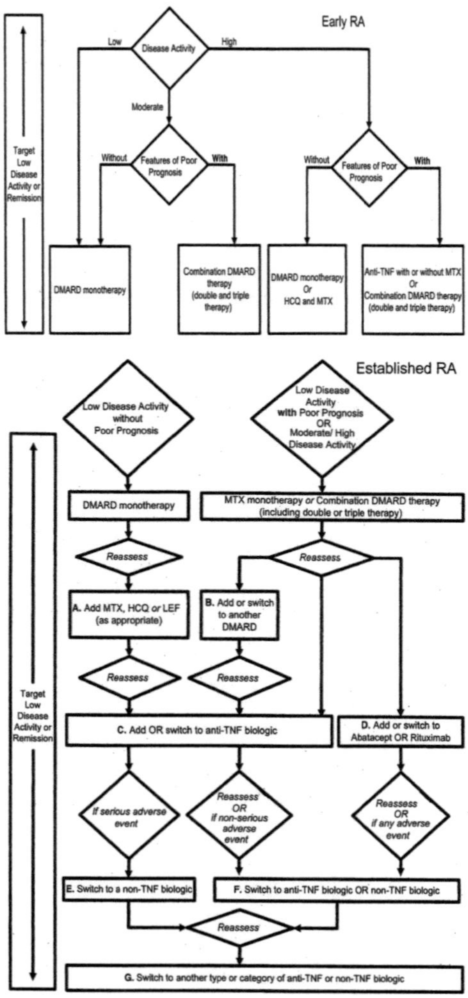

Figure 5. American College of Rheumatology 2012 Recommendation

http://dx.doi.org/10.5772/53321

On the other hand, the British National Institute for Health and Clinical Excellence (NICE) specifies the following guidance on usage (Figure 6) [21–27]:

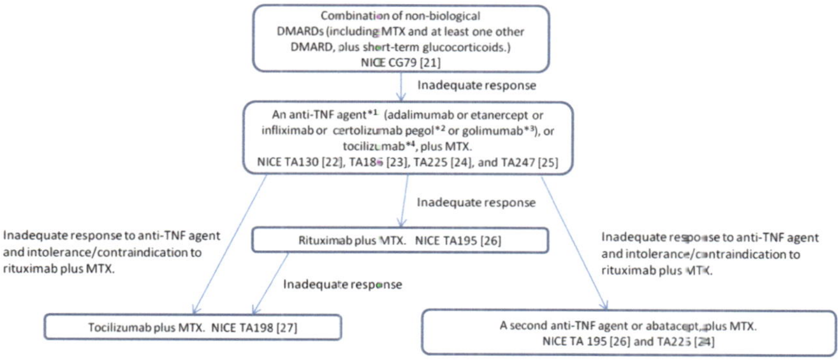

Figure 6. *1The annual cost of the biological agent is also specified and does not exceed £9,295 a year.*2If certolizumab pegol is the 1st Bio, there should be a system wherein the manufacturer provides the first 12 weeks for free [23]. *3If golimumab is used as the 1st Bio, compensation from the manufacturer is necessary so that the drug price of 50 mg and 100 mg is the same [24].*4Tocilizumab can be used as the 1st Bio with a discount provided by the manufacturer. Therefore, whichever biological agent is used first, the annual cost of any is £9,295 or less [27].NICE guidance on the treatment of patients with rheumatoid arthritis.

4. Selecting Biological Agents by Efficacy and Safety

Among TNF inhibitors, there are several biological agents to choose from, with no strict standards for which biological agent to use first in either the United States or the United Kingdom. Most physicians choose one based on their own experience. Recently however, data has begun to accumulate suggesting which usage is best.

Regarding efficacy, there is data indicating that etanercept is more effective than infliximab for active rheumatoid arthritis with high levels of anti-cyclic citrullinated peptide antibodies and rheumatoid factor [28]. In addition, among infliximab, adalimumab, and etanercept, it is reported that etanercept shows the highest efficacy in patients with high levels of anti-SS-A antibody [29].

With respect to adverse reactions, the occurrence of tuberculosis among patients treated with anti TNF agents has been shown to be low for the fusion protein preparation etanercept and high for the antibody preparations infliximab and adalimumab. It has been suggested that the reason for this could be that the antibody preparations, unlike the fusion protein preparation etanercept, simultaneously suppress the function of macrophages [30, 31].

Therefore, from the point of view of adverse reactions, etanercept may be the best choice for rheumatoid arthritis patients with a risk of tuberculosis.

The same could possibly be considered for tocilizumab, an IL-6 inhibitor which does not directly suppress macrophage function. A postmarketing survey of tocilizumab as used in a real-world clinical setting has shown an incidence of tuberculosis of 0.22% [32], which is lower than that of TNF inhibitors.

In comparative studies of related biological agents, almost no difference in efficacy was seen between infliximab and abatacept [33] or between adalimumab and abatacept [34]. However, in a study comparing adalimumab and tocilizumab, tocilizumab was shown to be more effective than adalimumab [35] (Table 2).

	ATTEST Study	AMPLE Study	ADACTA Study
Agents	Abatacept vs. Infliximab	Abatacept + MTX vs. Adalimumab + MTX	Tocilizumab vs. Abatacept
Primary endpoint	DAS28(ESR)	ACR20	DAS28(ESR)
Study period	1 year	1 year	24 weeks
Result	−2.88 vs.−2.25 (n.s)	64.8% vs. 63.4% (n.s)	−3.3 vs. −1.8 ($p < 0.0001$)

Table 2. Comparative study of related biological agents

Considered this way, the non-TNF cytokine inhibitor (IL-6 inhibitor) tocilizumab could be a biological agent with greater pharmacological effect than TNF inhibitors with fewer adverse reactions due to tuberculosis if used appropriately. Comparison of TNF and IL-6 shows mostly the same pharmacological effects due to cytokine redundancy. Examples of this include the induction of synovial proliferation, induction of inflammatory cytokines, and articular destruction.

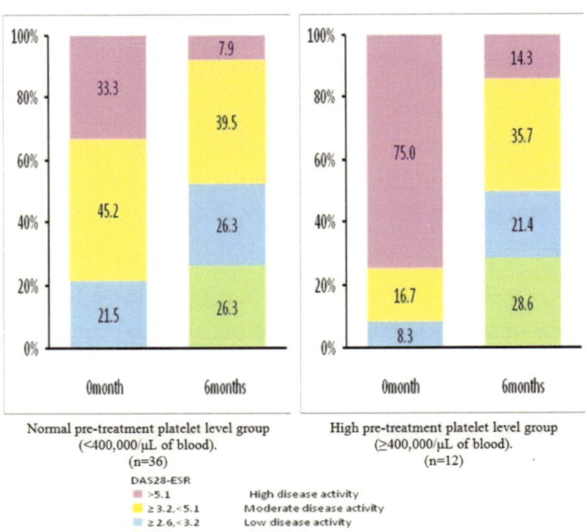

Figure 7. Degree of DAS28 remission with tocilizumab treatment (own data)

However, a characteristic effect of IL-6, which is stronger than that of TNF, is the induction of peripheral platelets in bone marrow megakaryocytes. The effect of IL-6 to induce C-reactive protein in hepatocytes is also thought to be stronger than the effect of TNF.

When the outcomes of cases in which tocilizumab was selected as the 1st Bio were compared in rheumatoid arthritis patients stratified by pre-treatment platelet levels, improvement in rheumatoid activity due to tocilizumab was found to be more marked in patients with high pre-treatment platelet levels (≥400,000 /μL of blood) than in those with normal platelet levels (Figure 7).

From these results, the effects of IL-6 are stronger than the effects of TNF in patients with rheumatoid arthritis of high activity and high platelet levels, which might be a good indication for the use of tocilizumab. In SCID-Hu-RA experimented mouse, which is implanted human RA synovium into back of the severe combined immune deficient (SCID) mouse, human RA synovium is markedly suppressed by tocilizumab treatment in compared with control mouse [36].Tocilizumab not only improves clinical symptoms of rheumatoid arthritis, but is also effective in improving pathological findings in rheumatoid arthritis (Figure 8).

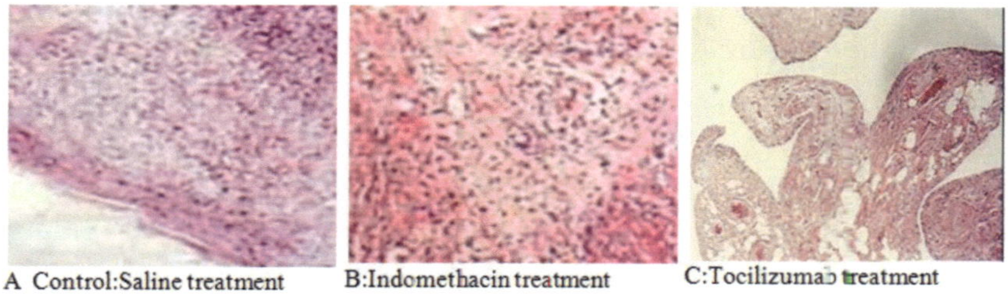

Figure 8. Typical changes in synovial membrane seen with tocilizumab treatment

Inflammatory cells in synovial membrane are suppressed by tocilizumab and replaced by fibrous tissue or adipose tissue.

5. Problems with Biological Agents

Biological agents are a very useful treatment for active rheumatoid arthritis, but there are still many problems which must be solved, including their high cost and the problem of adverse reactions such as infections. As described in the US recommendation and UK guidance, they should probably be used in patients who do not obtain symptomatic relief following treatment with DMARDs.

Author details

Hiroaki Matsuno*

Address all correspondence to: spr845x9@chime.ocn.ne.jp

Matsuno Clinic for Rheumatic Diseases, Japan

References

[1] Maini, R., St Clair, E. W., Breedveld, F., Furst, D., Kalden, J., Weisman, M., et al. (1999). Infliximab (chimeric anti-tumour necrosis factor alpha monoclonal antibody) versus placebo in rheumatoid arthritis patients receiving concomitant methotrexate: a randomised phase III trial. ATTRACT Study Group. *Lancet*, 354, 1932-9.

[2] St Clair, E. W., van der Heijde, D. M., Smolen, J. S., Maini, RN, Bathon, J. M., Emery, P., et al. (2004). Combination of infliximab and methotrexate therapy for early rheumatoid arthritis: a randomized, controlled trial. *Arthritis Rheum*, 50, 3432-43.

[3] Bathon, J. M., Martin, R. W., Fleischmann, R. M., Tesser, J. R., Schiff, M. H., Keystone, E. C., et al. (2000). A comparison of etanercept and methotrexate in patients with early rheumatoid arthritis. *N Engl J Med*, 343, 1586-93.

[4] Klareskog, L., van der Heijde, D., de Jager, J. P., Gough, A., Kalden, J., Malaise, M., et al. (2004). TEMPO (Trial of Etanercept and Methotrexate with Radiographic Patient Outcomes) study investigators. Therapeutic effect of the combination of etanercept and methotrexate compared with each treatment alone in patients with rheumatoid arthritis: double-blind randomised controlled trial. *Lancet*, 363, 675-81.

[5] Breedveld, F. C., Weisman, M. H., Kavanaugh, A. F., Cohen, S. B., Pavelka, K., van Vollenhoven, R., et al. (2006). The PREMIER study: A multicenter, randomized, double-blind clinical trial of combination therapy with adalimumab plus methotrexate versus methotrexate alone or adalimumab alone in patients with early, aggressive rheumatoid arthritis who had not had previous methotrexate treatment. *Arthritis Rheum*, 54, 26-37.

[6] Keystone, E. C., Kavanaugh, A. F., Sharp, J. T., Tannenbaum, H., Hua, Y., Teoh, L. S., et al. (2004). Radiographic, clinical, and functional outcomes of treatment with adalimumab (a human anti-tumor necrosis factor monoclonal antibody) in patients with active rheumatoid arthritis receiving concomitant methotrexate therapy: a randomized, placebo-controlled, 52-week trial. *Arthritis Rheum*, 50(5), 1400-11.

[7] Keystone, E. C., Genovese, M. C., Klareskog, L., Hsia, E. C., Hall, S. T., Miranda, P. C., et al. (2009). Golimumab, a human antibody to tumour necrosis factor α given by monthly subcutaneous injections, in active rheumatoid arthritis despite methotrexate therapy: the GO-FORWARD Study. *Ann Rheum Dis*, 68(6), 789-96.

[8] Smolen, J. S., Kay, J., Doyle, M. K., Landewe, R., Matteson, E. L., Wollenhaupt, J., et al. (2009). Golimumab in patients with active rheumatoid arthritis after treatment with tumour necrosis factor alpha inhibitors (GO-AFTER study): a multicentre, randomised, double-blind, placebo-controlled, phase III trial. *Lancet*, 374(9685), 210-21.

[9] Fleischmann, R., Vencovsky, J., van Vollenhoven, R. F., Borenstein, D., Box, J., Coteur, G., et al. (2009). Efficacy and safety of certolizumab pegol monotherapy every 4 weeks in patients with rheumatoid arthritis failing previous disease-modifying antirheumatic therapy: the FAST4WARD study. *Ann Rheum Dis*, 68(6), 805-11.

[10] Smolen, J., Landewe, R. B., Mease, P., Brzezicki, J., Mason, D., Luijtens, K., et al. (2009). Efficacy and safety of certolizumab pegol plus methotrexate in active rheumatoid arthritis: the RAPID 2 study. A randomised controlled trial. *Ann Rheum Dis*, 68(6), 797-804.

[11] Bresnihan, B., Alvaro-Gracia, J. M., Cobby, M., Doherty, M., Domljan, Z., Emery, P., et al. (1998). Treatment of rheumatoid arthritis with recombinant human interleukin-1 receptor antagonist. *Arthritis Rheum*, 41(12), 2196-204.

[12] Cohen, S., Hurd, E., Cush, J., Schiff, M., Weinblatt, ME, Moreland, L. W., et al. (2002). Treatment of rheumatoid arthritis with anakinra, a recombinant human interleukin-1 receptor antagonist, in combination with methotrexate: results of a twenty-four-week, multicenter, randomized, double-blind, placebo-controlled trial. *Arthritis Rheum*, 46(3), 614-24.

[13] Nishimoto, N., Hashimoto, J., Miyasaka, N., Yamamoto, K., Kawai, S., Takeuchi, T., et al. (2007). Study of active controlled monotherapy used for rheumatoid arthritis, an IL-6 inhibitor (SAMURAI): evidence of clinical and radiographic benefit from an x ray reader-blinded randomised controlled trial of tocilizumab. *Ann Rheum Dis*, 66(9), 1162-7.

[14] Smolen, J. S., Beaulieu, A., Rubbert-Roth, A., Ramos-Remus, C., Rovensky, J., Alecock, E., et al. (2008). Effect of interleukin-6 receptor inhibition with tocilizumab in patients with rheumatoid arthritis (OPTION study): a double-blind, placebo-controlled, randomised trial. *Lancet*, 371(9617), 987-97.

[15] Kremer, J. M., Genant, H. K., Moreland, L. W., Russell, AS, Emery, P., Abud-Mendoza, C., et al. (2006). Effects of abatacept in patients with methotrexate-resistant active rheumatoid arthritis: a randomized trial. *Ann Intern Med*, 144(12), 865-76.

[16] Genovese, M. C., Becker, J. C., Schiff, M., Luggen, M., Sherrer, Y., Kremer, J., et al. (2005). Abatacept for rheumatoid arthritis refractory to tumor necrosis factor alpha inhibition. *N Engl J Med*, 353(11), 1114-23.

[17] Cohen, S. B., Keystone, E., Genovese, M. C., Emery, P., Peterfy, C., Tak, P. P., et al. (2010). Continued inhibition of structural damage over 2 years in patients with rheumatoid arthritis treated with rituximab in combination with methotrexate. *Ann Rheum Dis*, 69(6), 1158-61.

[18] Emery, P., Deodhar, A., Rigby, W. F., Isaacs, JD, Combe, B., Racewicz, A. J., et al. (2010). Efficacy and safety of different doses and retreatment of rituximab: a randomised, placebo-controlled trial in patients who are biological naive with active rheumatoid arthritis and an inadequate response to methotrexate (Study Evaluating Rituximab's Efficacy in MTX iNadequate rEsponders (SERENE)). *Ann Rheum Dis*, 69(9), 1629-35.

[19] Smolen, J. S., Aletaha, D., Koeller, M., Weisman, M. H., & Emery, P. (2007). New therapies for treatment of rheumatoid arthritis. *Lancet*, 370(9602), 1861-74.

[20] Singh, J. A., Furst, D. E., Bharat, A., Curtis, J. R., Kavanaugh, A. F., Kremer, J. M., et al. (2012). 2012 update of the 2008 American College of Rheumatology recommendations for the use of disease-modifying antirheumatic drugs and biologic agents in the treatment of rheumatoid arthritis. *Arthritis Care Res (Hoboken)*, 64(5), 625-39.

[21] National Institute for Health and Clinical Excellence: NICE. (2012). http://publications.nice.org.uk/rheumatoid-arthritis-cg79, accessed September.

[22] National Institute for Health and Clinical Excellence: NICE. (2012). http://www.nice.org.uk/nicemedia/live/11867/37914/37914.pdf, accessed September.

[23] National Institute for Health and Clinical Excellence: NICE. (2012). http://www.nice.org.uk/nicemedia/live/12808/47544/47544.pdf, accessed September.

[24] National Institute for Health and Clinical Excellence: NICE. (2012). http://www.nice.org.uk/nicemedia/live/13490/54929/54929.pdf, accessed September.

[25] National Institute for Health and Clinical Excellence: NICE. (2012). http://publications.nice.org.uk/tocilizumab-for-the-treatment-of-rheumatoid-arthritis-rapid-review-of-technology-appraisal-guidance-ta247, accessed September.

[26] National Institute for Health and Clinical Excellence: NICE. (2012). http://www.nice.org.uk/nicemedia/live/13108/50413/50413.pdf, accessed September.

[27] National Institute for Health and Clinical Excellence: NICE. (2012). http://www.nice.org.uk/nicemedia/live/13669/58202/58202.pdf, accessed September.

[28] Potter, C., Hyrich, K. L., Tracey, A., Lunt, M., Plant, D., Symmons, D. P., et al. (2009). Association of rheumatoid factor and anti-cyclic citrullinated peptide positivity, but not carriage of shared epitope or PTPN22 susceptibility variants, with anti-tumour necrosis factor response in rheumatoid arthritis. *Ann Rheum Dis*, 68(1), 69-74.

[29] Matsudaira, R., Tamura, N., Sekiya, F., Ogasawara, M., Yamanaka, K., & Takasaki, Y. (2011). Anti-Ro/SSA antibodies are an independent factor associated with an insufficient response to tumor necrosis factor inhibitors in patients with rheumatoid arthritis. *J Rheumatol*, 38(11), 2346-54.

[30] Dixon, W. G., Hyrich, K. L., Watson, K. D., Lunt, M., Galloway, J., Ustianowski, A., et al. (2010). Drug-specific risk of tuberculosis in patients with rheumatoid arthritis

treated with anti-TNF therapy: results from the British Society for Rheumatology Biologics Register (BSRBR). *Ann Rheum Dis*, 69(3), 522-8.

[31] Singh, J. A., Noorbaloochi, S., & Singh, G. (2010). Golimumab for rheumatoid arthritis: a systematic review. *J Rheumatol*, 37(6), 1096-104.

[32] Koike, T., Harigai, M., Inokuma, S., Ishiguro, N., Ryu, J., Takeuchi, T., et al. (2011). Postmarketing surveillance of tocilizumab for rheumatoid arthritis in Japan: interim analysis of 3881 patients. *Ann Rheum Dis*, 70(12), 2148-51.

[33] Schiff, M., Keiserman, M., Codding, C., Songcharoen, S., Berman, A., Nayiager, S., et al. (2008). Efficacy and safety of abatacept or infliximab vs placebo in ATTEST: a phase III, multi-centre, randomised, double-blind, placebo-controlled study in patients with rheumatoid arthritis and an inadequate response to methotrexate. *Ann Rheum Dis*, 67(8), 1096-103.

[34] Schiff, M., Fleischmann, R., Weinblatt, M., Valente, R., van der Heijde, D., Citera, G., et al. (2012). Abatacept SC versus adalimumab on background methotrexate in RA: one year results from the AMPLE study. *Ann Rheum Dis*, 71(3), 60.

[35] Gabay, C., Emery, P., van Vollenhoven, R., Dikranian, A., Alten, R., Klearman, M., et al. (2012). Tocilizumab (TCZ) monotherapy is superior to adalimumab (ADA) monotherapy in reducing disease activity in patients with rheumatoid arthritis (RA): 24-week data from the phase 4 ADACTA trial. *Ann Rheum Dis*, 71(3), 152.

[36] Matsuno, H., Sawai, T., Nezuka, T., Uzuki, M., Tsuji, H., Nishimoto, N., et al. (1998). Treatment of rheumatoid synovitis with anti-reshaping human interleukin-6 receptor monoclonal antibody: use of rheumatoid arthritis tissue implants in the SCID mouse model. *Arthritis Rheum*, 41(11), 2014-21.

Chapter 6

Perioperative Surgical Site Infections and Complications in Elective Orthopedic Surgery in Patients with Rheumatoid Arthritis Treated with Anti-Tumor Necrosis Factor-Alpha Agents – Discontinue or Not, Clinical Dilemma

Koichiro Komiya and Nobuki Terada

Additional information is available at the end of the chapter

http://dx.doi.org/10.5772/54012

1. Introduction

Rheumatoid arthritis (RA) is characterized by the destruction of peripheral joints in which articular cartilage and subchondral bone are destroyed by chronic proliferative synovitis. This damage often leads to significant loss of joint function and impairs the ADL of patients with RA.

Most patients with RA are in use of traditional disease modifying antirheumatic drugs (DMARDs) to control disease activity, and among the traditional, non-biological DMARDs (nbDMARDs), methotrexate (MTX) is a first line and an anchor drug for the treatment of RA. Currently introduced biologic agents, especially anti-tumor necrosis factor-alpha (TNF-α) agents, have revolutionized the treatment of RA. TNF-α triggers the inflammatory cascade and stimulates the production of matrix degradable proteinases such as matrix metalloproteinases, which well known to play a major role in the proteolytic degradation of extracellular matrix macromolecules of cartilage and bone, which is a key step in joint destruction in RA. Anti-TNF-α agents are now in routine use for RA patients who have failed to respond to nbDMARDs, and have been demonstrated to improve the clinical symptoms and delay joint destruction dramatically. Unfortunately, despite of the administration of nbDMARDs and/or biologic agents, complete prevention of the destruction of the affected joints is still not achieved. Over the course of their lifetime, many patients with RA may require orthopaedic surgical interventions, such as total joint arthroplasty (TJA), arthrodeis, reconstructive surgeries, cervical stabilization, and so on.

For orthopaedic surgeons, post-operative surgical site infections (SSI) and delayed wound healing are major concerns, especially in TJA. Prosthetic infection is associated with prolonged antibacterial therapy and hospitalization, functional decline, depression, shorter prosthesis durability, which have great impact on morbidity, mortality and quality of life. The baseline infection risk is increased 13-fold in individuals with RA when compared with the general population [1]. In addition, receiving anti-TNF-α agents showed an increased risk of serious infections. Delayed wound healing or wound dehiscence is also believed to occur more frequently in patients with RA. Patients with RA are already predisposed to impaired wound healing as a result of reduction in skin thickness above that which is due to steroid use. Furthermore TNF-α is required for normal wound healing, and in experimental settings anti-TNF-α has been linked to poor wound healing [2]. Thus careful management of anti-rheumatic agents and their adverse effects in a perioperative period is essential. Among nbDMARDs, only MTX has been investigated prospectively and randomized manner, and demonstrated that continuation of MTX treatment did not increase the risk of either infections or surgical complications in elective orthopaedic surgery in patients with RA [3]. As for biologic anti-TNF-α agents, current national guidelines suggested that treatment with biologic agents should be discontinued during the perioperative period. Although discontinuation of anti-TNF-α agents during the perioperative period may have a positive effect on SSI and wound healing rates, but this is at the expense of increased risk of RA flare that could affect postoperative rehabilitation. However, there are no prospective clinical trials and few studies assessing the use of anti-TNF-α agents during the perioperative periods in RA patients undergoing elective orthopaedic surgery. In this chapter, we review the available literature related to perioperative complications, especially SSI, delayed wound healing and RA flare in elective orthopaedic surgery in patients with RA treated with anti-TNF-α agents, and discuss the perioperative management of anti-TNF-α agents, the clinical dilemma whether discontinue or not.

2. Risk of septic arthritis (SA) in RA patients

Individuals with RA are at an inherently increased risk of infection [1, 4]. Edwards et al. [1] reported that the incidence rate for SA was 12.9 times higher in subjects with RA than those without [95% confidence interval (CI) 10.1-16.5]. Doran et al. [4] performed a retrospective longitudinal cohort study and reported that the overall rate of infection per 100 person-years was higher in RA patients (19.64) than in non-RA patients (12.87), and the rate ratio for developing infections in patients with RA was 1.53 (95% CI 1.41-1.65). Infection sites that were associated with the highest rate ratio were the joints (rate ratio for SA 14.89 [95% CI 6.12-73.71]), bone (rate ratio for osteomyelitis 10.63 [95% CI 3.39-126.81]), and skin and soft tissues (rate ratio 3.28 [95% CI 2.67-4.07]) [4]. SA is a serious and severe condition for patients that can lead to irreversible joint destruction, and the incidence of SA in the general population is around 4-10/100,000/person-years [5, 6]. SA is lethal around 10% of a death rate [7]. In fact, infections requiring hospitalization were significantly more frequent in RA patients (9.57/100 person-years) than in non-RA patients (5.09/100 person-years) with rate ratio 1.88 (95% CI 1.71-2.07), and SA was also associated with a highest rate ratio of 21.66 (95% CI 7.37-257.61)] [4].

Accumulated data indicate that the risk factors for SA are increasing age, comorbidities (diabetes mellitus, chronic renal failure, chronic cardiac failure), joint prosthesis, skin infection and pre-existing joint damage [1, 8-10], but whether RA treatment with nbDMARDs, corticosteroids and biologics including anti-TNF-α agents increases the risk of SA is still unclear. DMARDs and biologics including anti-TNF-α agents are generally believed to be immunosuppressive and likely to increase the incidence of SA in patients with RA. But the data on these are very limited and sparse. Edwards et al. [1] performed a retrospective study using the United Kingdom General Practice Research Database to analyze the effect of DMARDs on developing SA in patients with RA. There was significantly increased risk of SA in individuals with RA prescribed DMARDs compared with those not prescribed DMARDs. The incidence rate ratios (IRR) for developing SA in the patients receiving DMARDs compared with receiving no DMARDs were different for different medications. Penicillamine (adjusted IRR 2.51, 95% CI 1.29-4.89, P=0.004), sulfasalazine (adjusted IRR 1.74, 95% CI 1.04-2.91, P=0.03) and prednisolone (adjusted IRR 2.94, 95% CI 1.93-4.46, P<0.001) were associated with an increased incidence of SA when compared with receiving no DMARDs [1]. The use of other DMARDs (including MTX) not showed such effect [1]. There was a number of individuals with RA developed SA without receiving DMARDs, thus they considered that the immune dysfunction associated with RA and the coexistent joint damage are more important risk factors than immunomodulatory therapies with DMARDs [1].

There is very limited information regarding the effect of anti-TNF-α therapy on the risk of SA. Galloway et al. [11] conducted a prospective observational study to evaluate the risk of SA in patients with RA treated with anti-TNF-α agents. They reported that incidence rates for SA were anti-TNF 4.2/1000/patient years (95% CI 3.6-4.8) and nbDMARDs 1.8/1000/patient years (95% CI 1.1-2.7). The adjusted hazard ratio (HR) for SA in the anti-TNF cohort was 2.3 (95% CI 1.2-4.4). The risk did not differ significantly between the three agents: infliximab (IFX), etanercept (ETN) and adalimumab (ADA). The hazard for SA in the anti-TNF cohort was greatest in the early months of therapy, as well as data from other cohorts [12], and the risk then decreased steadily over the remainder of the follow-up period [11]. One of the potential explanations for early increased risk is that it may reflect a true reduction in risk of joint infection in patients who achieve better control of their RA [11].

In summary of this section, patients with RA are at an increased risk of SA irrespective of therapy. Some DMARDs and corticosteroid increase the risk of SA. Exposure to anti-TNF therapy is also associated with an increased risk of SA and this risk was greatest in the first year of treatment. Thus, this increased risk of SA in RA may be due to not only as a consequence of the disease nature of RA but also treatment with some immunomodulatory agents. Current evidence does not support any one anti-TNF agent having a safer profile with regard to SA.

3. Risk of SSI in RA patients undergoing TJA

TJA is a major orthopaedic procedure for destructed joints. In RA, total knee arthroplasty (TKA) and total hip arthroplasty (THA) are the most common, promised surgical interventions for patients to recover from painful joints and impaired activities of daily life. However, prosthetic joint infection often requires revision of the infected prosthesis and prolonged intravenous antimicrobial therapy, and has a mortality rate of 2.7-18% [13]. Patients with RA have been identified to have a higher baseline risk of infectious diseases compared with general population. In addition, the immunosuppressive drugs used in the treatment of RA may further increase the risk of infection. Whether this increased baseline risk of infections in RA patients might influence the risk of deep infection after primary TJA is somewhat conflicting.

Wymenga et al. [14] conducted a multicenter prospective study to investigate the association between perioperative factors and SA after TKA and THA. At 1-year follow up, 9/362 patients (2.5%) after TKA and 17/2651 patients (0.64%) after THA were completed by SA. They reported that RA was a risk factor for SA for TKA (risk ratio 4.8; 95% CI 1.2-19), but they could not confirm this in THA. Schrama et al. [15] reported a retrospective study using the Norwegian Arthroplasty Register to examine the risk of revision arthroplasty due to infection in RA (6,629 procedures) compared with OA patients (102,157 procedures). The incidence of revision due to infection in TKA and THA were 0.7% (176/24,294 procedures) and 0.6% (534/84,492 procedures), respectively. The risk of revision for infection in RA patients with TKA was 1.6 (95% CI 1.06-2.38) times higher compared to OA patients, but there were no difference in THA. This discrepancy between TKA and THA were also reported by Wymenga et al. [14], and Schrama et al. mentioned that the vulnerable soft tissue envelope around the knee joint could make the TKA in RA patients more susceptible to infection, since the connective tissue disease RA and its potentially immunomodulating medication are risk factors for skin and soft tissue infections. Jamsen et al. [16] analyzed primary (40,135 procedures) and revision (3,014 procedures) knee arthroplasties in a large series of knee arthroplasties from Finnish Arthroplasty Register. In total, 387 reoperations were performed for the treatment of infection (0.90%; 95% CI 0.81-0.99). The adjusted HR for reoperation due to infection in primary and revision TKA in patients with RA were 1.86 (95% CI 1.31-2.63) and 1.01 (95% CI 0.44-2.34) compared with primary OA, respectively. Robertsson et al. [17] also reported using another large series of knee arthroplasties, the Swedish Knee Arthroplasty Register that the risk of revision for infection was significantly higher in RA patients compared to OA patients [risk ratio (RR) 1.4; 95% CI 1.1-1.9]. The data on influences of nbDMARDs on the risk of prosthetic infection in patients with RA were absent in these studies [14-17].

Bongartz et al. [13] conducted a retrospective study using the Mayo Clinic Total Joint Registry to examine the incidence and risk factors of prosthetic joint infection in RA patients (657 procedures; THA or TKA). 23 (3.7%) joint arthroplasties were complicated by infection. The risk of prosthetic joint infections were increased in RA patients (HR 4.08, 95% CI 1.35-12.33) compared with a matched cohort of OA patients. Revision arthroplasty (HR 2.99, 95% CI 1.02-8.75), previous prosthetic joint infection of the replaced joint (HR 5.49, 95% CI

1.87-16.14), and operation time (HR 1.36 per 60-minitue increase, 95% CI 1.02-1.81) were significant predictors of postoperative prosthetic joint infection. Based on the pharmacokinetic half-life and/or data on the biologic activity of each DMARD, perioperative DMARDs use was judged as either withheld or maintained. DMARDs were withheld perioperatively in 57% of procedures and stopping DMARDs therapy at the time of surgery lowered the risk of prosthesis infection (HR 0.65, 95% CI 0.09-4.95), but this was statistically not significant. There were 3 prosthesis infections in 38 patients who were treated with anti-TNF agents at the time of surgery as compared with no infection in 12 patients who stopped their anti-TNF therapy prior to surgery, but this difference was not statistically significant. Perioperative corticosteroid use was not associated with an increased risk of prosthesis infection.

Besides DMARDs, the risk of perioperative use of corticosteroids for prosthetic infection in patients with RA is controversial. Berbari et al. [18] conducted a case-control study to determine risk factors for the development of prosthetic joint infection. 462 episodes of prosthetic joint infection in 460 patients were used for analysis. Univariate analysis identified that RA, steroid therapy as risk factors for joint prosthetic infection with odds ratio (OR) of 2.0 (95% CI 1.3-3.0) and 2.0 (95% CI 1.3-3.1) respectively. Wilson et al. [19] reported that 67 (1.6%) out of the 4,171 TKA were complicated by infection. The incidence of infection in RA patients (2.2%; 45/2076) was significantly higher than in OA (1%; 16/1857) ($P<0.0001$). Despite the fact that a higher percentage of patients who had RA and infection had used steroids than had those who did not have an infection (75% compared with 46%), a history of oral use of steroids was not a significant risk factor.

While most of papers agreed with increased risk of prosthetic infection in RA patients, da Cunha et al. [20] conducted a retrospective study to compare the incidence of infections between RA and OA patients in THA and TKA, and reported that no significant difference was observed between the RA and OA groups regarding the rates of prosthesis infections (TKA 7.1% vs. 0% and THA 2.1% vs. 0%, respectively, both with $P>0.1$), incisional infections (TKA 14.3% vs. 3.3% and THA 4.3% vs. 1.3%, respectively, both with $P>0.1$), and systematic infections (TKA 7.1% vs. 3.6%, $P=0.92$ and THA 4.3% vs. 10.7%, $P>0.1$, respectively). They concluded that RA was not identified as a risk factor for perioperative infections in THA and TKA in their case series. The low incidence of infections in both groups may explain their findings. Although the data on usage and mean dose of DMARDs, biologics and corticosteroids were reported, the association between prosthesis infection and these drugs were not analyzed in this study.

Whether the use of nbDMARDs constitutes an independent risk factor for SSI remains unclear. Among nbDMARDs, only MTX had been investigated in a prospective and randomized study. Grennan et al. [3] reported that signs of infection or surgical complications occurred in two of 88 procedures (2%) in the group of MTX continuation, 11 of 72 procedures (15%) in the group of MTX discontinuation, and 24 of 228 procedures (10.5%) in the MTX naïve group. Furthermore, accumulated data support the perioperative use of MTX, and international 3E Initiative stated in the recommendation that MTX can be safely continued in the perioperative period in RA patients undergoing elective orthopaedic surgery [21].

In summary of this section, most of studies support the increased prevalence of TJA infection in RA patients. Among nbDMARDs, only MTX had been intensively investigated the influences of the perioperative use on the risk of SSI, and accumulated data support the safety of perioperative continuation of MTX undergoing elective orthopaedic surgery. We should be aware that TJA in RA patients is high-risk in infection and sufficient antibiotic prophylaxis should be taken with a careful follow-up.

4. Risk of SSI in RA patients treated with anti-TNF-α agents undergoing orthopaedic surgery

The information about the risk of SSI in RA patients treated with anti-TNF-α agents undergoing orthopedic surgery is very limited, and to date, there are only 14 studies on this matter.

We at first take up 4 studies those analyzed whether continuation of TNF blockers in perioperative period increases the risk of SSI in patients on anti-TNF therapy.

Talwalker et al. [22] performed a small retrospective study. 16 procedures in 11 patients (RA; n=10, psoriatic arthritis; n=1) on anti-TNF undergoing elective joint surgery were reviewed. TNF blockers were continued in group A (4 procedures), while in group B (12 procedures), they were withheld before surgery and restarted after the procedure. In group A, IFX was used in one operation, the patient receiving the injection 3 days before surgery while ETN was used in three patients. In group B, IFX was stopped nearly 4 weeks before surgery, whereas ADA and ETN was stopped at 2 weeks. The timings for restarting the drug were variable. Postoperatively, none of the patients in either group developed serious wound and systematic infections, but one flare up occurred in a patient receiving ETN in group B.

Wendling et al. [23] conducted a retrospective study with a sample size of 50 surgical procedures (foot and ankle; 13, hand and wrist; 11, TJA; 12, others; 14) in 30 patients with RA treated with TNF blockers. TNF blockers at the time of surgery was IFX (n=26), ETN (n=13), ADA (n=11), with a mean exposure of 12.1 months (range 1-42). TNF blockers were withheld before surgery in 18/50 patients, and for the rest, surgery was performed between two TNF blocker injections. Postoperatively, no infections occurred in either group whether TNF blocker was discontinued or not, but RA flares were observed in 6 cases (12%) and significantly associated with anti-TNF interruption before surgery (5 interruptions/6 cases of flare vs. 13 interruption/44 surgical procedures without flare; Fisher's exact value=0.02).

Den Broeder et al. [24] performed a large retrospective study. Two parallel cohorts were defined: cohort 1 did not use anti-TNF, cohort 2 used anti-TNF but had either stopped (2A) or continued anti-TNF preoperatively (2B), the cutoff point being set at 4 times the half-life time of the drug. In total, 1,219 procedures were performed (wrist/hand; 317, ankle/foot; 280, knee; 195, hip; 172, shoulder; 114, elbow; 102, other; 39). Crude infection risk in cohorts 1, 2A, and 2B were 4.0% (41/1023), 5.8% (6/104), and 8.7% (8/92), respectively. History of prior SSI or skin infection was found to be the strongest predictor for SSI (OR 13.8, 95% CI 5.2-36.7, P<0.0001), but perioperative use of anti-TNF was not significantly associated with an increase in SSI rates (OR 1.5, 95% CI 0.43-5.2, *P*=0.43). However, wound dehiscence occurred more frequently in patients that continued anti-TNF compared to patients that temporarily discontinued anti-TNF treatment (OR 11.2, 95% CI 1.4-90).

Bongartz et al. [13] conducted a retrospective, single-center, double cohort study that included all patients with RA who underwent THA or TKA at the Mayo Clinic Rochester between January 1996 and June 2004. 657 surgeries in 462 patients with RA were identified. There were 3 prosthesis infections in 38 patients who were treated with anti-TNF agents at the time of surgery as compared with no infection in 12 patients who stopped their anti-TNF therapy prior to surgery. However, the result did not reach statistical significance.

Secondary, we take up 7 studies which compare the perioperative risk of infection between patients on TNF blockers and those on nbDMARDs.

Bibbo et al. [25] reported a 12-month prospective study that compared foot and ankle surgery in 16 RA patients (mean age 50 years) on TNF blockers (group 1) (IFX; 5, ETN; 11) compared with 15 controls (mean age 60 years) on nbDMARDs (group 2). Patients on TNF blockers discontinued treatment prior to surgery (ETN; mean 2.6 days, IFX; mean 20.2 days) and resumed treatment postoperatively. Infectious complications occurred in two patients: one case of a superficial infection in a group 1 patient and one case of a deep infection (osteomyelitis) in a group 2 patient. Delayed wound healing occurred in three patients, all occurred in group 2. Bone healing complications occurred in three patients, all in group 2, comprised of two nonunions and one delayed union. When considered individually, the occurrence of an infectious or healing complication proved to be statistically similar between groups 1 and 2. However, when complications summed (infectious and healing complications), group 2 demonstrated a statistically higher overall complication rate (*P*=0.033, Fisher's exact test). They concluded that the use of TNF blockers may be safely undertaken in the perioperative period without increasing the risk of infectious or healing complications in the patients with RA undergoing elective foot and ankle surgery.

Hirano et al. [26] performed retrospective cohort study where adverse events of surgical wounds were compared between patients treated with TNF blockers (n=39) (IFX; 24, ETN; 15) and those on nbDMARDs (n=74). TKA is the commonest surgery followed by THA. Administration of TNF blockers was stopped prior to surgeries (IFX; mean 29.8 days, ETN; mean 9.6 days) and restarted after surgical wounds were completely healed. Adverse events of surgical wounds occurred after two operations in the TNF group (5.1%) and five operations in the nbDMARDs group (6.8%), which was not statistically significant difference by Fisher's exact test (*P*=1.0000). OR was 0.7459 (95% CI 0.1380-4.0336). Although most of adverse events of surgical wounds were wound dehiscence and continuation of discharge, postoperative infection occurred in one TKA in the TNF group. They concluded that the use of anti-TNF agents dose dot cause specific adverse events on surgical wounds after elective orthopedic surgeries in RA patients.

Kawakami et al. [27] performed a retrospective case-control study to identify perioperative complications associated the use of TNF blockers. RA patients on anti-TNF (64 procedures/49 patients) were compared to those on nbDMARDs (64 procedures/63 patients).

TKA is the commonest surgery followed by THA. TNF blockers (IFX; 35 and ETN; 29) were withheld 2-4 weeks prior to surgery according to the British Society for Rheumatology and the Japan College of Rheumatology guidelines (2-4 weeks for ETN, 4 weeks for IFX). Multivariate logistic regression analysis identified the use of TNF blockers (OR 21.80, 95% CI 1.231-386.1, *P*=0.036), prednisone dosage (OR 1.433, 95% CI 1.007-2.040, *P*=0.046), and disease duration (OR 1.169, 95% CI 1.030-1.326, *P*=0.015) as a risk factors for SSI. SSIs were developed 12.5% (8/64) in the anti-TNF group, whereas 2% (1/64) in the nbDMARDs group (*P*=0.016), but there was no delayed wound healing occurred in either groups. RA flare-ups during the perioperative periods were found in 17.2% (11/64) of anti-TNF group. These flare-ups were significantly increased in ETN group (31.0%, 9/29) compared with the IFX group (5.7%, 2/35) (*P*=0.009). Multivariate logistic regression analysis also revealed that the use of TNF blockers was the only risk factors for DVT (OR=2.83, 95% CI 1.10-7.25, *P*=0.03) in their study. DVT were developed 51% (23/45) in the anti-TNF group, whereas 26% (12/45) in the nbDMARDs group (*P*=0.015). They concluded that TNF blockers were likely cause SSI and DVT in RA patients undergoing elective orthopaedic surgery.

Momohara et al. [28] performed a retrospective study to identify risk factors for acute SSI after TJA (THA; 81, TKA; 339) in RA patients treated with biologics (48 patients, THA; 11, TKA; 37) and nbDMARDs (372 patients). In the biologics group, 19 (4.5%) received IFX, 23 (5.5%) received ETN, two (0.5%) received ADA, and four (1.0%) received tocilizumab (TCZ). Of the patients undergoing THA or TKA, 24 cases (5.7%) developed a superficial incisional SSI requiring the use of antibiotics and the three cases (0.7%) developed an organ/space SSI necessitating surgical treatment to remove the artificial joint prosthesis. Multivariate logistic regression analysis revealed that the use of biologics (OR=5.69; 95% CI 2.07-15.61, *P*=0.0007) and longer RA duration (OR=1.09; 95% CI 1.04-1.14, *P*=0.0003) were the only significant risk factors for acute SSI. Furthermore, multivariate logistic regression analysis of individual medication (nbDMARDs and biologics) adjusted for disease duration indicated that TNF blockers increased the risk of SSI (IFX OR=9.80; 95% CI 2.41-39.82, *P*=0.001; ETN OR=9.16; 95% CI 2.77-30.25, *P*=0.0003). They found that the use of biologics (IFX or ETN) and longer disease duration were associated with an increased risk of acute SSI in RA patients.

The Committee on Arthritis of the Japanese Orthopedic Association [29] investigated the prevalence of postoperative complications in patients with RA in teaching hospitals in Japan. The number of surgical procedures under treatment with biologic agent was 3,468 (IFX; 1,616, ETN; 1686, ADA; 41, TCZ; 102, abatacept; 23) and the prevalence of infection was 1.3% (46 procedures). For IFX, ETN, and TCZ, the mean times of withdrawal before surgery were 26.4, 14.1, and 19.8 days, respectively. The prevalence of infection was 1.0% (567 procedures) in 56,339 procedures under treatment with nbDMARDs. There were no significant differences between biologics and nbDMARDs groups with respect to the prevalence of infections (OR 1.32, 95% CI 0.98-1.79, *P*=0.07). In the joint arthroplasty group, the prevalence of infection was 2.1% (34/1,626 procedures) in biologics group and 1.0% (298/29,903 procedures) in nbDMARDs group. There was a significant difference between biologics and nbDMARDs groups (OR 2.12, 95% CI 1.48-3.03, *P*<0.0001). They concluded that the infection risk of joint arthroplasty in RA patients on anti-TNF therapy was more than twofold greater compared with those treated with nbDMARDS.

Kubota et al. [30] performed a retrospective study to analyze the influence of biological agents on delayed wound healing and the postoperative SSI in RA patients. The patients were divided into two groups, those treated with biologics (bio group; 276 joints) and not treated with biologic agents (non-bio group; 278 joints). Biologics administered in the bio group were IFX (n=14), ETN (n=236), ADA (n=8), and TCZ (n=18), and these agents were withheld 2-4 weeks before surgery. TKA is the commonest surgery followed by THA. In the bio group, postoperative superficial and deep infection developed in one and two joints, respectively. In the non-bio group, superficial infection developed in one joint, and deep infection was not observed. The incidence of SSIs did not differ significantly between the two groups (Mann-Whitney *U*-test, *P*=0.31251). Delayed wound healing occurred in 15 joints (5.4%) in the bio group (all the patients were treated with ETN), and 12 joints (4.3%) in the non-bio group, but the difference was not statistically significant (Mann-Whitney *U*-test, *P*=0.522). They concluded that the use of biologics may not affect the incidence of postoperative adverse events related to SSI and wound healing.

Hayata et al. [31] performed a retrospective study to investigate the complications of orthopeadic surgery for RA patients treated with IFX (52 patients). Commonest surgery was arthroscopic synovectomy (n=30), followed by TJA (n=16). The mean timing of surgery after infusion of IFX was 4 weeks. There were two cases (3.8%) of superficial wound infection (one case was foot arthroplasty and the other was spine surgery), but there was no deep wound infection. Furthermore, there is no correlation between infection and clinical factors including age, disease duration, preoperative CRP, MMP-3, rheumatoid arthritis particle-agglutination (RAPA) and the period until surgery after IFX infusion. They concluded that IFX did not increase the risk of either infection or surgical complications occurring in patients with RA within 1 year of orthopeadic surgery.

Thirdly, we take up 3 studies which compare the patients with postoperative infection and those without, to identify the association between anti-TNF therapy and the risk of infection.

Gilson et al. [32] carried out a retrospective case-control study using French RATIO registry to analyze the risk factors for TJA infections in patients receiving TNF blockers. 20 patients (18 with RA) treated with TNF blockers (IFX; 7, ETN; 5, ADA; 8) and presented with TJA infections were compared to controls (40 patients) without TJA infections on TNF blockers. TJA infections concerned principally the knee (n=12, 60%) and the hip (n=5, 25%). 8 cases (40%) versus 5 controls (13%) had undergone primary or revision TJA for the joint subsequently infected during the previous year (*P*=0.03). Of these procedures, TNF blockers were continued in 5 cases compared to 1 in the control group (*P*=0.08). Multivariate analysis demonstrated that the predictors of infection were primary TJA or TJA revision for the joint subsequently infected within the last year (OR 88.3, 95% CI 1.1-7071.6, *P*=0.04) and increased daily steroid intake (OR 5.0 per 5 mg/day increase, 95% CI 1.1-21.6, *P*=0.03). They concluded that TJA infection was rare but potentially severe in patients receiving TNF blockers. Important risk factors were primary TJA or TJA revision for the joint subsequently infected within the last year, particularly when TNF blockers were not interrupted before surgery, and the daily steroid intake.

Giles et al. [33] performed a retrospective study to investigate the association between anti-TNF therapy and the development of serious postoperative infection in RA patients undergoing orthopaedic surgery. 91 patients were identified as having at least one orthopedic procedure, and 10 of the 91 patients (11%) developed serious postoperative infection. The demographic features and RA therapies between infection group (n=10) and no infection group (n=81) were comparable. But infection group (7/10 patients; 70%) were significantly more likely treated with TNF-α blocker at the time of surgery compared with no infection group (28/81 patients; 35%) (P=0.041). Univariate analysis revealed that anti-TNF was significantly associated with the development of postoperative infections (OR 4.4, 95% CI 1.10-18.41). This association remained statistically significant after adjustment for age, sex, and disease duration (OR 4.6, 95% CI 1.1-20.0); prednisone use, diabetes, and serum rheumatoid factor status (OR 5.0, 95% CI 1.1-21.9); and all these 6 variables simultaneously (OR 5.3, 95% CI 1.1-24.9). They concluded that treatment with TNF blockers associated with increased risk of early infectious complications following orthopaedic surgery in patients with RA. They suggest that TNF blockers should be withheld prior to orthopaedic surgery.

Ruyssen-Witrand et al. [34] performed a systematic retrospective study to assess the complication rates after surgery in rheumatic patients treated with TNF blockers. 127 surgical procedures (107 orthopaedic procedures, 84.3%) performed in 92 rheumatic patients (71 RA patients, 77.2%) receiving TNF blockers. Orthopaedic procedures had a postoperative complication rate of 12% (n=13) with 5.6% (n=6) of infections, whereas 'clean' orthopedic procedures such as joint replacement or vertebral surgery had a complication rate of around 10% (n=4) with 7% (n=3) infections. Among the procedures where TNF blockers were discontinued more than 5 half-lives before surgery (36 procedures), there were 19.4% (7/36) complications compared to 18.4% (12/65) for procedures where anti-TNF therapy was interrupted less than 5 half-lives before or was not interrupted at all (P=0.48). If therapy was discontinued for more than 2 half-lives the complication rate was 17.6%, versus 30.0% if therapy was discontinued less than 2 half-lives before or was not discontinued (P=0.24). Thus, interrupting TNF blockers did not decrease the postoperative complications. No risk factors, either demographic or for severity, were statistically significant in predicting post-surgical complications. Analysis of treatments showed more complications with ADA (28.6%) than ETN (11.5%), but this was not statistically significant (P=0.18). The cumulative corticosteroid dose was higher in the group with postoperative complications, but this was not also statistically significant. The authors concluded that the postoperative complication rate is high in patients treated with TNF blockers, thus discontinuing TNF therapy before surgery should be considered.

In summary of this section, it is difficult to make definite conclusion on the association between anti-TNF therapy and SSI in RA patients undergoing orthopedic surgery due to the retrospective nature and small sample size of most of reported studies. In 4 studies [13, 22-24], perioperative continuation of anti-TNF therapy did not increase the risk of SSI, whereas in 3 studies [27-29], the risk of SSI was increased in anti-TNF therapy group, regardless of discontinuation of the therapy perioperatively. Another point of view, preoperative discontinuation of TNF blockers causes the reduction of effects of the agents at the operation date, thus the results of these studies may not show the accurate influences of TNF blockers on the risk of SSI. However, in the other four studies [25, 26, 30, 31], appropriate preoperative discontinuation of TNF blockers did not increase the risk of SSI compared with group on nbDMARDs. The risk factors for SSI, which most of RA patients undergoing TJA are considered to have, reported in 17 studies were the use of TNF blockers (OR 21.80 [27], OR 5.69 [28], and OR 4.4 [33]), prednisone dosage (OR 1.433) [27], increased daily steroid intake (OR 5.0 per 5mg/day increase) [32], longer disease duration (OR 1.169 [27] and OR 1.09 [28]), history of prior SSI or skin infection (OR 13.8) [24], primary or revision TJA for the joint subsequently infected within the last year (OR 88.3) [32], and "clean" surgical procedure such as TJA (OR 2.12) [29]. Thus, it may be preferable to perform TJA, if needed, before the induction of TNF blockers [32]. In cases of prosthetic surgery after induction of TNF blockers, their withdrawal during the perioperative period is highly recommended and steroid intake should be reduced as low as possible before surgery [32].

Further larger prospective studies are clearly needed to make clear the association between perioperative use of TNF blockers and SSI, and in clinical practice until these studies are done, we should discontinue TNF blockers and take a sufficient antibiotic prophylaxis with a careful follow-up.

5. Risk of wound healing complications in RA patients treated with anti-TNF-α agents

Patients with RA are already predisposed to impaired wound healing as a result of reduction in skin thickness [2, 35]. Thus, many orthopaedic surgeons consider the risk of wound healing complication to be high in RA patients, especially treated with TNF blockers [36]. Wound healing is a complex process and TNF-α is required for normal wound healing. An "acute" wound healing process generally includes haemostasis/inflammation, proliferation and tissue remodeling stages [37]. On the other hand, in a "chronic" wound, wound healing is impaired and is characterized by excessive inflammation, enhanced proteolysis, and reduced matrix deposition. Tarnuzzer et al. [38] demonstrated that the levels of TNF-α in fluid from "chronic" wounds were approximately 100-fold higher than those in fluid from an "acute" wound (mastectomy incision). However, the experimental data on the role of TNF-α in wound healing is still controversial. Mooney et al. [2] reported that local application of TNF-α increased wound disruption strength and eventually promoted wound healing, whereas Rapala et al. [39] and Salomon et al. [40] reported that local application of TNF-α down-regulated the synthesis of collagen and was detrimental to wound healing. Some studies analyzed the effect of blockade of TNF-α on wound healing. Mori et al. [41] reported that in TNF receptor p55-deficient mice, angiogenesis, collagen accumulation, and reepithelialization were up-regulated, and wound healing was accelerated eventually. Iglesias et al. [42] analyzed wound healing in SWISS-OF1 mice and reported that surgical wounds showed a higher degree of collagenization in ETN-treated versus untreated mice, with no difference in the time course of wound healing. They concluded that anti-TNF therapy did not affect wound healing. Streit et al. [37] reported a case series of patients with "chronic", therapy-resistant leg ulcers responded well to topical application of IFX. Ashcroft et al. [43] also reported that inhibiting TNF-α is a critical event in reversing the severely impaired wound healing.

Surgical wound in elective orthopaedic surgery is basically considered as "acute" wound. In the 9 of 17 studies taken up in section 4, the association between anti-TNF therapy and "acute" wound healing complications in RA patients were reported as follows. Den Broeder et al. [24] reported that wound dehiscence occurred more frequently in patients who continued anti-TNF therapy (9/92 cases, 9.8%) compared to those temporarily discontinued anti-TNF therapy (1/104 cases, 0.9%) (OR 11.2, 95% CI 1.4-90). Wendling et al. [23] reported that three cases (6%) of delayed wound healing were recorded in patients on TNF blockers (50 surgical procedures). Ruyssen-Witrand et al. [34] reported that postoperative wound healing complications occurred in 6 cases (4.7%) in patients treated with TNF blockers (127 surgical procedures). Kubota et al. [30] reported that delayed wound healing occurred in 15 joints (5.4%) in bio group and 12 joints (4.3%) in non-bio group, but the difference between two groups was not statistically significant. Hirano et al. [26] reported that adverse events of surgical wounds occurred after two operations (5.1%) in the TNF group (n=39) and five operations (6.8%) in the nbDMARDs group (n=74), but the difference between two groups was not statistically significant. Suzuki et al. [29] reported that delayed wound healing occurred in 14 cases (IFX; 2, ETN; 9, TCZ; 3) (0.4%) in biologics group (n=3,468). In the remaining 3 of 9 studies by Kawakami et al. [27], Momohara et al. [28], and Bibbo et al. [25], there was no delayed wound healing in patients with anti-TNF therapy.

In summary of this section, the role of TNF-α in wound healing is still controversial. Anti-TNF therapy seems to be preferable for improvement in healing of "chronic" wounds where the level of TNF-α is excessive compared with "acute" wounds. Thus, perioperative discontinuation of anti-TNF therapy is preferable to decrease the risk of wound healing complications, but reported data are controversial and insufficient to make clear conclusion about this matter.

6. Perioperative discontinuation of anti-TNF-α agents and risk of RA flare

For orthopaedic surgeons, one of the major concerns is whether perioperative discontinuation of TNF blockers results in flare up of the disease activity. Because RA flare may compromise postoperative rehabilitation, which strongly affect the result of orthopaedic surgery. However, the information about perioperative RA flare after discontinuation of anti-TNF therapy in perioperative period is very limited. Only some comments about the flare were reported in 3 of 17 studies taken up section 4. Talwalker et al. [22] reported that one flare up occurred postoperatively in a patient receiving ETN, but the flare up was well controlled once the drug was restarted. Wendling et al. [23] reported that postoperative RA flares were observed in 6 cases (12%) and significantly associated with anti-TNF interruption before surgery (5 interruptions/6 cases of flare vs. 13 interruption/44 cases without flare; Fisher's exact value=0.02). Kawakami et al. [27] reported that RA flares during the perioperative periods were found in 17.2% (11/64) of anti-TNF group. These flares were significantly increased in ETN group (31.0%, 9/29) compared with the IFX group (5.7%, 2/35) (*P*=0.009). The reason for increased risk of postoperative RA flare in ETN compared with IFX is unclear, but considered as follows. The half-life of IFX is longer than that of ETN, and in the IFX group, the surgery was usually performed in the middle of the 8-week treatment of period, and there was actually no withholding of anti-TNF therapy. Moreover, the function of IFX is based on an antigen-antibody reaction, whereas the function of ETN is a reversible connection response of ETN of TNF [27, 44].

On the other hand, intensive treatment with TNF blockers and MTX leads to clinical remission in approximately 20-50% of RA patients. This excellent clinical result raised a new problem, whether the patients with RA on TNF therapy can discontinue their therapy after acquisition of low disease activity (LDA). In the BeST study [45], 67% of RA patients treated early with combination of IFX and MTX were able to stop anti-TNF treatment. Brocq et al. [46] performed a small prospective cohort study to determine the time to relapse after cessation of TNF antagonist therapy. The mean disease duration was 11.3 years. Amongst the 20 patients, three quarter (75%) relapsed within the first 12 months with the mean time to relapse of 15 weeks. Saleem et al. [47] reported comparative data for patients treated early (n=27) versus late (n=20) with combination therapy of MTX and anti-TNF. All patients fulfilled the criteria of clinical remission for at least 6 months. Anti-TNF therapy was then discontinued, while remaining on MTX for 24 months. The primary outcome measure was a flare of the disease determined by an increase in Disease Activity Score (DAS). At 24 months, there were significantly more patients in the initial treatment group that had sustained remission compared with the delayed treatment group (59% vs. 15%, *P*=0.003). Shorter disease duration was found for be a predictor of sustained remission following cessation of TNF blockers. Tanaka et al. [48] conducted a multicenter study (remission induction by Remicade in RA; RRR study) to determine whether IFX might be discontinued after achievement of LDA in patient with RA and to evaluate progression of articular destruction during the discontinuation. 114 RA patients with RA who had received IFX treatment, and discontinued the drug after achieving DAS 28<3.2 (LDA) for >24 weeks, were studied. The mean disease duration of the 114 patients was 5.9 years, mean DAS28 5.5 and modified total Sharp score (mTSS) 63.3. 12 patients withdrew from the study. Out of the 102 patients, 56 patients (55%) remained to have DAS 28<3.2 (RRR-achieved group) and 44 patients (43%) reached DAS 28<2.6 at 1 year after discontinuing IFX. On the other hand, 29 patients flared within 1 year (mean duration 6.4 months) after the discontinuation and in 17 patients DAS28 was >3.2 at 1 year. Thus, the remission induction by IFX was failed in 46 patients (45%) at 1 year after the discontinuation (RRR-failed group). Yearly progression of mTSS (ΔTSS) remained <0.5 (structural remission) in 67% and 44% of the RRR-achieved and RRR-failed group, respectively. Patients for whom RRR was achieved were younger (49.5 vs. 56.1 years), their disease duration was shorter (4.8 vs. 7.8 years) and mTSS was lower (46.9 vs. 97.2) than for those whom RRR failed. DAS28 at RRR-study entry had the most marked correlation with the maintenance of LDA for 1 year after the discontinuation. They concluded that after attaining LDA by IFX, 55% of the patients with RA able to discontinue IFX for >1 year without progression of radiological articular progression. Klarenbeek et al. [49] conducted a study using five-year data of the BeSt study to determine the relapse rate after discontinuing treatment in patients with RA in sustained clinical remission, to identify predictors of relapse and evaluate treatment response after restarting treatment. 508 patients with recent-onset RA were randomized into four dynamic treatment strategies, aiming at DAS≦2.4. When DAS was <1.6 for≧6months, the last DMARD was tapered and discontinued. If DAS increased ≧1.6, the last DMARD was immediately reintroduced. 115/508 patients (23%) achieved drug-free remission during a five-year period. Of these 53/115 patients (46%) restarted treatment because the DAS≧1.6 after a median of 5 months, 59/115 patients (51%) remained drug-free remission for median duration of 23 months. To focus the group of initial combination with IFX (n=128), 36/128 patients (28%) achieved drug-free remission during a five-year period. Of these 15/36 patients (42%) restarted treatment, 21/36 patients (58%) remained drug-free remission. Of the 53 patients who restarted treatment, 39 (74%) again achieved remission 3-6 months after the restart without showing radiological progression during the relapse.

As mentioned above, after maintaining LDA by intensive treatment with TNF blockers, discontinuation of TNF blockers without disease flare, joint damage progression, and functional impairment is possible in some RA patients. Patients with shorter disease duration are more likely to remain in remission after discontinuing TNF blockers compared to their counterparts with established disease [45-48]. Furthermore, patients with longstanding disease are more likely to have orthopaedic surgical intervention, especially prosthetic surgery, compared to those with early disease. However, the significance of discontinuation of anti-TNF therapy in perioperative periods is different from the cessation after achievement of LDA. Because perioperative discontinuation of anti-TNF therapy is basically temporary, and the therapy is restarted promptly after confirmation of good wound healing and no evidence of infection. Therefore, if TNF blockers are withheld prior to surgery, those with longer disease duration need to be monitored carefully for features of relapse [36].

In summary of this section, perioperative discontinuation of anti-TNF therapy in elective orthopaedic surgery likely caused postoperative RA flare. The risk of postoperative flare was increased in ETN which had a shorter half-life compared with IFX, and also increased in the patients with long disease duration. Shortening the period of withholding anti-TNF therapy is desirable to prevent the postoperative flare, but shortening the duration of discontinuation may cause an increase in SSI and wound healing complications. This is the clinical dilemma for orthopaedic surgeons. Data on this matter also insufficient to make definite conclusion, thus further studies are clearly needed.

7. Recommended perioperative discontinuation period of anti-TNF-α agents in national guidelines

Although the conclusions about the influences of continuation of anti-TNF therapy in perioperative period on SSI, wound healing and RA flare are somewhat conflicting, but there are few studies which recommend the perioperative continuation of anti-TNF therapy positively. The national guidelines on each society recommend preoperative discontinuation of TNF blockers and show the preoperative off-period based on the half-life of each agents (Table 1).

	mean half-life (days)	2 half-lives (days)	3 half-lives (days)	5 half-lives (days)
Infliximab (IFX)	8-10	16-20	24-30	40-50
Etanercept (ETN)	4.3	8.6	12.9	21.5
Adalimumab (ADA)	14	28	42	70
Golimumab (GOL)	12	24	36	60
Certolizumab (CTZ)	14	28	42	70

Table 1. Mean half-lives of TNF blockers

The current American Society of Rheumatology (ACR) guidelines (2008) state that anti-TNF should not be used during the preoperative period, for at least 1week prior to and 1 week after surgery. It was recommended this decision should be further tempered by the pharmacokinetic properties of a given biologic agent (e.g., longer periods of time off therapy may be appropriate when using agents with longer half-lives.), and the type of surgery [50].

The recently updated British Society of Rheumatology (BSR) guidelines (2010) propose as follows. In RA patients on anti-TNF, the potential benefit of preventing postoperative infections by stopping treatment (different surgical procedures pose different risks of infection and wound healing) should be balanced against the risk of a perioperative flare in RA activity. If anti-TNF is to be stopped before surgery, consideration should be given TNF blockers three to five times the half-life of the relevant drug prior to surgery and should not be restarted after surgery until there is good wound healing and no evidence of infection [51].

The Club Rhumatismes et Inflammation (CRI) (French Society of Rheumatology) provides guidelines that based on drug half-lives and clinical settings. For minor surgery, in a sterile setting with minor risk infection, IFX, ADA and ETN should be withheld, respectively, at least 1 month, 3-4 weeks and 1-2 weeks. However, for surgery performed in a septic environment, the respective duration for interruption of IFX, ADA and ETN are 8, 4-6 and 2-3 weeks [52].

Recently updated the Board of Japan College of Rheumatology (JCR) guidelines (2012) caution that surgery should be delayed until a sufficient time had elapsed from the last administration of TNF-α antagonists (recommend to keep 2-4 weeks for ETN or 4 weeks for IFX with long half-life), because it is not clear whether or not TNF-α blockade interferes with the healing of wounds and prevention of postoperative infection. Treatment with TNF-α antagonists could be resumed after complete healing of the surgical wound and in the absence of any postoperative infection [53].

The Canadian Rheumatology Association (CRA) guidelines state that biologic DMARD should be held prior to surgical procedures. The timing for withholding biologic DMARD should be based on the individual patient, the nature of the surgery, and the pharmacokinetic properties of the agent. Biologic DMARD may be restarted postoperatively if there is no evidence of infection and wound healing is satisfactory [54].

In clinical practice, we should follow each one's national guidelines and medical circumstance of each country. We summarized concisely the recommendations of main national guidelines in Table 2.

	Recommended perioperative management of TNF blockers
American Society of Rheumatology (ACR)	*Discontinue for at least 1week prior to and 1 week after surgery (this decision should be further tempered by the pharmacokinetic properties of a given biologic agent and the type of surgery)
British Society of Rheumatology (BSR)	*Discontinuation should be balanced against the risk of a perioperative RA flare (three to five times the half-life of the relevant drug prior to surgery) *Should not be restarted after surgery until there is good wound healing and no evidence of infection
Club Rhumatismes et Inflammation (CRI)	*Minor surgery: discontinue for at least 1 month (infliximab), 3-4 weeks (adalimumab) and 1-2 weeks (etanercept) *Surgery in a septic environment: discontinue for 8 weeks (infliximab), 4-6 weeks (adalimumab) and 2-3 weeks(etanercept)
Japan College of Rheumatology (JCR)	*Discontinue for 2-4 weeks (etanercept) or 4 weeks (infliximab) *Could be resumed after complete healing of the surgical wound and in the absence of any postoperative infection
Canadian Rheumatology Association (CRA)	*Discontinuation should be based on the individual patient, the nature of the surgery, and the pharmacokinetic properties of the agent. *Restarted postoperatively if there is no evidence of infection and wound healing is satisfactory

Table 2. Recommendations for perioperative management of TNF blockers in national guidelines

8. Conclusions

It is difficult to draw definite conclusion on the influence of perioperative use of TNF blockers on the risk of SSI, wound healing and flare of disease activity in RA patients undergoing orthopaedic surgery, due to the retrospective nature and small sample size of most of past studies. Although we have a limitation in the review of the perioperative management of TNF blockers, it is seemed for us that perioperative discontinuation of anti-TNF therapy was preferable to decrease the risk of SSI and wound healing complication, whereas it likely caused the increased risk of RA flare. At present, the national guidelines on each society recommend preoperative discontinuation of TNF blockers.

The risk factors for SSIs, which most of RA patients undergoing TJA are considered to have, are the use of TNF blockers, increased daily steroid intake, older age and longer disease duration, history of prior SSI or skin infection, and "clear" surgical procedure such as TJA, thus it may be preferable to perform TJA, if needed, before the induction of TNF blockers. When withholding the anti-TNF therapy, the potential benefit of preventing SSI (different surgical procedures pose different risks of infection and wound healing) should be balanced against the risk of RA flare, and we should also take pharmacokinetic properties of the agents into consideration. Shortening the period of withholding anti-TNF therapy is desirable to prevent the postoperative flare, but it may cause an increase in SSI and wound healing complications. This is the clinical dilemma for orthopaedic surgeons. Further larger prospective studies are clearly needed to make definite conclusion of perioperative management of TNF blockers, and in clinical practice until these studies are done, we should follow each one's national guidelines and take a sufficient antibiotic prophylaxis with a careful follow-up.

Author details

Koichiro Komiya and Nobuki Terada

*Address all correspondence to: komiya@qb3.so-net.ne.jp

Department of Orthopaedic Surgery, Fujita Health University Second Hospital, Aichi, Japan

References

[1] Edwards CJ, Cooper C, Fisher D, Field M, van Staa TP, Arden NK. The importance of the disease process and disease-modifying antirheumatic drug treatment in the development of septic arthritis in patients with rheumatoid arthritis. Arthritis and Rheumatism 2007; 57(7): 1151-1157.

[2] Mooney DP, O'Reilly M, Gamelli RL. Tumor necrosis factor and wound healing. Annals of Surgery1990; 211(2): 124-129.

[3] Grennan DM, Gray J, Loudon J, Fear S. Methotrexate and early postoperative complications in patients with rheumatoid arthritis undergoing elective orthopaedic surgery. Annals of the Rheumatic Diseases 2001; 60(3): 214-217.

[4] Doran MF, Crowson CS, Pond GR, O'Fallon WM, Gabriel SE. Frequency of infection in patients with rheumatoid arthritis compared with controls: a population-based study. Arthritis and Rheumatism 2002; 46(9): 2287-2293.

[5] Weston VC, Jones AC, Bradbury N, Fawthrop F, Doherty M. Clinical features and outcome of septic arthritis in a single UK Health District 1982-1991. Annals of the Rheumatic Diseases 1999; 58(4): 214-219.

[6] Geirsson AJ, Statkevicius S, Vikingsson A. Septic arthritis in Iceland1990-2002: increasing incidence due to iatrogenic infections. Annals of the Rheumatic Diseases 2008; 67(5): 638-643.

[7] Gupta MN, Sturrock RD, Field M. A prospective 2-year study of 75 patients with adult-onset septic arthritis. Rheumatology (Oxford) 2001; 40(1): 24-30.

[8] Kaandorp CJ, Van Schaardenburg D, Krijnen P, Habbema JD, van de Laar MA. Risk factors for septic arthritis in patients with joint disease. A prospective study. Arthritis and Rheumatism 1995; 38(12): 1819-1825.

[9] Favero M, Schiavon F, Riato L, Carraro V, Punzi L. Rheumatoid arthritis is the major risk factor for septic arthritis in rheumatological settings. Autoimmunity Reviews 2008; 8(1): 59-61.

[10] Doran MF, Crowson CS, Pond GR, O'Fallon WM, Gabriel SE. Predictors for infection in rheumatoid arthritis. Arthritis and Rheumatism 2002; 46(9): 2294-2300.

[11] Galloway JB, Hyrich KL, Mercer LK, Dixon WG, Ustianowski AP, Helbert M, Watson KD, Lunt M, Symmons DP; BSR Biologics Register. Risk of septic arthritis in patients with rheumatoid arthritis and the effect of anti-TNF therapy: results from the British Society for Rheumatology Biologic Register. Annals of the Rheumatic Diseases 2011; 70(10): 1810-1814.

[12] Askling J, Dixon W. The safety of anti-tumour necrosis factor therapy in rheumatoid arthritis. Current Opinion in Rheumatology 2008; 20(2): 138-144.

[13] Bongartz T, Halligan CS, Osmon DR, Reinalda MS, Bamlet WR, Crowson CS, Hanssen AD, Matteson EL. Incidence and risk factors of prosthetic joint infection after total hip or knee replacement in patients with rheumatoid arthritis. Arthritis and Rheumatism 2008; 59(12): 1713-1720.

[14] Wymenga AB, van Horn JR, Theeuwes A, Muytjens HL, Slooff TJ. Perioperative factors associated with septic arthritis after arthroplasty. Prospective multicentre study of 362 knee and 2,651 hip operations. Acta Orthopaedica Scandinavica 1992; 63(6): 665-671.

[15] Schrama JC, Espehaug B, Hallan G, Engesaeter LB, Furnes O, Havelin LI, Fevang BT. Risk of revision for infection in primary total hip and knee arthroplasty in patients with rheumatoid arthritis compared with oateoarthritis: a prospective, population-based study on 108,786 hip and knee joint arthroplasties from the Norwegian Arthroplasty Register. Arthritis Care and Research 2010; 62(4): 473-479.

[16] Jamsen E, Huhtala H, Puolakka T, Moilanen T. Risk factors for infection after knee arthroplasty. A register-based analysis of 43,149 cases. The Journal of Bone and Joint Surgery (American Volume) 2009; 91(1): 38-47.

[17] Robertsson O, Knutson K, Lewold S, Lidgren L. The Swedish Knee Arthroplasty Register 1975-1997: an update with special emphasis on 41,223 knees operated on in 1988-1997. Acta Orthopaedica Scandinavica 2001; 72(5): 503-513.

[18] Berbari EF, Hanssen AD, Duffy MC, Steckelberg JM, Ilstrup DM, Harmsen WS, Osmon DR. Risk factors for prosthetic joint infection: case-control study. Clinical Infectious Disease 1998; 27(5): 1247-1254.

[19] Wilson MG, Kelly K, Thornhill TS. Infection as a complication of total knee-replacement arthroplasty. Risk factors and treatment in sixty-seven cases. The Journal of Bone and Joint Surgery (American Volume) 1990; 72(6): 878-883.

[20] da Cunha BM, de Oliveira SB, Santos-Neto L. Incidence of infectious complications in hip and knee arthroplasties in rheumatoid arthritis and osteoarthritis patients. Revista Brasileira de Rheumatologia 2011; 51(6): 609-615.

[21] Visser K, Katchamart W, Loza E, Martinez-Lopez JA, Salliot C, Trudeau J, Bombardier C, Carmona L, van der Heijde D, Bijlsma JW, Boumpas DT, Canhao H, Edwards CJ, Hamuryudan V, Kvien TK, Leeb BF, Martin-Mola EM, Mielants H, Muller-Ladner U, Murphy G, Ostergaad M, Pereira IA, Ramos-Remus C, Valentini G, Zochling J, Dougados M. Multinational evidence-based recommendations for the use of methotrexate in rheumatic disorders with a focus on rheumatoid arthritis: integrating systematic literature research and expert opinion of a broad international panel of rheumatologists in the 3E Initiative. Annals of the Rheumatic Diseases 2009; 68(7): 1086-1093.

[22] Talwalkar SC, Grennan DM, Gray J, Johnson P, Hayton MJ. Tumour necrosis factor alpha antagonists and early postoperative complications in patients with inflammatory joint disease undergoing elective orthopaedic surgery. Annals of the Rheumatic Diseases 2005; 64(4): 650-651.

[23] Wendling D, Balblanc JC, Brousse A, Lohse A, Lehuede G, Garbuio P, Toussirot E, Auge B, Jacques D. Surgery in patients receiving anti-tumor necrosis factor alpha treatment in rheumatoid arthritis: an observational study on 50 surgical procedures. Annals of the Rheumatic Diseases 2005; 64(9): 1378-1379.

[24] den Broeder AA, Creemers MC, Fransen J, de Jong E, de Rooij DJ, Wymenga A, de Waal-Malefijt M, van den Hoogen FH. Risk factors for surgical site infections and other complications in elective surgery in patients with rheumatoid arthritis with special attention for anti-tumor necrosis factor: a large retrospective study. The Journal of Rheumatology 2007; 34(4): 689-695.

[25] Bibbo C, Goldberg JW. Infectious and healing complications after elective orthopaedic foot and ankle surgery during tumor necrosis factor-alpha inhibition therapy. Foot and Ankle International. 2004; 25(5): 331-335.

[26] Hirano Y, Kojima T, Kanayama Y, Shioura T, Hayashi M, Kida D, Kaneko A, Eto Y, Ishiguro N. Influences of anti-tumour necrosis factor agents on postoperative recovery in patients with rheumatoid arthritis. Clinical Rheumatology 2010; 29(5): 495-500.

[27] Kawakami K, Ikari K, Kawamura K, Tsukahara S, Iwamoto T, Yano K, Sakuma Y, Tokita A, Momohara S. Complications and features after joint surgery in rheumatoid

arthritis patients treated with tumour necrosis factor-alpha blockers: perioperative interruption of tumour necrosis factor-alpha blockers decreases complications? Rheumatology (Oxford) 2010; 49(2): 341-347.

[28] Momohara S, Kawakami K, Iwamoto T, Yano K, Sakuma Y, Hiroshima R, Imamura H, Masuda I, Tokita A, Ikari K. Prosthetic joint infection after total hip or knee arthroplasty in rheumatoid arthritis patients treated with nonbiologic and biologic disease-modifying antirheumatic drugs. Modern Rheumatology 2011; 21(5): 469-475.

[29] Suzuki M, Nishida K, Soen S, Oda H, Inoue H, Kaneko A, Takagishi K, Tanaka T, Matsubara T, Mitsugi N, Mochida Y, Momohara S, Mori T, Suguro T. Risk of postoperative complications in rheumatoid arthritis relevant to treatment with biologic agents: a report from Committee on Arthritis of the Japanese Orthopaedic Association. Journal of Orthopaedic Sciense 2011; 16(6): 778-784.

[30] Kubota A, Nakamura T, Miyazaki Y, Sekiguchi M, Suguro T. Perioperative complications in elective surgery in patients with rheumatoid arthritis treated with biologics. Modern Rheumatology 2012; [Epub ahead of print].

[31] Hayata K, Kanbe K, Chiba J, Nakamura A, Inoue Y, Hobo K. Clinical factors related to the efficacy and complications of orthopedic surgery for rheumatoid arthritis with infliximab. International Journal of Rheumatic Disease 2011; 14(1): 31-36.

[32] Gilson M, Gossec L, Mariette X, Gherissi D, Guyot MH, Berthelot JM, Wendling D, Michelet C, Dellamonica P, Tubach F, Dougados M, Salmon D. Risk factors for total joint arthroplasty infection in patients receiving tumor necrosis factor α-blockers: a case-control study. Arthritis Research and Therapy 2010; 12(4): R145.

[33] Giles JT, Bartlett SJ, Gelber AC, Nanda S, Fontaine K, Ruffing V, Bathon JM. Tumor necrosis factor inhibitor therapy and risk of serious postoperative orthopaedic infection in rheumatoid arthritis. Arthritis and Rheumatism 2006; 55(2): 333-337.

[34] Ruyssen-Witrand A, Gossec L, Salliot C, Luc M, Duclos M, Guignard S, Dougados M. Complication rates of 127 surgical procedures performed in rheumatic patients receiving tumor necrosis factor alpha blockers. Clinical and Experimental Rheumatology 2007; 25(3): 430-436.

[35] Busti AJ, Hooper JS, Amaya CJ, Kazi S. Effects of perioperative anti-inflammatory and immunomodulating therapy on surgical wound healing. Pharmacotherapy 2005; 25(11): 1566-1591.

[36] Goh L, Jewell T, Laversuch C, Samanta A. Should anti-TNF therapy be discontinued in rheumatoid arthritis patients undergoing elective orthopaedic surgery? A systematic review of the evidence. Rheumatology International 2012; 32(1): 5-13.

[37] Streit M, Beleznay Z, Braathen LR. Topical application of the tumour necrosis factor-alpha antibody infliximab improves healing of chronic wounds. International Wound Journal 2006; 3(3): 171-179.

http://dx.doi.org/10.5772/54012

[38] Tarnuzzer RW, Schultz GS. Biochemical analysis of acute and chronic wound environments. Wound Repair and Regeneration 1996; 4(3): 321-325.

[39] Rapala K, Peltonen H, Heino J, Kujari H, Pujol JP, Niinikoski J, Laato M. Tumour necrosis factor-alpha selectivity modulates expression of collagen genes in rat granulation tissue. The European Journal of Surgery 1997; 163(3); 207-214.

[40] Salomon GD, Kasid A, Cromack DT, Director E, Talbolt TL, Sank A, Norton JA. The local effects of cachectin/tumor necrosis factor on wound healing. Annals of Surgery 1991; 214(2): 175-180.

[41] Mori R, Kondo T, Ohshima T, Ishida Y, Mukaida N. Accelerated wound healing in tumor necrosis factor receptor p55-deficient mice with reduced leukocyte infiltration. FASEB Journal 2002; 16(9): 963-974.

[42] Iglesias E, O'Valle F, Salvatierra J, Aneiros-Fernandez J, Cantero-Hinojosa J, Hernandez-Cortez P. Effect of blockade of tumor necrosis factor-alpha with etanercept on surgical wound healing in SWISS-OF1 mice. The Journal of Rheumatology 2009; 36(10): 2144-2148.

[43] Ashcroft GS, Jeong MJ, Ashworth JJ, Hardman M, Jin W, Moutsopoulos N, Wild T, McCartney-Francis N, Sim D, McGrady G, Song XY, Wahl SM. Tumor necrosis factor-alpha (TNF-α) is a therapeutic target for impaired cutaneous wound healing. Wound Repair and Regeneration 2012; 20(1): 38-49.

[44] Scallon B, Cai A, Solowski N, Rosenberg A, Song XY, Shealy D, Wagner C. Binding and functional comparisons of two types of tumor necrosis factor antagonists. The Journal of Pharmacology and Experimental Therapeutics 2002; 301(2): 418-426.

[45] Goekoop-Ruiterman YP, de Vries-Bouwstra JK, Allaart CF, van Zeben D, Kerstens PJ, Hazes JM, Zwinderman AH, Ronday HK, Han KH, Westedt ML, Gerards AH, van Groenendael JH, Lems WF, van Krugten MV, Breedveld FC, Dijkmans BA. Clinical and radiographic outcomes of four different treatment strategies in patients with early rheumatoid arthritis (the BeSt study): a randomized, controlled trial. Arthritis and Rheumatism 2005; 52(11): 3381-3390.

[46] Brocq O, Millasseau E, Albert C, Grisot C, Flory P, Roux CH, Euller-Zieqler L. Effect of discontinuing TNFalpha antagonist therapy in patients with remission of rheumatoid arthritis. Joint, Bone, Spine 2009; 76(4): 350-355.

[47] Saleem B, Keen H, Goeb V, Parmar R, Nizam S, Hensor EM, Churchman SM, Quinn M, Wakefield R, Conaghan PG, Ponchel F, Emery P. Patients with RA in remission on TNF blockers: when and in whom can TNF blocker therapy be stopped? Annals of the Rheumatic Diseases 2010; 69(9): 1636-1642.

[48] Tanaka Y, Takeuchi T, Mimori T, Saito K, Nawata M, Kameda H, Nojima T, Miyasaka N, koike T; RRR study investigators. Discontinuing of Infliximab after attaining low disease activity in patients with rheumatoid arthritis: RRR (remission induction by Remicade in RA) study. Annals of the Rheumatic Diseases 2010; 69(7): 1286-1291.

[49] Klarenbeek NB, van der Kooij SM, Guler-Yuksel M, van Groenendael JH, Han KH, Kerstens PJ, Huizinga TW, Dijkmans BA, Allaart CF. Discontinuing treatment in patients with rheumatoid arthritis in sustained clinical remission: exploratory analyses from the BeSt study. Annals of the Rheumatic Diseases 2011; 70(2): 315-319.

[50] Saag KG, Teng GG, Patkar NM, Anuntiyo J, Finney C, Curtis JR, Paulus HE, Mudano A, Pisu M, Elkins-Melton M, Outman R, Allison JJ, Suarez Almazor M, Bridges SL Jr, Chatham WW, Hochberg M, MacLean C, Mikuls T, Moreland LW, O'Dell J, Turkiewicz AM, Furst DE; American College of Rheumatology. American College of Rheumatology 2008 recommendations for the use of nonbiologic and biologic disease-modifying anti-rheumatic drugs in rheumatoid arthritis. Arthritis and Rheumatism 2008; 59 (6): 762-784.

[51] Ding T, Ledingham J, Luqmani R, Westlake S, Hyrich K, Lunt M, Kiely P, Bukhari M, Abernethy R, Bosworth A, Ostor A, Gadsby K, McKenna F, Finney D, Dixey J, Deighton C; Standards, Audit and Guidelines Working Group of BSR Clinical Affairs Committee; BHPR. BSR and BHPR rheumatoid arthritis guidelines on safety of anti-TNF therapies. Rheumatology (Oxford) 2010; 49(11): 2217-2219.

[52] Pham T, Claudepierre P, Deprez X, Fautrel B, Goupille P, Hilliquin P, Masson C, Morel J, Puechal X, Saraux A, Schaeverbeke T, Mariette X, Sibilia J; Club Rhumatismes et Inflammation, French Society of rheumatology. Anti-TNF-alpha therapy and safety monitoring. Clinical tool guide elaborated by the Club Rhumatismes et Inflammations (CRI), section of the French Society of Rheumatology (Societe Francaise de Rhumatologie, SFR). Joint, Bone, Spine 2005; 72 (Suppl 1): S1-58.

[53] Koike R, Takeuchi T, Eguchi K, Miyasaka N; Japan College of Rheumatology. Update on the Japanese guidelines for the use of infliximab and etanercept in rheumatoid arthritis. Modern Rheumatology 2007; 17(6): 451-458.

[54] Bombardier C, Hazlewood GS, Akhavan P, Schieir O, Dooley A, Haraoui B, Khraishi M, Leclercq SA, Legare J, Mosher DP, Pencharz J, Pope JE, Thomson J, Thorne C, Zummer M, Gardam MA, Askling J, Bykerek V. Canadian Rheumatology Association Recommendations for the Pharmacological Management of Rheumatoid Arthritis with Traditional and Biologic Disease-modifying Antirheumatic Drugs: Part II Safety. The journal of Rheumatology 2012; 39(8): 1583-1602.

Chapter 7

Extraskeletal Manifestations in Rheumatoid Arthritis - Clinical Cases

Katarzyna Romanowska-Próchnicka,
Przemysław Rzodkiewicz, Marzena Olesińska,
Dariusz Szukiewicz and Sławomir Maśliński

Additional information is available at the end of the chapter

http://dx.doi.org/10.5772/53739

1. Introduction

Rheumatoid arthritis (RA) is a chronic, autoimmune disease, which attacks the joints but also may cause extra-articular complications. The disease can present itself in a variety of ways. It depends on many factors, including the presence of rheumatoid factor, presence and rate of anti-CCP, number of swollen and painful joints (over 20 in the beginning of the disease), levels of inflammatory markers (ESR, CRP), patient's young age, occurrence of rheumatoid nodules. Patients who present the above criteria, especially with early, polyarticular onset of the disease, have usually aggressive, progressive and destructive course of the disease manifested by extra-articular manifestations. Proper primary treatment in the early stage of RA may reduce the number of swollen joints and severity of inflammation, slow the progression of joint deformations and decrease the amount of erosions. However, it does not completely preserve the occurrence of extra-articular complications. A lot of these complications can be observed in patients with long lasting RA, with recurrent exacerbations, undertreated or non compliant. Many of RA symptoms can also be seen in other diseases. That is why the recognition of the disease in many times is difficult.

In this paper we provide overview of major extra-articular complications of RA, describing its incidence and clinical features. To illustrate the complexity, variety of course and most common diagnostic problems, descriptions of four case studies are also included.

2. Non joint related complications of rheumatoid arthritis

Because there is no agreed classification of complications accompanying RA, this paper includes not only extra articular manifestations but also non-articular complications of RA.

2.1. Rheumatoid anemia

Normocytic or microcytic anemia is a relatively common feature of RA. The development of anemia is related to the effects of proinflammatory cytokines: tumor necrosis factor alpha (TNF-α), interferon gamma (IFN-γ), interleukin-1 (IL-1), and interleukin-6 (IL-6) [1].

Anemia in RA is a result of iron deficiency, related to increased hepcidin production, which is a recognized key factor of this disease. Hepcidin is a peptide hormone produced by the liver. It inhibits intestinal iron absorption, iron release from macrophages and hepatocytes and placental iron transport [2]. As a result, these mechanisms decrease iron delivery. The main mediator of hepcidin increase in inflammation is IL-6 [2]. The IL-6–dependent STAT-3 pathway and the unfolded protein response–associated cyclic AMP response element-binding protein-H (CREBH) pathway are responsible for the signal transduction pathways that regulate hepcidin during inflammation and endoplastic reticulum stress [3].

Another factor regulating hepcidin level during inflammation is IL-1. It has been shown that hepatocytes can be stimulated directly by the cytokines IL-6, IL-1α, and IL-1β to produce hepcidin [4]. Moreover, IL-1 induces hypoferremia [5], up-regulates ferritin [6], and plays a primary role in the anemia of chronic inflammation [7].

It has been shown that increased TNF–α levels correlate with systemic iron deficiency [8]. Levels of TNF-α were found to be significantly higher in anemic compared to non-anemic patients [9]. TNF–α is a pro-inflammatory cytokine that decreases iron level through mechanisms that are independent of the induction of hepcidin [10]. Experiments with laboratory animals shown that treatment with TNF-α down-regulate mucosal transfer of iron [11]. Duodenal ferritin levels are induced in these animals, providing for iron storage during the acute phase response [12]. This mechanism would prevent dietary iron exsorption across the mucosa to circulation [13]. Treatment of macrophages with TNF-α, surprisingly is associated with a rise in intracellular free or labile iron that is required for activation of the transcription factor NF-κB [14]. NF-κB is an important regulator of cellular responses to stimuli such as stress. Reduction of intracellular iron by chelation has an inhibitory effect on NF-κB induction of TNF-α and other cytokines [15,16]. Further studies of the TNF-α mechanism are needed to better understand its reciprocal relationship with iron and control of the NF-κB inflammatory response [13].

It is considered that IFN-γ can also modulate iron status. Recent In vitro studies suggest that IFN-γ may modulate hepcidin induction by M. tuberculosis infected macrophages [17]. In vivo studies have shown that a high iron diet will reduce IFN-γ [18], implicating its role in the deleterious effects that iron-loading can have on the immune response. IFN-γ is a key modulator of macrophage iron status and immune functions [13]. In vitro studies show that IFN-γ could induce nitric oxide production–mediated apoptosis process, which might be involved in the pathogenesis of anemia in RA patients [19]. There is evidence suggesting that increased local IFN- γ production in bone marrow may be implicated in the pathogenesis of anemia seen in up to 50% of patients with RA [20].

The best way of correcting anemia is to control systemic disease by treatment with disease-modifying antirheumatic drugs (DMARDs). It has been shown that treatment with infliximab and methotrexate significantly improves hemoglobin level among anemic RA patients when compared to treatment with placebo and methotrexate [21]. In trials of tocilizumab in RA substantial increase of hemoglobin levels was shown in patients with anemia in comparison to patients without the disease [22]. In patients with persistent anemia, an erythropoietin therapy may be considered. Erythropoietin therapy might be used if hormone level in serum is lower than 500 mU/ml [23].

2.2. Rheumatoid nodules

Rheumatoid nodules (RN) are the most common extraskeletal manifestations of RA. RN occur in approximately 20-35% of seropositive patients [24]. It does not depend on the severity of inflammation. Rheumatoid nodules usually appear in patient with long lasting and active inflammation process in RA (average disease duration of eleven years) [33]. However, 11% of patients have RN in early stage of the disease, sometimes even earlier than inflammation process in the joints. RN affects males more than females. Nodules are formed most frequently in soft tissues, skin colored, painless, movable. However, they can also be painful and attached to the structure below tendons and bursae. They gain size from 2 mm to a couple of centimeters in diameter. They appear in extensor parts of limbs in the proximal area of interphalangeal and metacarpophalangeal joints, proximal forearm, elbows, foots and ankles [25]. The nodules can occur not only subcutaneous but also internally – in lungs [26] and other internal organs (heart [27], liver [28], pancreas [29], kidney [30]).

In histopathology, rheumatoid nodules contain massive areas of sharply defined necrobiosis, specifically eosinophilic necrobiotic granuloma in the centere, surrounded by a palisade of macrophages and fibroblasts, and a peripheral vascular area containing T lymphocytes and macrophages. Nodules have collagen degeneration and common fibrosis. Usually there are inflammatory components (tuberculoid and sarcoid reactions) [31]. Immunohistochemical studies of a rheumatoid nodules (RN) suggest that it is a Th1 granuloma with focal vasculitis. According to Hodkinson, patients with rheumatoid nodules have increased level of circulating Th1 and IL-12, IL-2, and VEGF levels and IL-8, than those without RN [32].

Etiology of RN is unknown, but there are series of studies suggesting that nodules are an effect of repeated trauma in the local tissue, which induce local vascular damage, and increase the level of proangiogenesis factors and cause granulation of tissue formations [32].

Nodules are usually asymptomatic but sometimes there is inflammation, ulceration, deeper nodules can have fistula. In this case a surgical and antibiotic treatment is required. Although RNs are a cosmetic issue and usually do not need medical treatment. Nodules can enlarge, recur or persist indefinitely. Sometimes nodules undergo remission after colchicine, hydroxychloroquine and D-penicillamine [34]. There are two (Ching et al. and Baan et al.)

double-blind randomized studies with corticosteroids injections and placebo [35,36]. Ching et al. injected 24 nodules in 11 patients and concluded that it is a safe and effective way of treating rheumatoid nodules [36]. Baan et al. has a similar conclusion. Surgical removal of the nodules may be considered if they limit joint motion [35].

2.3. Thrombocytosis

Thrombocytosis is one of the most common extra-articular manifestations of RA and is often correlated with the disease activity. Thrombocytosis is a manifestation observed in 40% of active patients with rheumatoid arthritis, it usually occurs during the active clinical stages of RA.

Thrombocytes or platelets are cytoplasmic fragments shed from mature megakaryocytes. These cells are implicated in the pathophysiology of a number of connective tissue disorders, including RA. Presence of platelets was documented in synovium [37] and synovial fluid of RA patients [38]. Activation of platelets in RA was observed in number of studies [39-42]. Platelet alpha granules contains number of biologically active substances, which released in response to activation, may contribute to the inflammatory cascade. Thrombocytes are a source of a number of substances e.g. P-selectin, platelet-derived growth factor, CTAP-III, acidic and basic fibroblast growth factor, epidermal growth factor, transforming growth factor beta, which may influence inflammation [43]. Positive correlation between P-selectine, platelets number and RA activity was observed [39].

Recent studies indicate that proinflammatory cytokines, playing a role in disease development, may have also megakaryocytopoetic/thrombopoetic properties [43]. Persistent overproduction of certain thrombocytopoietic factors can induce megakaryocytopoiesis and thrombocytopoiesis [44]. The megakaryocytopoiesis and inflammatory cascade of RA share hematopoietic cytokines and respond to a number of colony-stimulating factors. Progenitors of osteoclasts are important cells during the development of erosion [45]. Megakaryocytopoiesis – is a complex process of development of megakaryocytes from pluripotent stem cells. The process includes a number of events: cell division, endoreplication, abortive mitosis, and maturation which may result in the biogenesis of platelets [43]. Megakaryocytes and platelet production are dependent on the interactions of hematopoietic stem/progenitor cells, the bone marrow stromal microenvironment and intracellular events and are influenced by certain interleukins, colony-stimulating factors (CSF), and hormones which stimulate proliferation and differentiation at different stages [46]. Each day, approximately two hundred milliards of platelets are released into the circulation of healthy adults [43].

The main proinflammatory cytokines of RA, TNF-α and IL-1β, could contribute to the production of thrombocytes. Although not primarily involved in the production of thrombocytes in the marrow, TNF-α and IL-1 can influence on thrombocytosis during inflammation by inducing synthesis and secretion of megakaryocytopoietic cytokines (i.e. stem cell factor, granulocyte colony-stimulating factor, IL-6, IL-11, and leukemia inhibitory factor) [rewieved by 43]. Interleukin-1 is also a potent inducer of IL-6 megakaryopoiesis stimulatory cytokine [47].

IL-4 important anti inflammatory cytokine may also play dual regulatory role in thrombopoiesis of RA. It functions as a downregulator of megakaryocytopoiesis [48], but also interacts with other cytokines, costimulating the growth of hematopoietic precursors [49-51]. It was shown that IL-4 increases along with IL-1 and IL-6 in patients with active RA complicated by thrombocytosis [43, 52 and 53].

Roles of different pleiotropic megakaryocytopoietic cytokines have been investigated in patients with thrombocytosis secondary to RA. Among those cytokines, IL-6 predominates in the stimulation of megakaryopoiesis [54]. Moreover, IL-6 may be responsible for the higher TPO in inflammatory events [55]. IL-6 and thrombopoietin (TPO) may be responsible for the development of reactive thrombocytosis in RA [52, 53 and 56]. Thrombopoietin (TPO) is the main regulator hormone of platelet production. The binding of TPO to its receptor influences all stages of megakaryocyte development and thrombocytosis both in vivo and in vitro [57]. Enhanced megakaryocyte and platelet mass can act as negative feedback to the megakaryocytopoiesis via receptor-mediated uptake and catabolism of the TPO [57]. Therefore, TPO, proinflammatory cytokines, anti-inflammatory mediators, megakaryocyte mass, and platelets themselves act in concert to regulate megakaryocytopoiesis of RA. Platelets can also be activated, and the growth hormones secreted from their alpha granules may actively contribute to the tissue inflammation associated with RA [39-42].

2.4. Pulmonary involvement

Pulmonary involvement includes pleurisy/ pleural effusion, rheumatoid nodules, interstitial involvement, pulmonary vasculitis - pulmonary hypertension, airways involvement (obliterative bronchiolitis), drug-induced lung diseases.

Patients with RA have different prevalence of lung involvement. Estimated prevalence depends on the method of detection. For example, the incidence of lung involvement based on X-rays occurs in 1-12% of patients [58]. Next the functional test of lung capacity reveals 5-15% prevalence of restrictive lung disease [59]. However a reduction in the capacity of the lung to diffuse carbon monoxide was observed in more than 50% of the patients with RA [60]. The high-resolution computer tomography (HRCT) is the most sensitive detector of pulmonary changes in RA patients. The prevalence of lung involvement is up to 80% in RA patients [60].

Pleurisy/pleural effusion are the most common manifestations of the lung disease in RA. The prevalence is about 5- 20% of patients with rheumatoid arthritis [61]. The occurrence is significantly higher when considering postmortem studies - 40% - 75% [62]. Pleurisy appears in patients with active RA, more frequently in males than females. The amount of pleural effusion is usually small, and most of the patients do not require pleural puncture. The fluid is present over a couple of weeks. It resolves usually after corticosteroids therapy and DMARD's therapy. Sometimes when the amount of the fluid is high and the patient has symptoms of pulmonary insufficiency (short of breath, chest pain, cough) the thoracentesis is needed. Each time any infections and malignancy should be excluded in the first place.

Pulmonary rheumatoid nodules are usually coexisting with subcutaneous rheumatoid nodules and occur in patients with positive rheumatoid factor. Prevalence is different. It depends on a radiological method. Rheumatoid nodules are detected by X-ray in 0,2% of RA [63] patients and in 4% by HRCT [64]. Males are affected more often than females. Pulmonary nodules can be single or multiple, usually are asymptomatic. They appear in periphery right middle lobe or both upper lobes, gain from a couple of millimeters to a couple of centimeters in diameter [65]. In most cases a patient requires biopsy and malignancy exclusion. In histological examinations the pulmonary nodules look similar to the subcutaneous nodules. They are characterized by a central zone of fibrinoid necrosis, surrounded by a layer of palisading mononuclear cells within an outer zone of vascular granulation tissue, lymphocytes, plasma cells, and fibroblasts [66, 67].

In 1953 Caplan [68] described coexistence of rheumatoid nodules and pneumoconiosis in chest radiographs of coal miners suffering from RA. X-rays show that the nodules are about 0.5 centimeter up to a couple of centimeters in diameter, and also a massive fibrosis. Nodules can collapse or calcify [68]. The course of the disease is sudden, it can regress or progress. It develops especially in miners working in anthracite coal-mines and in people exposed to silica and asbestos [69]. Prevalence is higher among patients with silicosis. In Caplan's syndrome, a hypergammaglobilinemia with high level of alpha 2- globulin and a hipoalbuminemia may occur [70]. Unge et al. investigated thirteen cases of Caplan's syndrome by chest X-ray, rheumatic and immunological tests, heart and lung physiology and pathological-anatomical specimens. No positive correlation was found between exposure time to silica, radiological findings and the level of rheumatoid factor. There was also no correlation found between the degree of rheumatic inflammations and pulmonary progress. The hypothesis that silica acts as an adjuvant was not reflected in rheumatic parameters [71]. Patients with Caplan's syndrome require DMARD's therapy. In case of a progression in the lungs, the corticosteroid therapy is needed.

Interstitial lung disease is one of the lung manifestations in RA patients. According to the recent American Thoracic Society (ATS)/European Respiratory Society consensus classification, idiopathic interstitial pneumonias (IIPs) include seven clinico-radiologic-pathologic entities:

- idiopathic pulmonary fibrosis (IPF),
- usual interstitial pneumonia (UIP),
- nonspecific interstitial pneumonia (NSIP),
- cryptogenic organizing pneumonia,
- acute interstitial pneumonia,
- respiratory bronchiolitis-associated ILD,
- desquamative interstitial pneumonia,
- lymphoid interstitial pneumonia[72]

Hyun-Kyung Lee et al. performed a retrospective study at Asian Medical Center to investigate the histopathologic patterns of interstitial lung diseases in patients with RA and their correlation with clinical features and outcome [73]. UIP was the most common (55.6% in 10/18 patients) of the lung involvement in RA patients. NSIP was second popular (33.3% in 6/18). UIP was determine as fibrosis (fibrotic lesion and honeycombing). NSIP was divided in 3 histopatholgic subgroups. First group was distinguished with interstitial inflammation, second group, with both inflammations, and fibrosis, and third group, primarily with fibrosis. The UIP group had worse diagnosis than the NCIS group [73].

Clinical features of pulmonary fibrosis in RA patients are similar to those of idiopathic pulmonary fibrosis. 90% of pulmonary fibrosis patients have earlier joints diseases. Males with seropositive RA are more exposed than females [74]. Patients with pulmonary fibrosis in RA reveal both lymphocytic alveolitis and neutrophilic inflammation with or without pulmonary fibrosis in bronchoalveolar lavage (BAL). This study showed increased levels of CD4 and CD4:CD8 ratio in lymphocytic alveolitis [75].

The pathogensis of pulmonary fibrosis depends on two types of factors – RA-independent and RA-associated. The RA independent factors are linked with tobacco usage and alpha-1 antitrypsin level. The RA-associated factors combine with genetical predisposition of HLA gene occurrence and the cytokines level, especially proinflammatory cytokines by alveolar macrophages, in particular TNF-α [76].

Patients with pulmonary fibrosis have a different course of the disease. Some cases have a slowly progressing disease, some have stable course, while others show a rapidly deteriorating process of the disease. Severe loss of pulmonary functions is rare [77].

Drug induced pulmonary involvement in patients with RA can occur after methotrexate therapy, gold salts, D-pecicilammine, sufasalzine.

Methotrexate – pneumtonitis (MTX pneumonitis) is not a common complication but a lifetreating one. The data about the prevalence of MTX pneumonitis in RA shows a great variation. Several retrospective and prospective studies have reported prevalence rates between 0.3% and 11.6% [78]. The methotrexate complications can occur with a dose of 7.5 mg per week, as early as 1 month after initiation of therapy, and as late as two years therapy [79]. The clinical presentation of methotrexate – pneumonitis is nonspecific. In general, patients have a nonproductive cough, dyspnoe, fever, pleuric chest pain. Physical examination often reveals bilateral inspiratory crackles. Laboratory findings may include mild leukocytosis or eosinophilia. The X-rays could be normal or could reveal interstitial lung diseases. The high resolution tomography (HRCT) reveals "ground glass". The pathology of the methotrexate - pneumonitis is unknown. However a toxic drug reaction is suggested by the accumulation of methotrexate in lung tissue. Age, sex, cumulative or weekly dose of methotrexate and the disease duration, are not associated with the development of MTX-pneumonitis. Recent studies suggest 5 conditions that induce an increased risk of the development of MTX- complication: diabetes mellitus, hypoalbuminemia, rheumatoid pleuropulmonary involvement, previous use of disease-modifying agents (gold, sulfasalazine, or penicillamine), older age [79]. Patients who are suspected of MTX-induced lung toxicity should cancel methotrexate therapy. Most of the patients improve without any other intervention, but in some cases the corticosteridotherapy is needed.

The treatment of interstitial fibrosis in RA is variable because of variable course of pulmonary involvement. Generally, high daily doses of steroids are beneficial in some patients. In some cases immunosuppressive (azathioprine or cyclophosphamid) agent should be added to steroid therapy. Raghu et al. reported a prospective double-blind, randomized, placebo-controlled clinical trial with azathioprine combined with prednisone in the treatment of idiopathic pulmonary fibrosis. This study shows the efficacy of azathioprine associated with prednisone and both the frequency and risk of side effects are lower than those of cyclophosphamide [80].

2.5. Amyloidosis

Secondary amyloidosis is potentially a life treatening complication of RA. The prevalence estimates from 7% to 26% in RA patients [81]. Amyloidosis is worldwide and prevalence depends on demographic location. For example, a study from Finland of the autopsy records of 1666 patients with RA revealed a prevalence of amyloidosis of 5.8% [82]. SAA1 gene polymorphism increases frequency of amyloidosis. The frequency of SAA1 genotype is higher among Japanese, Chinese, and white Australians than in other races. The frequency of SAA1 in Japanese is about 40% [83].

Amyloidosis is characterized by extracellular tissue deposition of fibrils that are composed of fragments of serum amyloid A (SAA) protein produced by hepatocytes. Secondary amyloidosis occurs during chronic inflammations. In developing countries secondary amyloidosis coexist with chronic, infectious diseases, tuberculosis, leprosy, bronchiectasis, chronic osteomyelitis, and chronic pyelonephritis. In industrialized countries, noninfectious diseases such as rheumatoid arthritis (23-51%), juvenile idiopathic arthritis (7-48%) and ankylosing spondylitis (0-12%) may cause amyloidosis [84, 85]. It occurs in patients with RA, who have long and very active aggressive course of disease. Amyloidosis is related to the acute phase of inflammation and elevated serum SAA1 level. SAA synthesis and secretion by hepatocytes is mediated by cytokines, mainly IL-1, TNF-α and IL-6 [86].

The diagnosis of secondary amyloidosis is based on histological examination of tissue from fat tissue, upper gastro intestinal duct or rectum. The most common presentation in amyloid is renal. Renal involvement in RA patient with amyloidosis is approximately 90% of all. Almost every patient with renal involvement has proteinuria. In some cases a renal insufficiency (high level of creatynina and low level of GFR) may appear. Amyloidosis is associated with the occurrence of nephrotic syndrome (proteinuria> 3.5 g, hypoalbuminaemia, vascular edema of lower limb). The amyloid can be present in spleen and liver. However, even severe damage of liver and spleen is usually asymptomatic. Heart involvement occurs in 10% patients with RA. This is shown as poor diagnostic factor.

Survival rate of patients diagnosed with amyloidosis in RA is approximately 4-5 years [87]. The clinical risk factors associated with a poor survival are: female gender, older age, reduced serum albumin, and increased serum creatinine concentration [88].

First aim in treatment of amyloidosis in RA is to decrease the level of serum amyloid A, by means of inflammation processes suppression. The effective DMARD's therapy and biologic therapy can cause decreased level of inflammation and reduce probability of amyloidosis. First drug therapy in amyloidosis is based on immunosupresive agents (cyclophosphamide [89], methotrexate [90], and azathioprine [91]), which improve the prognosis. According to Nakamura et al. cyclophosphamide therapy is more effective than methotrexate therapy in secondary amyloidosis in RA patients [92]. Biologic agents (anty TNF-α therapy) and inhibitor IL-6 decrease the level of serum Amyloid A by decreasing the polymorphism SAA1 gene. T. Nakamura performed a study about efficacy of etanercept in patients with AA amyloidosis secondary to rheumatoid arthritis. The conclusion of this study is that etanercept is safe and effective even in patient on hemodialysis [93]. The latest Nakamura study proved that etanercept treatment was more effective than cyclophsphamide treatment [94]. Eprodisate is a new class of antiamyloid compounds for treating AA amyloidosis, which results in a significant delay in progression to hemodialysis or end-stage renal disease in AA amyloidosis [95].

2.6. Sjögren's syndrome

Sjögren's syndrome (SS) is a chronic autoimmune inflammatory disease that affects lacrimal and salivary glands causing mucous dryness [96]. The symptoms are related to diminished lacrimal and salivary gland function and frequently present with keratoconjunctivitis sicca, xeropthalmia, xerostomia, sialadenitis, cervical caries and infections. SS can cause also systemic manifestations. They are subdivided into nonvisceral (skin, arthralgia, myalgia) and visceral (lung, heart, kidney, gastrointestinal, endocrine, central and peripheral nervous system).

Sjögren's syndrome is called secondary SS (sSS) when it is associated with other autoimmune disorders such as scleroderma and RA [97]. Sjögren's syndrome definition was developed by the team of experts from Europe and America, "European American consensus group criteria" (EACG) that requires for recognition criteria:

- Subcjective ocular symtoms: symptoms of dry eyes over 3 months, forgein body sensation in the eyes,
- Subjective oral symtoms: symtoms of dry mouth over 3 months, swollen salivary glands
- Objcective ocular signs: Abnormal Schirmer Test (tears flow less then 5 mm in 5 minutes)
- Objective oral signs: unstimulated whole salivary flow less then 1.5 ml in 15 minutes, abnormal parotid sialography, abnormal salivary scintigraphy
- Positive histopathological examination of lymphocytic infiltration at salivary glands, at least one focus score,
- Positive antibody titers antiSSA/SSB.

The SS diagnosis requires a presence of one subcjective symptom plus 2 of the 3 objective criteria [98].

The development of SS secondary to RA occurs on a different genetic background (HLA DR4). A distinct set of therapeutic responses suggest different pathogenetic processes [99, 100]. SS secondary to RA seems to be a complication of this disorder: the sicca syndrome is less serious, Ab to Ro/SSA and La/SSB are present less frequently and the evolution of SS is closely linked to that of RA. SS secondary to RA usually is subclinical and requires specific tests for its diagnosis [99, 101].

As the physiopathology of these two diseases is distinctive, it is possible to suggest that patients with RA and secondary SS have two different diseases [96]. In primary SS there is an important role of B cells and type I interferon [97,102] in contrast to the predominance of Th17 cytokines in RA [103]. It was suggested that decreased expression of TGF-α1 observed in patients with SS secondary to RA might promote joint destruction [101]. The concentration of TGF-α1 was significantly higher in patients with RA than in those with SS accompanying RA and in control group. The highest serum TGF-α1 concentrations were found in patients with most severe joint damage, as evidenced by Steinbrocker stage. TGF-α1 is cytokine that prevents inappropriate autoimmune responses [101].

The exact prevalence of sSS in RA varies considerably, depending on the definition of sSS, disease duration of RA and geographic region [102]. It has been demonstrated in Spain that patients with RA duration up to 10 years have had a prevalence of secondary SS of 17% and after 30 years it was as high as 25% [103]. Another study of early arthritis in the UK confirmed the dependence of the prevalence of sSS on disease duration [104], but this relationship was not confirmed in the study from Norway [105]. However, significant correlation was found between reduced salivary production and RA disease activity [105]. Geographical variation was shown in a comparative study between Greek and British RA patients, sSS was demonstrated in 43% and 17%, respectively [106]. The prevalence of sSS may reflect geographical factors, but could also be due to the range of anti-TNF therapy [101].

The high prevalence of dry eyes in RA patients without fulfilling the diagnostic criteria for secondary SS has been noticed by Fujita et al. [107] who found it in 90% of non-SS RA patients. In his study only 10% of patients had Secondary SS. The correlation between secondary SS and disease activity was also studied. It was found that RA activity had no significant correlation with the presence of dry eyes. However there was some correlation to patients diagnosed with secondary SS [106]. Antero et al. could not find a higher RA activity measured by DAS-28 in patients with secondary SS when compared to the ones without it during the studies of Brazilian population. Neither secondary SS occurrence, nor eye sicca subjective and objective findings have any relation to the disease duration [101]. The presence of sicca symptoms was high in the studied population, although only 24% of patients met the criteria of secondary SS [101]. Ocular symptoms of dryness were more common than oral ones in RA patients [101]. The impact of sSS on RA is illustrated by a twofold increased risk of non-Hodgin's lymphoma compared to RA patients without sSS [108], and there is a tendency of increased mortality in RA patients with sSS compared to RA patients without sSS [109,110].

A therapy for the Secondary Sjögren's syndrome with RA can be divided into four separate aeras. First is to manage the dryness in the eyes and mouth as well as the skin and other mucosal surface. Next is to treat non-visceral manifestations such as arthralgia and myalgia, chronic fatigue syndrome. These symptoms are generally treated with salicylates, nonsteroidal agents, and hydroxychloroquine [111]. Patients with SS have a low tolerance of NSAIDs resulting from dysphagia, secondary to decreased saliva flow and increased frequency of gastro-oesophageal reflux disease. Usually patients with RA and SS use low doses of steroids and hydroxychloroquine to reduce arthaligia and myalgia. For visceral involvement, including vasculitic skin lesions, pneumonitis, neuropathy, and nephritis, corticosteroids are used with the dosage of 0.5 mg per one kilogram body mass. Drugs such as hydroxychloroquine, azathioprine, and methotrexate are used to help the corticosteroids [112]. Methotrexate seems to be more useful than azathioprine in Seconadry Sjögren's syndrome with RA [113]. The biological agent used in SS is rituximab. The recent studies show a significant decrease in fatigue, however no significant changes in secondary endpoints assessing glandular manifestations (unstimulated salivary flow rate and Shirmer's test results) [114, 115]. For life-threatening complications the cyclophosphamide therapy is needed. Lymphocytic aggressive manifestations, including lymphoma in SS with RA, require interdisciplinary help - hematologists.

2.7. Vasculitis

Rheumatoid vasculitis is a rare but most serious systemic complication of rheumatoid arthritis. It typically affects small and medium-size vessels. It occurs almost exclusively in patients with seropositive nodular RA who suffer from RA for at least 10 years and is associated with poor prognosis [116-118]. 40% of patients die within 5 years as well as significant mortality due to both organ damage from vasculities and consequences of the treatment [119-121]. Althought diagnostic criteria for systemic rheumatoid vasculitis were originally described in 1984 by Scott et al. [122], no validated definition of vasculities exist. Recent studies suggest that rheumatoid factor, anti-cyclic citrullinated polypeptide (CCP) positivity, male gender, tobacco use, rheumatoid nodules, and older onset or long disease duration confer added risk of vasculities [116]. Patients with the Felty`s syndrome are also prone to vasculitis [121].

There appears to be a genetic predisposition toward developing rheumatoid vasculitis. RA studies focused mainly on the third hypervariable region of HLA-DRB1 called the shared epitope. Recent studies suggest a relationship between rheumatoid vasculitis and three specific genotypes of the HLA-DRB1 shared epitope: *0401/*0401, *0401/*0404, and *0101/*0401 [118]. Research performed by the Mayo Clinic described a new correlation of HLA-C3 with rheumatoid vasculitis [123]. Strong correlation of smoking with the development of rheumatoid vasculitis was also discovered [123]. Other studies have also supported this relation, not only in rheumatoid vasculitis but also in other extra-articular manifestations [124]. Higher levels of anti-cyclic citrullinated polypeptide (CCP) antibodies levels were observed in patients with RA, who have systemic vasculities [125]. The presence of anti-CCP antibodies in patients with RA is linked to a progressive joint damage and severe extra-articular manifestations [121, 125]. During the studies of evaluating anti-CCP and RA vasculitis, antibodies were detected in 93% of patients with systemic RA vasculitis and only in 7% of patients with primary systemic small vessel vasculitis [121, 125]. However many patients with RA who have circulating or tissue-deposited immune complexes and high levels of autoantibodies do not develop vasculitis [124]. Systemic inflammation accompanying the development of RA promotes early and aggressive atherosclerotic vascular disease which may present similar to vasculitis manifestations. In such case, histopathologic confirmation of vasculitis is required [124]. Characteristic histopathology confirmation of vasculitis is generally necessary for a diagnosis of rheumatoid vasculitis. Other clinical and laboratory features are often supportive and may be used to assist a follow-up [124].

Pathologic features of rheumatoid vasculitis include mononuclear cells or neutrophilic infiltration of the vessel wall of small and medium vessels. Features of vessel wall destruction are often found, including necrosis, leukocytoclasis, and disruption of the internal and external elastic lamina. An important observation is that inflammation of more than three cell layers of the vessel is a significant feature to distinguish rheumatoid vasculitis from RA without vasculitis [124,126]. RA vasculitis may involve a number of body organs. Manifestations differ depending on involved part of the body. The most common sites of involvement are the skin and peripheral nerves. Cutaneous manifestations of rheumatoid vasculitis include palpable purpura, focal digital lesions, nodules, ulcers, digital necrosis and pyoderma. Peripheral nervous system involvement may be represented by distal sensory or motor neuropathy, mononeuritis multiplex. Central nervous system involvement may result in transient ischemic attack, stroke, or seizure. Vasculitis development in the eye manifestates in corneal ulceration and scleromalacia. Pulmonary involvement includes fibrosing alveolitis and alveolar hemorrhage. Vasculitis in major organs is much less common but can lead to significant morbidity and mortality, including myocardial infarction, bowel ischemia, and renal failure [124].

High incidence of cardiovascular-related deaths is observed in patients with RA. Dawson et al. noted that 31 % of the RA patients had an estimated pulmonary artery systolic pressure of 30 mmHg or more, and 21% of all the RA patients had pulmonary hypertension [127]. Severe pulmonary hypertension in patients with RA is not common and usually is associated with other collagen-vascular diseases such as progressive systemic sclerosis, syndrome of calcinosis, Raynaud's phenomenon, esophageal dysfunction, sclerodactyly and telangiectasia [128]. Pulmonary hypertension might be considered as primary or secondary. Primary pulmonary hypertension is often clinically silent until well advanced. It has a very poor prognosis and a median survival of only 2–3 years [129]. Secondary pulmonary hypertension progresses slower than the primary form. Treatment of pulmonary hypertension initially needs to be directed at the underlying cause. In RA, the pulmonary hypertension is usually a result of RA-associated lung disease and implies a poor prognosis.

A number of structural abnormalities have been reported in RA patients population. Aortic root enlargement, pericardial effusion, mitral valve abnormalities and impaired left ventricular function are more common in patients with RA than in control groups [127]. It has been noted that RA patients have an increased number of abnormalities related to the function of the left ventricle [130]. Impairment of left ventricular function may cause elevation of pressure on the left atrium which results in raises of the pulmonary artery pressure. Mild to moderate primary pulmonary hypertension is a common case in the RA population. Dawson et al. identified that 31% of hospital RA patients have pulmonary hypertension on echocardiography. In these patients no significant symptoms, signs, ECG or structural echocardiographic changes were apparent, probably because of early stage of disease [127]. Shortness of breath as a result of cartiorespiratory disesase in RA may appear because of constraints arising from RA. It was suggested that number of deaths that have been previously linked to ischaemic heart disease, may really have had been due to primary pulmonary hypertension [127].

A treatment of vasculitis depends on the degree of organ system involvement. Mild rheumatoid vasculitis involving the skin or peripheral nerves can be treated with prednisone (30-200mg/day) and methotrexate (10-25 mg/week) or azathioprine (50-150 mg/day). More serious organ system involvement may require treatment with higher-dose steroids and cyclophosphamide or biologic agents [124]. Management of patients with RA vasculitis should take into account the increased risk of comorbidities in particular from cardiovascular disease [121].

2.8. Pericarditis and myocarditis

Pericarditis is one of the most common extraskeletal manifestations in RA. It occurs in 30-50% of the patients [131]. The highest occurrence of the disease is observed in male patients with destructive and nodular RA [132]. It occurs seldom, require echocardiographic diagnostics which may show asymptomatic pericardial involvement. Symptoms can also include chest pains and pericardial effusion. Prognosis of RA patients with pericarditis depends on age, cardiac status. The prognosis is best when diagnosed in the first year [133]. Majority of patients develop pericarditis after arthritis begins, however pericarditis may also manifest before diagnosis of RA. Early diagnosis of RA is then relevant, and effective treatment improves the outcome of patients with RA [134]. Treatment with non-steroidal anti-inflammatory drugs, corticosteroids and/or other immunosuppressive drugs seems appropriate in the majority of patients with a definite diagnosis of RA-associated pericarditis, and in severe cases, pericardiectomy is required [135].

Patients with RA have a two to five times increased risk of developing severe and premature cardiocascular disease [136]. Relationship between cardiocascular risk and inflammation has been suggested. Endothelial dysfunction, reduced arterial elasticy and compressibility and increased atherosclerotic burden observed in RA support this theory [137-139]. Diffused necrotizing or granulomatous myocarditis may be a cause of cardiomyopathy. Postmortem histological studies showed cardiomyopathy in 3-30% of RA parients [131]. Pathogenesis includes myocyte injury, local and systemic cytokine-mediated immune responses, cell activation with cellular infiltration, oedema and necrosis [130]. It was hypothesized that elevated proinflammatory cytokines such as TNF-α, IL-1, IL-6 observed in RA may be associated with concomitant myocardial tissue injury [141]. These mechanisms occur to involve simultaneous activation of collagenolytic enzymes, MMPs [142]. Increased T2-ER observed in RA patients reflects ongoing inflammatory injury and persistence of tissue oedema in RA myocardium [141].

3. Case reports

These cases are included to illustrate the complexity, variety of course, complications and most common diagnostical problems with the rheumatoid arthritis.

3.1. Case nr. 1

A 26 years old female with 14 years history of seropositive rheumatoid arthritis. She has very aggressive course of disease. While diagnosed rheumatoid arthritis she had elevated rheumatoid factor – 1030 IU/ml, highly positive level of anti-citrullinated protein/peptide antibodies (ACPA) – 1137 U/ml, elevated level of inflammations factors - CRP, ESR. Furthermore she had objective factors of inflammations in the joints - overgrowth of synovium and infiltrations in joints cavity detected in ultrasound. The aggressive course of the disease correlates with progress in radiological changes in the joints. Radiogram of the hands shows Fourth Degree in Larsen Scale - it means that in the joints space there are severe erosions, with no joint space left and the original bone outlines are partly presented [143]. Radiograms of the legs show Second Degree in Larsen Scale - it means that in the joints space there are only one or several small erosions and diameter of the joints space is more than 1mm [143]. Therefore the patient required many surgical procedures. She underwent linear osteotomy of metatarsal bones of right foot in 2007 and had stabilizations of the left and right wrist with reconstruction of extensor palmaris of the second and third finger in the left hand in 2007. Then she received endoprosthesis of MCP II-III bones of the right hand in 2010. .

Physical examination showed symetric polyarthritis involving arms, wrists, metacarpophalangeal joints, proximal interphalangeal joints, knees, ankles and feet, 18- tender joints, 12– swollen joints, morning stiffness >120min, Disease Activity Score 28 (DAS28)- 6,67

She was treated with a variety of disease modifying antirheumatic drugs (DMARD's) over the years –sulfasalazine - in 2003 - 2007, chloroquine – in 2003-2007, cyclosporine – in 02.2009-04.2009 - with not good clinical response. After that she was treated with methotrexate. At first she was taking 7,5 mg i.m/week between 13.06.2007 - 18.09.2007. She showed intolerance to the drug – leucopenia. Next trial with methotrexate was in 17.03.2008 – 16.09.2008. She was treated with the dose of 10 mg -15 per os. She presented intolerance to the drug again- high level of liver enzymes, nausea. Methotrexate therapy was discontinued definitely. Next she received leflunomide – 20 mg/day from 04.02.2009 to 06.04.2009, also showing bad tolerance - leucopenia, high level of liver enzymes. After the DMARD's therapy failed, she was treated with anti TNF-α - etanercept 50mg sc/week for almost 2 years. In the end the patient did not show enough clinical response (difference between courses DAS28 < 1,2) and the therapy was canceled. Then she took tocilizumab - 480mg i.v./month – monotherapy - 6 courses, good response. Her Disease Activity Score 28 (DAS28) went near remission 2,98.

This case shows the patient in early age with very aggressive course of disease. She had high level of rheumatoid factor and anti-CCP antibody. She developed high level of radiological changes in joints and required surgical procedures. Her other risk factor of aggressive rheumatoid arthritis is poor response to disease modifying antirheumatic drugs and anti TNF-α.

This is a classical example of patient who has statistically high level of risk factor to develop destructive course of rheumatoid arthritis.

The most important thing in diagnostic process is to recognize a patient with high risk of aggressive course of the disease. Next the patient should receive appropriate treatment that includes combined therapy of at least two different DMARD's (disease modifying antirheumatic drugs) and in case of ineffectiveness of this therapy – also biologic agents. In case of seropositive RA with methotrexate intolerance patient should receive anti-TNF-α therapy in monotherapy (etanercept or adalibumab). If this therapy is not successful patient should be receiving inhibitor IL-6 – tocilizumab or fusion protein bind CTLA-4 - abatacept. This treatment can slow down or even stop the progression of the disease [144].

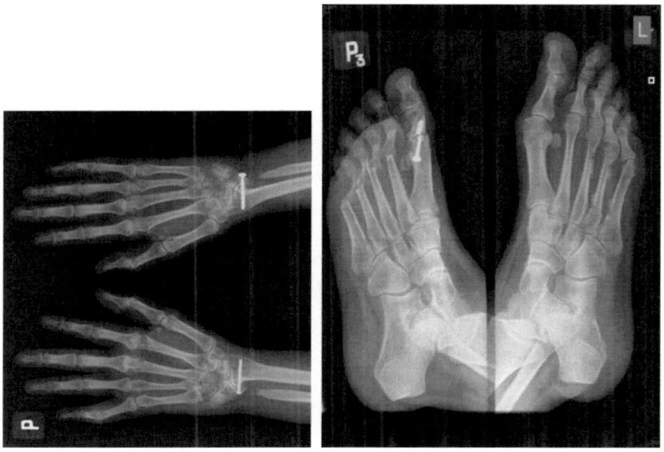

Figure 1. Case nr.1. A 26-year old woman with 14 years of rheumatoid arthritis. She underwent linear osteotomy of metatarsal bones of right foot in 2007 and had stabilizations of the left and right wrist with reconstruction of extensor palmaris of the second and third finger in the left hand in 2007. Then she received endoprosthesis of MCP II-III bones of the right hand in 2010.

Radiological changes are the visual outcome of the progressive rheumatoid arthritis. Thus, developed erosions in the joints in early stage of the disease prove joints destruction and probability of functional disability. There are predictive factors of long-term radiographic outcomes in early rheumatoid arthritis. N. Courvoisier performed a long-term study of 10 years to investigate predictive factors of radiographic outcome in RA and found the best independent predictive factor of the 10-year radiographic score to be baseline erosion score [145]. According to N. Courvoisier high level of erythrocyte sedimentation rate (ESR), presence and level of IgA rheumatoid factor, presence of an anti-citrullinated protein antibody (ACPA), serum level of matrix metalloproteinase-3 and radiographic score at baseline are the most important factors to predict which patients will develop severe form of rheumatoid arthritis. Interesting conclusion from this research work was that several demographic and clinical parameters, such as sex, age and number of tender or swollen joints, have not been shown to be independent prognostic factors [145].

3.2. Case nr. 2

A 48-year old female diagnosed with seropositive rheumatoid arthritis in 2004. Since 2004 the patient was treated with prednisolone, at the highest dose of 15mg/day. She has also received nonsteroidal anti-inflammatory drugs (NSAIDs) - paracetamol, ibuprofen, naproxen, diclofenac, recently ketoprofen. Since 2005 she has not taken any disease modifying antirheumatic drugs (DMARD's), although methotrexate and sulfasalazine were prescribed. The patient on her own decided to stop the treatment and did not cooperate with physicians.

In the spring of 2012 patient was admitted to the Department of Systemic Connective Tissue Diseases in Institute of Rheumatology with big flare-ups. Assessed Disease Activity Score 28 (DAS 28) was 7.22 (22 painful joints, 13 swollen joints, VAS-80, ESR-34mm/h). She has elevated rheumatoid factor - 681IU/ml, highly positive level of anti-citrullinated protein/peptide antibodies (ACPA) – 263,5U/ml. Physical examination revealed numerous rheumatoid nodules, with diameter range from 2 to 3 cm. The nodules were located on the extensor parts of the proximal interphalangeal and metacarpophalangeal joints and around wrists and ankles and elbows. The radiographs showed advanced changes from rheumatoid arthritis, ankylosis, joints subluxations, the highest degree of radiological V, according to Larsen - it means mutilating changes, where the original bony outlines have been destroyed [143].

In therapy the patient received the reference dose of methotrexate (25mg per week), the dose of glucocorticosteroids was reduced to 7,5mg/ day, and the dose of ketoprofen was reduced to 100mg per day. Patient was admitted to the Department one month after the start of the therapy. Disease Activity Score 28 went down to 3,3 (2 painful joints, 1 swollen joint, VAS- 55.) Inflammatory parameters were reduced (ESR-8mm/h, CRP- 3 mg/dl).

The purpose of the presentation of this case is to show a patient with aggressive natural course of disease, advanced articular changes and extra-articular complications - rheumatoid nodules. Rheumatoid nodules are benign structures, that relate to positive rheumatoid factor in 90%. Although there is no correlation between nodules, rheumatoid arthritis progression and severity of this disease, patients with rheumatoid nodules are recommended to take more aggressive treatment. Rheumatoid nodules are a cosmetic issue and do not require treatment, however complications can occur. There is high probability of infection, ulceration or even gangrene. Sometimes the internal nodules cause fistula. In this case there is a need for the surgical procedure. When nodules are painful, limit the motion or damage the underling structures, the injection of corticosteroids can reduce these symptoms. Conventional treatment (DMARD's) usually reduce or even completely resolve rheumatoid nodules. There are however published cases of accelerated rheumatoid nodules, that respond differently to the conventional treatment. In 1986 Kremer and Lee described the occurrence of such nodules during a study of a long-term methotrexate therapy [146]. Three patients had an increasing number of nodules during a therapy of methotrexate. Since then there has been a lot more descriptions of complications of methotrexate therapy. Usually patients complain of small, painful nodules on the hands – metacarpophalangeal and proximal interphalangeal joints, feet and ears. These observations were confirmed by Ahmed and coworkers. They arranged double blind study with methotrexate and azathioprine with patient with rheumatoid arthritis. Study showed an 8% incidence of methotrexate–induce accelerated rheumatoid nodules with arthritis improved and none of azathioprine [147]. Combined therapy- methotrexate and one of the following drugs: hydroxychloroquine [148], D-penicillamine [149], colchicine [150] or sulfasalazine [151] reduce probability of incidence of accelerated rheumatoid nodules. There are also case reports of another drug which have been implicated in occurrence of accelerated rheumatoid nodules. Anti-TNF-α therapy with etanercept can cause appearance of rheumatoid nodules.

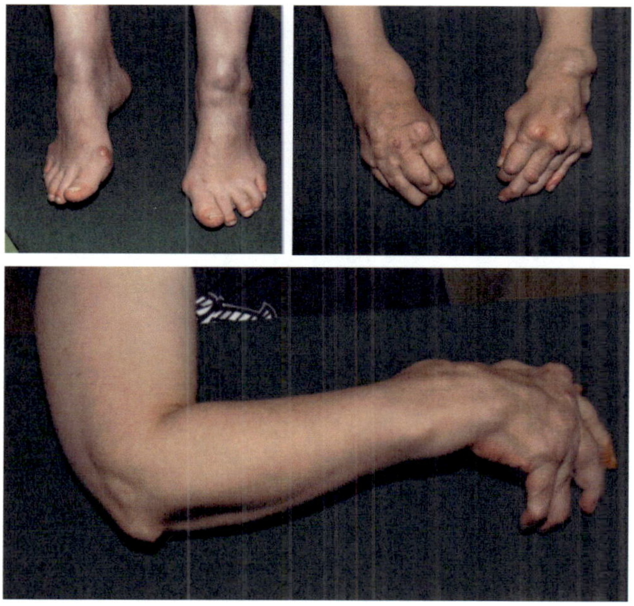

Figure 2. Case nr.2. A 48-year old female diagnosed with seropositive rheumatoid arthritis. She has numerous rheumatoid nodules.

The case report described above shows a patient with numerous rheumatoid nodules. This case is not related to the complications of methotrexate therapy, this is a typical case, where methotrexate decreased the size of nodules. However, there is an example of patient with very advanced clinical stage of rheumatoid arthritis (anykylosis in the hands during 7 years natural course of the RA). In the era of disease modifying antirheumatic drugs and biological treatment such case should never have happened. Patients who are quickly diagnosed with RA, should receive appropriate treatment within three months from the diagnosis. First step is DMARD's therapy. After three months of combined therapy (two different DMARD's including methotrexate 25mg/week [152]), patients require anti–TNF-α therapy combined with methotrexate. If this treatment fails, patients with seropositive RA should undergo an anti CD20 therapy – rituximab [153]. If the patients are seronegative RA, they should receive another biological agent (inhibitor IL-6, or anti IL-1 or fusion protein bind CTLA-4) [144]. Only this way patients with RA are able to significantly reduce the chance of disease progression.

3.3. Case nr. 3

A 68 year old patient, diagnosed with seropositive rheumatoid arthritis in 1978. In 2007 the patient was diagnosed with kidney failure based on the functional parameters of kidney: (creatinine 2.1 mg/dl, urea 150mg/dl, GFR-60) - renal insufficiency, (proteinuria over 3.5 grams/day, hypoalbuminemia, edema of lower limbs) - nephritic syndrome. Biopsy obtained from adipose tissue showed amyloidosis associated with RA. The patient has been hospitalized at the Institute of Rheumatology since 2008. She was admitted from Nefrology Department with severe microcytic anemia (Hb-7,6 g/dl, MCV- 83fL) after blood transfusion. She received 4 units of blood and she was qualified to erytropoietin treatment. She has also big exacerbation of rheumatoid inflammations (ESR- 107mm/h, CRP-86mg/l), Diseases Activity Score 28 (DAS28)- 6,69 (9-swollen joins, 9-painful joins, VAS-64). The patient was diagnosed with secondary Sjogren's syndrome based on dry mouth and eyes, positive Schirmer test - keratocjuctivitis sicca and histopathological examination - focus score of 2. The radiographs show advanced changes of rheumatoid arthritis with presence of erosions and joint subluxations - the highest degree of radiological V, according to Larsen- it means mutilating changes, where the original bony outlines have been destroyed [143]. She was treated with small doses of glucocorticosteroids and cyclophosphamid. The patient tolerated well the first 2 grams of cyclophosphamid treatment. Further therapy went with complications. After the patient fell down on the left shin, she has had abscess. Staphyloccocus aureus grew in bacteriological sowing. Patient received antibioticotherapy, cytostatic treatment was stopped. After one month of antibiotic therapy, the Staphyloccocus was still present in the sowing from endoprosthetic knee. She took antibiotics for over six months. In 2010 the patient received cytostatic treatment one more time. There was no bacteria present anymore. After administering the second gram of cyclofosfamid there was an increase of renal insufficiency, therefore the cyclostatic treatment was terminated. Over a 34-year period of time, the patient received various disease modifying antirheumatic drugs (DMARD's) - sulfasalazine, hydroxychloroquinee, cyclosporine, gold salts - with no therapeutic effect. Patient does not tolerate methotrexate, azathioprine and cyclophosphamid. Currently patient is treated with anti-TNF-α monotherapy with good tolerance, low inflammatory parameters and stabilization of kidney functions.

The description of this case is to show an aggressive course of disease with multiple exacerbations. The patient was treated with different drugs, which were ineffective or had side effects and in the end showed multiple organ damage. The most dangerous is renal failure caused by amyloidosis. In secondary amyloidosis AA renal involvement is observed in approximately 90% of all cases. Serum amyloid A (SSA) is responsible for amyloid deposits in involved organ. Concentration of amyloid A is proportional to inflammations process. Amyloidosis is diagnosed after about 17 years (4-40) of active rheumatoid arthritis [154]. Amyloid deposits concentrate in the renal capsule, particularly in mezangium, in the Bowman's capsule, but also in the renal pelvis, perynchema and in renal vessels. 95% of patients with secondary amyloidosis have proteinuria [155], nephritic syndrome or a different kind of kidney failure (hematuria, defect of renal pelvis or urinal infections). Main aim of the therapy in systemic amyloidosis is reducing and eliminating existing protein production or prohibiting further deposition of amyloid fibrils in organs.

The easiest way to reduce serum amyloid A is to reduce inflammations process by reducing CRP level by use DMARD's therapy [156] or anti -TNF-α therapy [157] TNF-α inhibitor achieved therapeutic success by reducing level of serum IL-6 [158,159]. Low level of serum IL-6 stops the synthesis of acute-phase proteins, systemic inflammation is suppressed, and SAA levels are lowered by decreasing polimorphism SAA1 gene. This supresses hepatocytes leading to reduction of amyloid deposits. New alternative is inhibitor IL-6- tociluzumab, a drug that directly inhibits polimorphism SAA1 gene [160,161].

Another way to stop amyloidosis is to reduce amyloidogenesis by stabilizing amyloid deposits in tissues. This aim can be achieved by interactions between amyloidogenic proteins and glycosaminoglycans promote fibril. There is a drug – eprodisate - which stops binding of SAA protein to precursor, next prohibiting polymerization of amyloid fibrils and deposition of the fibrils in tissues [162]. In 2007, Dember and coworkers published a multicenter, randomized, double blind, placebo-controlled trial to evaluate the efficacy and safety of eprodisate in patients with AA amyloidosis and kidney involvement. Eprodisate slow progression in the renal, stabilize renal functions and stop progression of amyloid deposits [95].

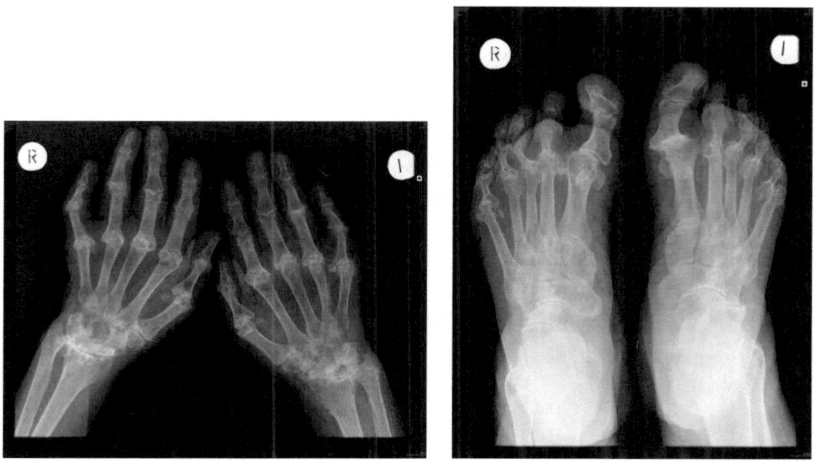

Figure 3. Case nr 3. A 68 year old patient, diagnosed with seropositive rheumatoid arthritis, secondary amylosicosis. Advanced changes in joins, the highest degree of radiological V, according to Larsen

The patient described above received the appropriate treatment. Rheumatoid arthritis and secondary amyloidosis required first classic treatment - DMARD's therapy (first drug in this case is cyclophosphamid) with glucocorticosteroids, next in case of this treatment's failure - anti-TNF-α therapy or inhibitors IL-6.

3.4. Case nr. 4

A 45 year old female was diagnosed with seropositive rheumatoid arthritis in 2000. She was treated with sulfasalazine, hydroxychlorochine and low dose of prednisolone.

On the December of 2006 the patient was admitted to the Department of Pulmonology with dyspnea and chest pain. Pleuritis with pleural effusion and degraded mass in the right lung were revealed based on chest X-ray. Bronchoscopy with cytology was taken. The result excluded bacterial infections and tuberculosis (cultures, PCR). Patient did not consent to pleural puncture. Tuberculostatic treatment was induced without influence on described lung changes. After 6 months pleural puncture was performed aspirating 1100ml of effusion fluid. The fluid had 46% of lymphocyte, very low level of glucose and highly positive rheumatoid factor, suggesting inflammation associated with RA exacerbation. Further investigations excluded heart failure and lung cancer. CT scan showed pleural effusion and mass (1,8 centimeters) suggested rheumatoid nodule in the third segment of right lung. The biopsy confirmed the diagnosis.

Patient was admitted to the Department of Rheumatology. Physical examination showed exacerbation of RA: 13 swollen joints, 11 painful, VAS - 68, ESR - 15mm/h and DAS28 - 5.8. Laboratory test revealed positive rheumatoid factor. Radiograms showed third degree in Larsen Scale (marked erosions in the joint surfaces). Other connective tissue diseases were excluded. The patient received 40mg/ day of methylprednisolone and methotrexate. The treatment was ineffective. Although the patient felt better, there were decreased swollen and painful joins with the same amount of fluid effusion. The treatment was switched to sulfasalzine, hydroxychloroquine and mehotrexate. It turned out that the patient does not tolerate methotrexate. On April of 2008 the patient was started on leflunamid treatment with good tolerance. The disease activity decreased to medium-low (DAS28 = 3.04). The inflammation in the lungs stabilized with a tendency to decrease in the amount of fluid in the pleural cavity.

This case shows that the image of RA can vary. A patient with rheumatoid arthritis requires an interdisciplinary care and multi-diagnosis. Therapies should be directed not only toward the treatment of arthritis, but also treatment of exacerbation of respiratory failure.

Pleural involvement is the most common manifestation of lung disease in rheumatoid arthritis. The prevalence is estimated to 5-20% patients with rheumatoid arthritis [61]. Other lung manifestations in rheumatoid arthritis are: rheumatoid nodules, interstitial lung diseases (heterogeneous group of disease depending of damage to the lung by inflammation or fibrosis), pulmonary hypertension, methotrexate induced lung diseases.

Traditional treatment of lung involvement in rheumatoid arthritis is corticosteroids. When there is pleural involvement, the treatment includes drainage of recurrent symptomatic effusion and oral corticosteroids, and treatment for the underlying rheumatoid arthritis. Next alternative treatment, especially for lung fibrosis, are cyclophosphamide [163], cyclosporine, azathioprine [163], and hydroxychloroquine [80]. Some case studies by Antoniou KM et al. suggest that infliximab may have an effect on interstitial lung diseases associated with rheumatoid arthritis. This study showed that infliximab can lead to stabilization or improvement of symptoms, lung function and lung image in X-rays [164].

http://dx.doi.org/10.5772/53739

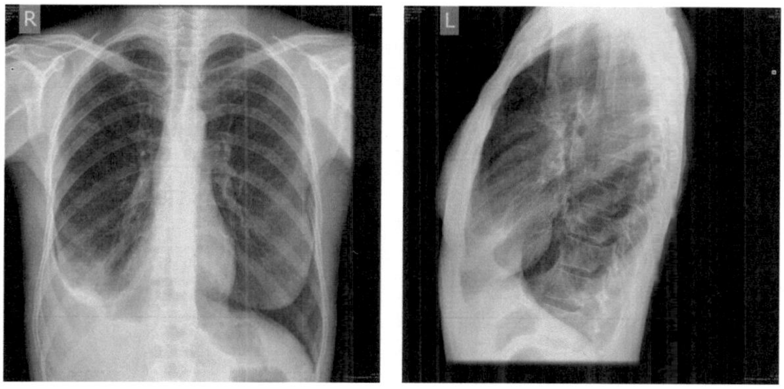

Figure 4. Case nr 4. A 45 year old female was diagnosed with seropositive rheumatoid arthritis, and lung involvement. X-rays showed right pleural effusion and in upper-middle side of right lung there was 1.6 centimetres mass looked like rheumatoid nodule.

4. Conclusion

Rheumatoid arthritis' course may vary. The occurrence of extraskeletal manifestations requires different diagnostic procedures and treatment. Many of extrasceletal manifestations are associated with more active or aggressive course of RA. Currently there are no predictors for extrasceletal manifestations which may suggest their presence in course of disease, although they are associated with risk factors like smoking, age, sex, level if inflammatory mediators, presence of rheumatoid factor, antinuclear antibodies and genetic factors. Extraskelatal features of RA are common and generally linked with aggressive course of disease. They need to be recognized early and treated in proper way.

Author details

Katarzyna Romanowska-Próchnicka[1,3], Przemysław Rzodkiewicz[2,3], Marzena Olesińska[1], Dariusz Szukiewicz[3] and Sławomir Maśliński[3]

1 Department and Polyclinic of Systemic Connective Tissue Diseases, Institute of Rheumatology, Warsaw, Poland

2 Department of Biochemistry and Molecular Biology, Institute of Rheumatology, Warsaw, Poland

3 Department of General and Experimental Pathology, Warsaw Medical University, Warsaw, Poland

References

[1] Masson C. Rheumatoid anemia. Joint Bone Spine. 2011;78(2):131-7.

[2] Nemeth E, Rivera S, Gabayan V, Keller C, Taudorf S, Pedersen BK, Ganz T. IL-6 mediates hypoferremia of inflammation by inducing the synthesis of the iron regulatory hormone hepcidin. J Clin Invest. 2004;113(9):1271-6.

[3] Shin DY, Chung J, Joe Y, Pae HO, Chang KC, Cho GJ, Ryter SW, Chung HT. Pretreatment with CO-releasing molecules suppresses hepcidin expression during inflammation and endoplasmic reticulum stress through inhibition of the STAT3 and CREBH pathways. Blood. 2012;119(11):2523-32.

[4] Lee P, Peng H, Gelbart T, Wang L, Beutler E. Regulation of hepcidin transcription by interleukin-1 and interleukin-6. Proc Natl Acad Sci U S A. 2005;102(6):1906-10.

[5] Alvarez-Hernández X, Liceaga J, McKay IC, Brock JH. Induction of hypoferremia and modulation of macrophage iron metabolism by tumor necrosis factor. Lab Invest. 1989;61(3):319-22.

[6] Torti FM, Torti SV. Regulation of ferritin genes and protein. Blood. 2002; 99(10): 3505-16.

[7] Maury CP, Andersson LC, Teppo AM, Partanen S, Juvonen E. Mechanism of anaemia in rheumatoid arthritis: demonstration of raised interleukin 1 beta concentrations in anaemic patients and of interleukin 1 mediated suppression of normal erythropoiesis and proliferation of human erythroleukaemia (HEL) cells in vitro. Ann Rheum Dis. 1988; 47(12):972-8.

[8] Atkinson SH, Rockett KA, Morgan G, Bejon PA, Sirugo G, O'Connell MA, Hanchard N, Kwiatkowski DP, Prentice AM. Tumor necrosis factor SNP haplotypes are associated with iron deficiency anemia in West African children. Blood. 2008;112(10): 4276-83.

[9] Keithi-Reddy SR, Addabbo F, Patel TV, Mittal BV, Goligorsky MS, Singh AK. Association of anemia and erythropoiesis stimulating agents with inflammatory biomarkers in chronic kidney disease. Kidney Int. 2008;74(6):782-90.

[10] Sharma N, Laftah AH, Brookes MJ, Cooper B, Iqbal T, Tselepis C. A role for tumour necrosis factor alpha in human small bowel iron transport. Biochem J. 2005;390(Pt 2): 437-46.

[11] Laftah AH, Sharma N, Brookes MJ, McKie AT, Simpson RJ, Iqbal TH, Tselepis C. Tumour necrosis factor alpha causes hypoferraemia and reduced intestinal iron absorption in mice. Biochem J. 2006;397(1):61-7.

[12] Torti FM, Torti SV. Regulation of ferritin genes and protein. Blood. 2002; 99:3505–16.

[13] Wessling-Resnick M. Iron homeostasis and the inflammatory response. Annu Rev Nutr. 2010;30:105-22.

[14] Xiong S, She H, Takeuchi H, Han B, Engelhardt JF, Barton CH, Zandi E, Giulivi C, Tsukamoto H. Signaling role of intracellular iron in NF-kappaB activation. J Biol Chem. 2003;278(20):17646-54.

[15] Schmidt PJ, Toran PT, Giannetti AM, Bjorkman PJ, Andrews NC. The transferrin receptor modulates Hfe-dependent regulation of hepcidin expression. Cell Metab. 2008; 7:205–14.

[16] Tsukamoto H. Iron regulation of hepatic macrophage TNFalpha expression. Free Radic Biol Med. 2002; 32:309–13.

[17] Omara FO, Blakley BR. The effects of iron deficiency and iron overload on cell-mediated immunity in the mouse. Br J Nutr. 1994; 72:899–909.

[18] Sow FB, Alvarez GR, Gross RP, Satoskar AR, Schlesinger LS, Zwilling BS, Lafuse WP. Role of STAT1, NF-kappaB, and C/EBPbeta in the macrophage transcriptional regulation of hepcidin by mycobacterial infection and IFN-gamma. J Leukoc Biol. 2009;86(5):1247-58.

[19] Kheansaard W, Mas-Oo-di S, Nilganuwong S, Tanyong DI. Interferon-gamma induced nitric oxide-mediated apoptosis of anemia of chronic disease in rheumatoid arthritis. Rheumatol Int. 2012;DOI 10.1007/s00296-011-2307-y. http://www.springerlink.com/content/h36027236338r151/?MUD=MP (accessed 13 August 2012)

[20] Papadaki HA, Kritikos HD, Valatas V, Boumpas DT, Eliopoulos GD. Anemia of chronic disease in rheumatoid arthritis is associated with increased apoptosis of bone marrow erythroid cells: improvement following anti-tumor necrosis factor-alpha antibody therapy. Blood. 2002 Jul 15;100(2):474-82.

[21] Doyle MK, Rahman MU, Han C, Han J, Giles J, Bingham CO 3rd, Bathon J. Treatment with infliximab plus methotrexate improves anemia in patients with rheumatoid arthritis independent of improvement in other clinical outcome measures-a pooled analysis from three large, multicenter, double-blind, randomized clinical trials. Semin Arthritis Rheum. 2009;39(2):123-31.

[22] Genovese MC, McKay JD, Nasonov EL, Mysler EF, da Silva NA, Alecock E, Woodworth T, Gomez-Reino JJ. Interleukin-6 receptor inhibition with tocilizumab reduces disease activity in rheumatoid arthritis with inadequate response to disease-modifying antirheumatic drugs: the tocilizumab in combination with traditional disease-modifying antirheumatic drug therapy study. Arthritis Rheum. 2008;58(10):2968-80.

[23] Moreno Lopez R, Sicilia Aladren B, Gomollon Garcia F. Use of agents stimulating erythropoiesis in digestive diseases. World J Gastroenterol. 2009;15(37):4675-85.

[24] Magro CM, Crowson AN. The spectrum of cutaneous lesions in rheumatoid arthritis. A clinical and pathological study of 43 patients. J Cutan Pathol 2003; 30:1-10.

[25] Sayah A, English JC 3rd: Rheumatoid arthritis. A review of the cutaneous manifestations. J Am Acad Dermatol 2005; 53:91-209.

[26] Tserkezoglou A, Metakidis S, Papastamatiou-Tsimara H, Zoitopoulos M. Solitary rheumatoid nodule of the pleura and rheumatoid pleural effusion. Thorax 1978;33:769-772, 1978

[27] Suriani RJ, Lansman S, Konstadt S. Intracardiac rheumatoid nodule presenting as a left atrail mass. Am Heart J 1994;127:463-465.

[28] Smits JG, Kooijman CD. Rheumatoid nodules in liver. Histopathology 1986;10:1211-1213.

[29] Riedlinger WF, Lairmore TC, Balfe DM, Dehner LP. Tumefactive necrobiotic granulomas (nodulosis) of the pancreas in an adult with long-standing rheumatoid arthritis. Int J Surg Pathol 2005;13:207-210.

[30] Schned AR, Moran M, Selikowitz SM, Taylor TH. Multiple rheumatoid nodules of the renal cortex. Arch Intern Med 1990;150:891-893.

[31] Miyasaka N, Sato K, Yamamoto K, Nishioka K. Immunological and immunohistochemical analysis of rheumatoid nodules. Ann Rheum Dis 1989;48:220-226.

[32] Hodkinson B, Meyer PW, Musenge E, Ally M, Anderson R, Tikly M. Exaggerated circulating Th-1 cytokine response in early rheumatoid arthritis patients with nodules. Cytokine. 2012;29. DOI 10.1016/j.cyto.2012.06.190 http://www.sciencedirect.com/science/article/pii/S1043466612004358 (accessed 13 August 2012)

[33] Gorman JD, David-Vaudey E, Pai M, Lum RF, Criswell LA. Lack of association of the HLA-DRB1 shared epitope with rheumatoid nodules: an individual patient data meta-analysis of 3,272 Caucasian patients with rheumatoid arthritis. Arthritis Rheum 2004;50:753–62.

[34] Diniz Mdos S, Almeida LM, Machado-Pinto J, Alves MF, Alvares MC Rheumatoid nodules: evaluation of the therapeutic response to intralesional fluorouracil and triamcinolone. [8rticle in English, Portuguese] An Bras Dermatol. 2011 Nov-Dec;86(6): 1236-8

[35] Baan H, Haagsma CJ, van de Laar MA. Corticosteroid injections reduce size of rheumatoid nodules. Clin Rheumatol. 2006 Feb;25(1):21-3. Epub 2005 Sep 15.

[36] Ching DW, Petrie JP, Klemp P, Jones JG. Injection therapy of superficial rheumatoid nodules. Br J Rheumatol. 1992 Nov;31(11):775-7.

[37] Palmer DG, Hogg N, Revell PA. Lymphocytes, polymorphonuclear leukocytes, macrophages and platelets in synovium involved by rheumatoid arthritis. A study with monoclonal antibodies. Pathology. 1986;18(4):431-7.

[38] Endresen GK. Investigation of blood platelets in synovial fluid from patients with rheumatoid arthritis. Scand J Rheumatol. 1981;10(3):204-8.

[39] Ertenli I, Kiraz S, Arici M, Haznedaroglu IC, Calguneri M, Celik I, Kirazli S P-selectin as a circulating molecular marker in rheumatoid arthritis with thrombocytosis. J Rheum 1998;25:1054–1058.

[40] Smith AF, Castor CW. Connective tissue activation. XII. Platelet abnormalities in patients with rheumatoid arthritis. J Rheumatol 1978;5:177–183.

[41] Zeller J, Weissbarth E, Mielke BH, Deicher H. Serotonin content of platelets in inflammatory rheumatoid diseases. Arthritis Rheum 1983;26:532–540.

[42] Endresen GK. Evidence for activation of platelets in the synovial fluid from patients with rheumatoid arthritis. Rheumatol Int 1989;9:19–24.

[43] Ertenli I, Kiraz S, Ozturk MA, Haznedaroglu I, Celik I, Calguneri M.Pathologic thrombopoiesis of rheumatoid arthritis. Rheumatol Int. 2003;23(2):49-60.

[44] Hollen CW, Henthorn J, Koziol JA, Burstein SA. Elevated serum interleukin-6 levels in patients with reactive thrombocytosis. Br J Haematol 1991;79:286–290.

[45] Manolagas SC, Jilka RL. Bone marrow, cytokines, and bone remodeling – emerging insights into the pathophysiology of osteoporosis. N Eng J Med. 1995; 332:305–311

[46] Hoffman R. The role of other hematopoietic growth factors and the marrow microenvironment in megakaryocytopoiesis. In: Kuter DJ, Hunt P, Sheridan W, Zucker-Franklin D. (ed.) Thrombopoiesis and thrombopoietins: molecular, cellular, preclinical and clinical biology. Humana, Totowa, 1997 pp 165–178.

[47] Warren MK, Conroy LB, Rose JS. The role of interleukin 6 and interleukin 1 in megakaryocyte development. Exp Hematol 1989:17:1095–1099.

[48] Sonoda J, Kuzuyama Y, Tanaka S, Yokota S, Maekawa T, Clark SC, Abe. Human interleukin 4 inhibits proliferation of megakaryocyte progenitor cells in culture. Blood 1993;81:624–630

[49] Mizel SB The interleukins. FASEB J 1989;3:2379–2388.

[50] Peschel C, Paul WE, Ohara J, Green I Effects of B cell stimulatory factor-1/interleukin-4 on hematopoietic progenitor cells. Blood 1987;70:254–263

[51] Rennick D, Yang G, Muller-Sieburg C, Smith C, Arai N, Takabe Y, Gemmell L. Interleukin 4 (B-cell stimulating factor 1) can enhance or antagonize the factor-dependent growth of hematopoietic progenitor cells. Proc Natl Acad Sci U S A 1987;84:6889–6893.

[52] Haznedaroglu IC, Ertenli I, Ozcebe OI, Kiraz S, Ozdemir O, Sayinalp N, Dundar SV, Calguneri M, Kirazli S. Megakaryocyte-related interleukins in reactive thrombocytosis versus autonomous thrombocytemia. Acta Haematol 1996;95:107–111.

[53] Ertenli I, Haznedaroglu IC, Kiraz S, Celik I, Calguneri M, Kirazli S. Cytokines affecting megakaryocytopoiesis in rheumatoid arthritis with thrombocytosis. Rheumatol Int 1996;16:5–8.

[54] Okamoto H, Yamamura M, Morita Y, Harada S, Makino H, Ota Z. The synovial expression and serum levels of interleukin-6, interleukin-11, leukemia inhibitory factor, and oncostatin M in rheumatoid arthritis. Arthritis Rheum 1997;40:1096–1105.

[55] Kaser A, Brandacher G, Steurer W, Kaser S, Offner FA, Zoller H, Theurl I, Widder W, Molnar C, Ludwiczek O, Atkins MB, Mier JW, Tilg. H Interleukin-6 stimulates thrombopoiesis through thrombopoietin: role in inflammatory thrombocytosis. Blood 2001;98:2720–2725

[56] Kiraz S, Ertenli I, Ozturk MA, Haznedaroglu IC, Celik I, Kiraz S, Calguneri M. Bloodstream thrombopoietin in rheumatoid arthritis with thrombocytosis. Clin Rheumatol 2002;21:453–456

[57] Kaushansky K. Thrombopoietin. N Engl J Med 1998;339:746–754.

[58] Dong Soon K. Interstitial lung disease in rheumatoid arthritis: recent advances. Pulm Med 2005; 12:346–353.

[59] Michel JJ, Turesson C, Lemster B, Atkins SR, Iclozan C, Bongartz T, Wasko MC, Matteson EL, Vallejo AN. CD56-expressing T cells that have features of senescence are expanded in rheumatoid arthritis. Arthritis Rheum. 2007;56(1):43-57.

[60] Dawson JK, Fewins HE, Desmond J, Lynch MP, Graham DR. Fibrosing alveolitis in patients with rheumatoid arthritis as assessed by high resolution computed tomography, chest radiography, and pulmonary function tests. Thorax. 2001;56(8):622-7.

[61] Joseph J, Sahn SA. Connective tissue diseases and the pleura. Chest 1993;104:262-270.

[62] Tanoue LT. Pulmonary manifestations of rheumatoid arthritis. Clin Chest Med 1998; 19:667–685.

[63] Walker WC, Wright V. Pulmonary lesions and rheumatoid arthritis. Medicine 1968; 47:501–520.

[64] Anaya JM, Diethelm L, Ortiz LA, Gutierrez M, Citera G, Welsh RA, Espinoza LR. Pulmonary involvement in rheumatoid arthritis. Semin Arthritis Rheum. 1995;24(4): 242-54.

[65] Yousem SA, Colby TV, Carrington CB. Lung biopsy in rheumatoid arthritis. Am Rev Respir Dis 1985;131:770-777.

[66] Hakala M, Paakko P, Huhti E, Tarkka M, Sutinen S. Open lung biopsy of patients with rheumatoid arthritis. Clin Rheumatol. 1990;9(4):452-60.

[67] Ziff M: The rheumatoid nodule. Arthritis Rheum 1990;33:761-766.

[68] Schreiber J, Koschel D, Kekow J, Waldburg N, Goette A, Merget R Rheumatoid pneumoconiosis (Caplan's syndrome). Eur J Intern Med. 2010;21(3):168-72.

[69] Ondrasik M. Caplan's syndrome. Baillieres Clin Rheumatol. 1989;3(1):205-10.

[70] Payne RB. Serum protein fractions in rheumatoid pneumoconiosis without arthritis. J Clin Pathol 1962; 15: 475-7.

[71] Unge G, Mellner C. Caplan's syndrome - a clinical study of 13 cases. Scand J Respir Dis. 1975;56(6):287-91.

[72] American Thoracic Society and European Respiratory Society. American Thoracic Society/European Respiratory Society international multidisciplinary consensus classification of idiopathic interstitial pneumonias. Am J Respir Crit Care Med 2002; 165, 277-304.

[73] Lee HK, Kim DS, Yoo B, Seo JB, Rho JY, Colby TV, Kitaichi M. Histopathologic pattern and clinical features of rheumatoid arthritis-associated interstitial lung disease. Chest. 2005;127(6):2019-27.

[74] Kelly CA. Rheumatoid arthritis: classical lung disease. Balliere's Clin Rheum 1993;7:1-16.

[75] Kolarz G, Scherak O, Popp W, Ritschka L, Thumb N, Wottawa A, Zwick H. Bronchoalveolar lavage in rheumatoid arthritis. Br J Rheumatol. 1993;32(7):556-61.

[76] Rochester CL, Elias J. Cytokines and cytokine networking in the pathogenesis of interstitial and fibrotic lung disorders. Semin Respir Med 1993;14:389-416.

[77] Schwarz MI, King TE. Interstitial Lung Disease (2 ed). Philadelphia, PA, Mosby Yearbook, 1993

[78] Barrera P, Van Ede A, Laan RF, Van Riel PL, Boerbooms AM, Van De Putte LB. Methotrexate re-lated pulmonary complications in rheumatoid arthritis. Ann Rheum Dis 1994;53:434 – 9.

[79] Lock BJ, Eggert M, Cooper JA Jr. Infiltrative lung disease due to noncytotoxic agents. Clin Chest Med. 2004;25(1):47-52.

[80] Raghu G, Depaso WJ, Cain K, Hammar SP, Wetzel CE, Dreis DF, Hutchinson J, Pardee NE, Winterbauer RH. Azathioprine combined with prednisone in the treatment of idiopathic pulmonary fibrosis: a prospective double-blind, randomized, placebo-controlled clinical trial. Am Rev Respir Dis 1991;144:291-296.

[81] Kobayashi H, Tada S, Fuchigami T, Okuda Y, Takasugi K, Matsumoto T, Iida M, Aoyagi K, Iwashita A, Daimaru Y, Fujishima M. Secondary amyloidosis in patients with rheumatoid arthritis: diagnostic and prognostic value of gastroduodenal biopsy. Br J Rheumatol. 1996;35(1):44-9.

[82] MEDSCAPE. Dhawan R. Chief Editor: Diamond HS. AA(inflammtory amyloidosis). Medscaape references 2011. http://emedicine.medscape.com/article/335559-overview (accessed 22 August 2012)

[83] Yamada T, Okuda Y, Takasugi K, Wang L, Marks D, Benson MD, Kluve-Beckerman B. An allele of serum amyloid A1 associated with amyloidosis in both Japanese and Caucasians. Amyloid. 2003;10:7–11.

[84] Lachmann HJ, Goodman HJ, Gilbertson JA, Gallimore JR, Sabin CA, Gillmore JD, Hawkins PN. Natural history and outcome in systemic AA amyloidosis. N Engl J Med. 2007;356(23):2361-71.

[85] Silva L, Sampaio L, Terroso G, Almeida G, Lucas R, Rios E, Bernardes JM, Bernardo A, Mariz E, Brito I, Pinto J, Maia C, Brito JS, Ventura FS. Amyloidosis secondary to rheumatic diseases - 16 cases. Acta Reumatol Port. Oct-Dec 2010;35(5):518-23.

[86] Husby G, Marhaug G, Dowton B, Sletten K, Sipe JD. Serum amyloid A (SAA): biochemistry, genetics and the pathogenesis of AA amyloidosis. Amyloid. 1994;1:119–37.

[87] Tanaka F, Migita K, Honda S, Fukuda T, Mine M, Nakamura T, Yamasaki S, Ida H, Kawakami A, Origuchi T, Eguchi K. Clinical outcome and survival of secondary (AA) amyloidosis. Clin Exp Rheumatol. 2003;21:343–6.

[88] Kitahama M, Koseki Y, Sakurai T, Kamatani N, Terai C. Female is a risk factor for developing AA-amyloidosis in patients with rheumatoid arthritis. Arthritis Rheum. 2007;56(Suppl):410–1.

[89] Nakamura T, Yamamura Y, Tomoda K, Tsukano M, Shono M, Baba S. Efficacy of cyclophosphamide combined with prednisolone in patients with AA amyloidosis secondary to rheumatoid arthritis. Clin Rheumatol. 2003;22:371–5.

[90] Fiter J, Nolla JM, Valverde J, Roig ED. Methotrexate treatment of amyloidosis secondary to rheumatoid arthritis. Rev Clin Esp. 1995;195:390–2.

[91] Shapiro DL, Spiera H. Regression of the nephrotic syndrome in rheumatoid arthritis and amyloidosis treated with azathioprine. A case report. Arthritis Rheum. 1995;38:1851–4.

[92] Nakamura T, Higashi S, Tomoda K, Tsukano M, Baba S, Shono M. Significance of SAA1.3 allele genotype in Japanese patients with amyloidosis secondary to rheumatoid arthritis. Rheumatology. 2006;45:43–9.

[93] Nakamura T, Higashi S, Tomoda K, Tsukano M, Baba S. Efficacy of etanercept in patients with AA amyloidosis secondary to rheumatoid arthritis Clinical and Experimental Rheumatology 2007; 25: 518-522.

[94] Nakamura T, Higashi SI, Tomoda K, Tsukano M, Shono M. Effectiveness of etanercept vs cyclophosphamide as treatment for patients with amyloid Aamyloidosis secondary to rheumatoid arthritis. Rheumatology (Oxford). 2012. doi: 10.1093/rheumatology/kes190 http://rheumatology.oxfordjournals.org/content/early/2012/08/09/rheumatology.kes190.long (accessed 20 August 2012)

[95] Dember LM, Hawkins PN, Hanzenberg BPC, Gorevic PD, Merlini GM, Butrimiene I, Livneh A, Lesnyak O, Puechal X, Lachmann HJ, Obici L, Balshaw R, Garceau D, Hauck W, Skinner M. Eprodisate for the treatment of renal disease in AA amyloidosis. N Engl J Med. 2007;356:2349–60.

[96] Antero DC, Parra AG, Miyazaki FH, Gehlen M, Skare TL. Secondary Sjögren's syndrome and disease activity of rheumatoid arthritis. Rev Assoc Med Bras. 2011;57(3): 319-22.

[97] Fox RI, Liu AY. Sjogren's syndrome in dermatology. Clin Dermatol. 2006;24:393-413.

[98] Seror R, Ravaud P, Bowman SJ, Baron G, Tzioufas A, Theander E, Gottenberg JE, Bootsma H, Mariette X, Vitali C. EULAR Sjogren's syndrome disease activity index: development of a consensus systemic disease activity index for primary Sjogren's syndrome. Ann Rheum Dis. 2010; 69 (6) :1103-1109.

[99] Fox RI. Sjogren's syndrome. Lancet 2005;366:321–331.

[100] Mattey DL, Gonzalez-Gay MA, Hajeer AH, Dababneh A, Thomson W, Garcia-Porrua C, Ollier WE. Association between HLA-DRB1*15 and secondary SS in patients with RA. J Rheumatol 2000;27(11):2611–2616.

[101] Mieliauskaite D, Venalis P, Dumalakiene I, Venalis A, Distler J. Relationship between serum levels of TGF-beta1 and clinical parameters in patients with rheumatoid arthritis and Sjögren's syndrome secondary to rheumatoid arthritis. Autoimmunity. 2009;42(4):356-8.

[102] Haga HJ, Naderi Y, Moreno AM, Peen E. A study of the prevalence of sicca symptoms and secondary Sjögren's syndrome in patients with rheumatoid arthritis, and its association to disease activity and treatment profile. Int J Rheum Dis. 2012;15(3): 284-8.

[103] Carmona L, Gozalez-Alvaro I, Balsa A, Angel Belmonte M, Tena X, Sanmarti R. Rheumatoid arthritis in Spain: occurrence of extra-articular manifestations and estimates of disease severity. Ann Rheum Dis. 2003;62:897-900.

[104] Young A, Koduri G. Extra-articular manifestations and complications of rheumatoid arthritis. Best Pract Res Clin Rheumatol. 2007; 21:909-27.

[105] Uhlig T, Kvien TK, Jensen JL, Axéll T. Sicca symptons, saliva and tear production and disease variables in 636 patients with rheumatoid arthritis. Ann Rheum Dis. 1999;58:415-22.

[106] Drosos AA, Lanchbury JS, Panayi GS. Rheumatoid arthritis in Greek and British patients. A comparative clinical, radiology and serology study. Arthritis Rheum 1992;35, 745–748.

[107] Fujita N, Igarashi T,Kurai T, Sakane N, Yoshino S, Takahasi H. Correlation between dry eye and rheumatoid arthritis activity. Ophthalmology 2005:140:808-13.

[108] Kauppi M, Pukkala E, Isomaki H. Elevated incidence of hematologic malignancies in patients with Sjogren's syndrome compared with rheumatoid arthritis (Finland). Cancer Causes Control 1997;8, 201–4.

[109] Martens PB, Pillemer SR, Jacobsson LT, O'Fallon WM, Matteson EL. Survivorship in a population based cohort of patients with Sjögren's syndrome, 1976-1992. J Rheumatol. 1999;26(6):1296-300.

[110] Turesson C, O'Fallon WM, Crowson CS, Gabriel SE, Matteson EL. Occurrence of extraarticular disease manifestations is associated with excess mortality in a community based cohort of patients with rheumatoid arthritis. J Rheumatol. 2002 ;29(1):62-7.

[111] Fox RI, Dixon R, Guarrasi V, Krubel S. Treatment of primary Sjögren's syndrome with hydroxychloroquine: a retrospective, open-label study. Lupus 1996; 5 (suppl 1): 31–36.

[112] Skopouli FN, Jagiello P, Tsifetaki N, Moutsopoulos HM. Methotrexate in primary Sjögren's syndrome. Clin Exp Rheumatol 1996; 14: 555–58.

[113] Price EJ, Rigby SP, Clancy U, Venables PJ. A double blind placebo controlled trial of azathioprine in the treatment of primary Sjögren's syndrome. J Rheumatol 1998; 25: 896–99.

[114] Meijer JM, Meiners P, Vissink A, Spijkervet FK, Abdulahad W, Kamminga N, Brouwer E, Kallenberg CG, Bootsma H. Effectiveness of rituximab treatment in primary Sjogren's syndrome: A randomized, double-blind, placebo,controlled trial. Arthritis Rheum. 2010;62:960-968

[115] Gottenberg JE, Guillevin L, Lambotte O, Combe B, Allanore Y, Cantagrel A, Larroche C, Soubrier M, Bouillet L, Dougados M, Fain O, Farge D, Kyndt X, Lortholary O, Masson C, Moura B, Remy P, Thomas T, Wendling D, Anaya JM, Sibilia J, Mariette X. Tolerance and short term efficacy of rituximab in 43 patients with systemic autoimmune diseases. Ann Rheum Dis. 2005;64:913-920.

[116] Voskuyl AE, Zwinderman AH, Westedt ML, Vandenbroucke JP, Breedveld FC, Hazes JM. Factors associated with the development of vasculitis in rheumatoid arthritis: results of a case-control study. Ann Rheum Dis. 1996;55(3):190-2.

[117] Turesson C, O'Fallon WM, Crowson CS, Gabriel SE, Matteson EL. Extra-articular disease manifestations in rheumatoid arthritis: incidence trends and risk factors over 46 years. Ann Rheum Dis. 2003;62(8):722-7.

[118] Gorman JD, David-Vaudey E, Pai M, Lum RF, Criswell LA. Particular HLA-DRB1 shared epitope genotypes are strongly associated with rheumatoid vasculitis. Arthritis Rheum. 2004;50(11):3476-84.

[119] Erhardt CC, Mumford PA, Venables PJ, Maini RN. Factors predicting a poor life prognosis in rheumatoid arthritis: an eight year prospective study. Ann Rheum Dis. 1989;48(1):7-13.

[120] Puechal X, Said G, Hilliquin P, Coste J, Job-Deslandre C, Lacroix C, Menkes CJ. Peripheral neuropathy with necrotizing vasculitis in rheumatoid arthritis. A clinicopathologic and prognostic study of thirty-two patients. Arthritis Rheum. 1995;38(11): 1618-29.

[121] Turesson C, Matteson EL. Vasculitis in rheumatoid arthritis. Curr Opin Rheumatol. 2009;21(1):35-40.

[122] Scott DG, Bacon PA, Tribe CR. Systemic rheumatoid vasculitis: a clinical and laboratory study of 50 cases. Medicine 1981;60:288–297.

[123] Turesson C, Schaid DJ, Weyand CM, Jacobsson LT, Goronzy JJ, Petersson IF, Dechant SA, Nyahll-Wahlin BM, Truedsson L, Sturfelt G, Matteson EL. Association of HLA-C3 and smoking with vasculitis in patients with rheumatoid arthritis. Arthritis Rheum 2006;54:2776–2783.

[124] Bartels CM, Bridges AJ. Rheumatoid vasculitis: vanishing menace or target for new treatments? Curr Rheumatol Rep. 2010;12(6):414-9.

[125] Turesson C, Jacobsson LT, Sturfelt G, Matteson EL, Mathsson L, Ronnelid J. Rheumatoid factor and antibodies to cyclic citrullinated peptides are associated with severe extra-articular manifestations in rheumatoid arthritis. Ann Rheum Dis. 2007;66(1): 59-64.

[126] Voskuyl AE, van Duinen SG, Zwinderman AH, Breedveld FC, Hazes JM. The diagnostic value of perivascular infiltrates in muscle biopsy specimens for the assessment of rheumatoid vasculitis. Ann Rheum Dis 1998;57:114–117.

[127] Dawson JK, Goodson NG, Graham DR, Lynch MP. Raised pulmonary artery pressures measured with Doppler echocardiography in rheumatoid arthritis patients. Rheumatology (Oxford). 2000;39(12):1320-5.

[128] Lehrman SG, Hollander RC. Severe pulmonary hypertension in a patient with rheumatoid arthritis--response to nifedipine. West J Med. 1986;145(2):242-4.

[129] D'Alonzo GE, Barst RJ, Ayres SM. Survival in patients with primary pulmonary hypertension: results from a National Prospective Registry. Ann Intern Med 1991;115: 343–9.

[130] Wislowska M, Sypula S, Kowalik I. Echocardiographic findings, 24-hour electrocardiographic Holter monitoring in patients with rheumatoid arthritis according to Steinbrocker's criteria, functional index, value of Waaler–Rose titre and duration of disease. Clin Rheumatol1998;17:369–77.

[131] Hurd ER. Extraarticular manifestations of rheumatoid arthritis. Sem Arthritis Rheum 1979;8:151–76.

[132] Voskuyl AE, Zwinderman AH, Westedt ML, Vandenbroucke JP, Breedveld FC, Hazes JMW. Factors associated with the development of vasculitis in rheumatoid arthritis: results of a case control study. Ann Rheum Dis 1996;55:190–92.

[133] Hara KS, Ballard DJ, Ilstrup DM, Connolly DC, Vollertsen RS. Rheumatoid pericarditis: clinical features and survival. Medicine 1990;69:81–91.

[134] Van der Heide A, Jacobs JW, Bijlsma JW, Heurkens AH, van Booma-Frankfort C, van der Veen MJ, Haanen HC, Hofman DM, van Albada-Kuipers GA, ter Borg EJ, Brus HL, Dinant HJ, Kruize AA, Schenk Y. The effectiveness of early treatment with sec-

ond line anti-rheumatic drugs; a randomized, controlled trial. Ann Int Med 1996;124:699–707.

[135] Voskuyl AE. The heart and cardiovascular manifestations in rheumatoid arthritis. Rheumatology (Oxford). 2006;45 Suppl 4:iv4-7.

[136] Douglas KMJ, Pace AV, Treharne GJ, Saratzis A, Nightingale P, Erb N, Banks MJ, Kitas GD. Excess recurrent cardiac events in rheumatoid arthritis patients with acute coronary syndrome. Ann Rheum Dis. 2006;65:348–53.

[137] Hurlimann D, Forster A, Noll G, Enseleit F, Chenevard R, Distler O, Béchir M, Spieker LE, Neidhart M, Michel BA, Gay RE, Lüscher TF, Gay S, Ruschitzka F. Anti-tumor necrosis factor-alpha treatment improves endothelial function in patients with rheumatoid arthritis. Circulation. 2002;22;106(17):2184-7.

[138] Park YB, Ahn CW, Choi HK, Lee SH, In BH, Lee HC, Nam CM, Lee SK. Atherosclerosis in rheumatoid arthritis: morphologic evidence obtained by carotid ultrasound. Arthritis Rheum. 2002;46(7):1714-9.

[139] Kumeda Y, Inaba M, Goto H, Nagata M, Henmi Y, Furumitsu Y, Ishimura E, Inui K, Yutani Y, Miki T, Shoji T, Nishizawa Y. Increased thickness of the arterial intima-media detected by ultrasonography in patients with rheumatoid arthritis. Arthritis Rheum. 2002;46(6):1489-97.

[140] Liu PP, Mason JW. Advances in the understanding of myocarditis. Circulation. 2001;104(9):1076-82.

[141] Puntmann VO, Taylor PC, Barr A, Schnackenburg B, Jahnke C, Paetsch I. Towards understanding the phenotypes of myocardial involvement in the presence of self-limiting and sustained systemic inflammation: a magnetic resonance imaging study. Rheumatology (Oxford). 2010r;49(3):528-35.

[142] Weber KT. Cardiac interstitium in health and disease: the fibrillar collagen network. J Am Coll Cardiol. 1989;13(7):1637-52.

[143] Sokka T. Radiographic Scoring in Rheumatoid Arthritis A Short Introduction to the Methods Bulletin of the NYU Hospital for Joint Diseases 2008;66(2):166-8

[144] Smolen JS, Landewe R, Breedveld FC, Dougados M, Emery P, Gaujoux-Viala C, Gorter S, Knevel R, Nam J, Schoels M, Aletaha D, Buch M, Gossec L, Huizinga T, Bijlsma JW, Burmester G, Combe B, Cutolo M, Gabay C, Gomez-Reino J, Kouloumas M, Kvien TK, Martin-Mola E, McInnes I, Pavelka K, van Riel P, Scholte M, Scott DL, Sokka T, Valesini G, van Vollenhoven R, Winthrop KL, Wong J, Zink A, van der Heijde D. EULAR recommendations for the management of rheumatoid arthritis with synthetic and biological disease-modifying antirheumatic drugs. Ann Rheum Dis. 2010;69(6):964-75.

[145] Courvoisier N, Dougados M, Cantagrel A, Goupille P, Meyer O, Sibilia J, Daures JP, Combe B. Prognostic Factors of 10-year Radiographic Outcome in Early Rheumatoid Arthritis: A Prospective Study. Arthritis Res Ther. 2008;10(5).

[146] Kremer JM, Lee JK: The safety and efficacy of the use of methotrexate in long-term therapy for rheumatoid arthritis. Arthritis Rheum 1986;29:822- 831.

[147] Ahmed SS, Arnett FC, Smith CA, Ahn C, Reveille JD. The HLA-DRB1*0401 allele and the development of methotrexate-induced accelerated rheumatoid nodulosis: a follow-up study of 79 Caucasian patients with rheumatoid arthritis. Medicine (Baltimore). 2001;80(4):271-8.

[148] Combe B, Guttierrez M, Anaya JM, Sany J. Possible efficacy of hydroxychloroquine on accelerated nodulosis during methotrexate therapy for rheumatoid arthritis. J Rheumatol 1999;20:755-756.

[149] Dash S, Seibold JR, Tiku ML. Successful treatment of methotrexate induced nodulosis with D-penicillamine. J Rheumatol 1999;26:1396-1369.

[150] Abraham Z, Rozenbaum M, Rosner I: Colchicine therapy for low-dosemethotrexate-induced accelerated nodulosis in rheumatoid arthritis patient. J Dermatol 1999;26:691-694.

[151] Chatham WW: Methotrexate associated rheumatoid nodulosis: Improvement with addition of sulfasalazine. Arthritis Rheum 1992;35:S148.

[152] Visser K, van der Heijde D. Optimal dosage and route of administration of methotrexate in rheumatoid arthritis: a systematic review of the literature. Ann Rheum Dis. 2009;68(7):1094-9.

[153] Paul P. Tak A Personalized Medicine Approach to Biologic Treatment of Rheumatoid Arthritis A Preliminary Treatment Algorithm 05/15/2012; Rheumatology. 2012;51(4): 600-609.

[154] Wiland P, Wojtala R, Goodacre J, Szechinski J. The prevalence of subclinical amyloidosis in Polish patients with rheumatoid arthritis. Clin Rheumatol. 2004, 23, 193–198.

[155] Bergesio F, Ciciani AM, Santostefano M, Brugnano R, Manganaro M, Palladini G, Di Palma AM, Gallo M, Tosi PL, Salvadori M; Immunopathology Group, Italian Society of Nephrology. Renal involvement in systemic amyloidosis--an Italian retrospective study on epidemiological and clinical data at diagnosis. Nephrol Dial Transplant. 2007;22(6):1608-18.

[156] Gillmore JD, Hawkins PN. Amyloidosis. In: Handbook of systemic autoimmune diseases. Eds: J.C. Mason, Ch.D. Pusey. Elsevier, New York 2008, 388–396.

[157] Kuroda T, Wada Y, Kobayashi D, Murakami S, Sakai T, Hirose S, Tanabe N, Saeki T, Nakano M, Narita I. Effective anti-TNF-alpha therapy can induce rapid resolution and sustained decrease of gastroduodenal mucosal amyloid deposits in reactive amyloidosis associated with rheumatoid arthritis. J Rheumatol. 2009;36(11):2409-15.

[158] Gottenberg JE, Merle-Vincent F, Bentaberry F, Allanore Y, Berenbaum F, Fautrel B, Combe B, Durbach A, Sibilia J, Dougados M, Mariette X. Anti-tumor necrosis factor alpha therapy in fifteen patients with AA amyloidosis secondary to inflammatory ar-

thritides: a followup report of tolerability and efficacy. Arthritis Rheum. 2003;48(7): 2019-24.

[159] Perry M.E., Stirling A., Hunter J.A. Effect of etanercept on serum amyloid A protein (SAA) levels in patients with AA amyloidosis complicating infl ammatory arthritis. Clin Rheumatol. 2008, 27, 923–925.

[160] Okuda Y, Takasugi K. Successful use of a humanized anti -interleukin -6 receptor antibody, tocilizumab to treat amyloid A amyloidosis complicating juvenile idiopathic arthritis. Arthritis Rheum. 2006, 54, 2997–3000.

[161] Sato H, Sakai T, Sugaya T, Otaki Y, Aoki K, Ishii K, Horizono H, Otani H, Abe A, Yamada N, Ishikawa H, Nakazono K, Murasawa A, Gejyo F. Tocilizumab dramatically ameliorated life-threatening diarrhea due to secondary amyloidosis associated with rheumatoid arthritis. Clin Rheumatol. 2009;28(9):1113-6.

[162] Hazenberg BP, Bijzet J, Limburg PC, Skinner M, Hawkins PN, Butrimiene I, Livneh A, Lesnyak O, Nasonov EL, Filipowicz-Sosnowska A, Gül A, Merlini G, Wiland P, Ozdogan H, Gorevic PD, Maïz HB, Benson MD, Direskeneli H, Kaarela K, Garceau D, Hauck W, Van Rijswijk MH. Diagnostic performance of amyloid A protein quantification in fat tissue of patients with clinical AA amyloidosis. Amyloid. 2007;14(2): 133-40.

[163] Raghu G, Depaso WJ, Cain K, Hammar SP, Wetzel CE, Dreis DF, Hutchinson J, Pardee NE, Winterbauer RH. Azathioprine combined with prednisone in the treatment of idiopathic pulmonary fibrosis: a prospective double-blind, randomized, placebo-controlled clinical trial. Am Rev Respir Dis. 1991;144(2):291-6.

[164] Antoniou KM, Mamoulaki M, Malagari K, Kritikos HD, Bouros D, Siafakas NM, Boumpas DT. Infliximab therapy in pulmonary fibrosis associated with collagen vascular disease. Clin Exp Rheumatol. 2007;25(1):23-8.

Chapter 8

Small Molecule DMARD Therapy and Its Position in RA Treatment

Hiroaki Matsuno

Additional information is available at the end of the chapter

http://dx.doi.org/10.5772/53320

1. Introduction

Small molecule disease-modifying antirheumatic drugs (DMARDs) played a central role in drug therapy for rheumatoid arthritis (RA) before biological preparations (biologics) came into extensive use for the treatment of this disease. Unlike non-steroidal anti-inflammatory drugs (NSAIDs) and steroids, which primarily alleviate the symptoms of RA such as pain and inflammation, DMARDs are known to suppress the progression of RA through their action against immunological abnormalities.

To review the history of the clinical positioning of DMARD therapy, until the beginning of the 1990s, DMARDs were used only in patients showing signs of disease progression (e.g., bone erosion) after NSAIDs or steroid treatment within the framework of pyramid therapy [1]. During the 1990s through the 2000s, the strategy and goals of RA therapy have undergone marked changes following the introduction of methotrexate (MTX) as another treatment option, the expansion of MTX as an anchor drug [2,3,4], endorsement of the usefulness of combined drug therapy involving DMARDs [5], the introduction of biologics into RA treatment [6,7,8], and other advances. In 2002, the American College of Rheumatology (ACR) released its Guidelines on RA Management, clearly indicating DMARDs as first-line drugs for the treatment of RA. As a result, NSAIDs and steroids came to be positioned as auxiliary means of treating RA [9].

The small molecule DMARDs that have been used frequently in Western countries are MTX, sulphasalazine (SASP), hydroxychloroquine (HCQ), leflunomide (LFN), and minocycline (MIN). In Japan, where the repertoire of drugs clinically available differs from that in Western countries, HCQ and MIN are not indicated for RA under the national health policy, and bucillamine (BUC) has been a more popular small molecule DMARD than these 2 drugs.

The use of biologics such as TNF inhibitors began to spread around the world within several years of their clinical introduction as drugs that exert rapid action and are expected to improve long-term prognosis and to allow patients with RA to maintain physical function [10]. During the 2000s, revisions of the guidelines on RA treatment and criteria for diagnosis of RA were accelerated in various countries, with the goal of treatment shifting from symptom control (anti-inflammatory analgesia) and delayed disease progression to achievement of disease remission and suppression of disease progression. As an accumulation of clinical trial data became available revealing from a long-term perspective the advantageous effects of biologics not found in small molecule DMARDs, including suppression of progression of bone destruction and physical dysfunction [11,12], biologics began to replace small molecule DMARDs, primarily in patients anticipated to have a poor prognosis and those with rapidly advancing disease. In addition, introduction of biologics into therapy at an early stage of active RA has been recommended in some guidelines because of the benefits expected from this kind of drug for maintaining long-term quality of life in many patients [13].

Nonetheless, there are still several open issues involved in the use of biologics, including:

1. presence of a considerable percentage of patients who fail to respond to treatment with biologics[14],
2. heavy economic burdens for individuals and the community due to high drug prices [15],
3. risk of serious adverse reactions (e.g., infection) in some patients [16,17], and so on.

These issues represent obstacles to the establishment of biologics as a predominant means of treatment for RA. In recent years, several reports have been published in the United States and Europe providing data intended to serve as evidence for the view that treatment with a combination of 3 small molecule DMARDs is expected to improve long-term prognosis of RA to an extent comparable with biologics. Following these reports, in Western countries, the guidelines/guidance on RA treatment have been further reviewed, resulting in restatement of the position that small molecule DMARDs are first-line drugs, and a clear statement that combination therapy with small molecule DMARDs should be tried before the therapy with biologics [18]. This chapter will describe the popular small molecule DMARDs currently used for treatment of RA and present a discussion regarding the current position of small molecule DMARDs in RA treatment guidelines/guidance, as well as its background. In addition, 2 new small molecule DMARDs, tofacitinib and iguratimod, are discussed.

2. Popular small molecule DMARDs

DMARDs is the collective term for a set of drugs known to suppress the progression of RA via action against immunological abnormalities. These drugs do not exhibit the rapid action on symptoms, i.e., inflammation and pain, exerted by NSAIDs and steroids.

DMARDs are additionally capable of delaying the progression of bone destruction, but it is rare that remission of RA can be achieved by DMARD mono-therapy in patients with established RA. DMARDs are generally slow in action, taking 1 to 3 months until manifestation of their effects. The response to these drugs varies greatly among individuals, and a number of patients fail to respond to treatment with DMARDs. Furthermore, patients whose disease activity is initially controlled by DMARDs sometimes cease to respond to the drugs (relapse) during prolonged use. Another characteristic of DMARDs is a high incidence of adverse reactions, with the incidence of adverse events with each DMARD being between 20% and 50%. If adverse reactions are mild, treatment with DAMARDs can be often continued by means of dose reduction or symptomatic treatment, but the risk that patients will develop life-threatening serious adverse reactions, including hematological disorders, renal disorder, and interstitial pneumonia, is common.

Some DMARDs are immune suppressors that are also used for control of host rejection of grafts and treatment of cancer, including MTX, LFN, tacrolimus (TAC), cyclosporine, azathioprine, and cyclophosphamide. The class also includes immune modulating agents, such as SASP, BUC, d-penicillamine, gold compound, and others, as well as HCQ, an anti-malaria agent, and MIN, an antibiotic (Table1).

Here, the popular DMARDs used clinically are described. BUC is approved as a DMARD for treatment of RA only in Japan and Korea, and currently, the use of BUC is almost exclusively confined to Japan, where this drug is still used in quantities as large as SASP, second to MTX among the approved DMARDs.

3. Methotrexate (MTX)

MTX is a folic acid antagonist. The drug has been reported to exert immunosuppressive activity through its action (suppression of proliferation) on immune competent cells by means of DNA synthesis inhibition, and to exert anti-inflammatory activity by inducing pooling of adenosine [19]. Details are unknown about the mechanism of its antirheumatic activity, but the drug has shown excellent efficacy and long duration, and it is the most frequently used small molecule DMARD in the world as an anchor drug for RA treatment [3,4]. The most recent guidelines recommend early initiation of treatment with MTX as a first-line drug in patients with factors associated with poor prognosis such as positive ACPA, bone erosion, extra-articular symptoms, or restricted physical function [18]. Among the antirheumatic drugs, MTX tends to exert its effects relatively early (within 1 to 2 months) and these effects include suppression of joint destruction [20,21].

Drug	Approximate time to benefit	Usual maintenance dose	Toxicities requiring monitoring
Hydroxychloroquine	2-6 months	200 mg twice a day	Macular damage
Sulfasalazine	1-3 months	1,000 mg 2-3 times a day	Myelosuppression
Methotrexate	1-2 months	Oral 7.5-20 mg/week; injectable 7.5-20mg/week	Myelosuppression, hepatic fibrosis, cirrhosis, pulmonary infiltrates or fibrosis
Leflunomide	4-12 weeks (skewed earlier)	20 mg/day in a single dose, if tolerated; otherwise, 10 mg/day	Diarrhea, alopecia, rash, headache, theoretical risk of immunosuppression infection
Bucillamine	1-3 months	100-200 mg a day	Myelosuppression, hepatotoxicity, proteinuria
Tacrolimus	6-12weeks	3 mg a day	Renal insufficiency, anemia, hypertension, Impaired glucose tolerance
Azathioprine	2-3 months	50-150 mg/day	Myelosuppression, hepatotoxicity, lymphoproliferative disorders
D-penicillamine	3-6 months	250-750 mg/day	Myelosuppression, proteinuria
Gold, oral	4-6 months	3 mg twice a day	Myelosuppression, proteinuria
Gold, intramuscular	3-6 months	25-50 mg intramuscularly every 2-4 weeks	Myelosuppression, proteinuria
Minocycline	1-3 months	100 mg twice a day	Hyperpigmentation, dizziness, vaginal yeast infections
Cyclosporine	6-12weeks	2.5-4 mg/kg/day	Renal insufficiency, anemia, hypertension, Impaired glucose tolerance

Table 1 summary of small molecule DMARDs

Adverse reactions to MTX include infection, stomatitis, glossitis, nausea, hepatic dysfunction [22], and others. It is known that these adverse reactions are more likely to appear in patients with compromised renal function and in elderly patients, and that they can be reduced by concomitant use of folic acid or leucovorin [23,24,25]. Interstitial pneumonia and bone marrow suppression are known as serious adverse reactions. Interstitial pneumonia can develop suddenly and is sometimes intractable [26]. Marrow suppression involves impaired hematopoiesis. Both of these reactions are serious and require hospitalization. As a rule, MTX is administered once weekly via an oral or parenteral route at an initial dose level of 7.5 to 15 mg, with the dose being gradually increased up to 25 mg/week if responses are insufficient. In Japan, MTX is only administered orally, at an initial dose level of 6 mg/week. The dose is gradually increased up to 16 mg if responses are insufficient. The weekly dose level may be divided into 1 to 3 doses in 1 or 2 days. It is known that the effects of MTX are strengthened by concomitant use of biologics [27].

4. Sulphasalazine (SASP)

This drug exerts action relatively rapidly (in 1 to 2 months) among the DMARDs. Like MTX, SASP has been reported to exert anti-inflammatory activity by inducing pooling of adenosine [28], and to have immunomodulating effects as well, e.g., suppression of antibody production [29]. The antirheumatic activity of SASP has not been sufficiently clarified, but because it suppresses joint destruction [20], it is considered as an option for treatment of RA with MTX. As compared to other DMARDs, SASP can be characterized by low nephrotoxicity, and the risk for teratogenicity in pregnant women is also considered to be lower with SASP than with other DMARDs. Adverse reactions to SASP include liver disorder, drug eruption, bone marrow disorders, and others. Because the incidence of gastrointestinal disorders as an adverse reaction is high with the bulk form of SASP, it is usually administered in the form of an enteric-coated tablet for the treatment of RA. In Western countries, this drug is usually recommended for treatment at a dose level of 2 to 3 mg/day, while in Japan, the upper limit of the dose level is set at 1 mg/day.

5. Leflunomide (LFN)

LFN is a metabolic antagonist capable of suppressing the proliferation of T lymphocytes through pyrimidine synthesis inhibition [20]. This drug has been reported to suppress joint destruction. It is characterized by the long half-life of its active form. Adverse reactions to LFN include infection, diarrhea, bone marrow disorders, hypertension, liver disorder, nausea, alopecia, and others. Interstitial pneumonia is an adverse reaction that requires utmost caution and is potentially fatal. LFN has been reported to be teratogenic [30,31]. For a couple planning pregnancy, it is necessary for both partners to take cholestyramine to eliminate the active metabolites of LFN completely. Because of the long the half-life of the active metabolite *in vivo*, the drug is administered at a loading dose level (100 mg) for the first 3 days, followed by administration at a constant dose level (20 mg/day).

6. Hydroxychloroquine (HCQ)

HCQ was used as an anti-malaria agent before it was used as an antirheumatic drug [32]. The anti-malaria activity of HCQ is considered to have no relationship to its antirheumatic activity. HCQ is believed to suppress antigen presentation by elevating the pH of the cytoplasmic compartment of antigen-presenting macrophages [33]. More recently, it was reported that HCQ acts on the toll-like receptor to manifest effects on the immune system [34]. The efficacy of HCQ is less than that of MTX, but HCQ has an excellent safety profile. For this reason, HCQ is used for the treatment of mild RA [35]. Uncombined HCQ treatment does not suppress the progression of bone destruction. Although the tolerability is high, adverse reactions such as nausea and dizziness occasionally appear. Furthermore, the drug has a high affinity for the retina and thus exerts high ocular toxicity. This is the reason that use of the drug is not approved in some countries. Although retinal disorders induced by HCQ are irreversible and if severe can lead to blindness, recovery from retinal disorders is sometimes possible if they are detected early. HCQ is also used occasionally for treatment of articular and skin symptoms of SLE. For the treatment of RA, the drug is administered at a dose of 400 mg/day.

7. Minocycline (MIN)

The US Food and Drug Administration (FDA) has not approved MIN for treatment of RA. However, a slow efficacy of this drug against RA has been shown in some double-blind trials [36,37,38,39]. Although the usefulness of this drug as a means of treatment for RA is low, it has evidenced effects at early stages of RA. Compounds of the tetracycline family are known to suppress matrix metalloproteinase [40], and this action is believed to suppress narrowing of the joint space in patients with RA. The activity of MIN as an antibiotic is considered to have no relationship to its antirheumatic activity.

8. Bucillamine (BUC)

BUC has been approved as a means of RA treatment in only Japan and Korea. As noted, at present, its use is almost exclusively confined to Japan. BUC is used as frequently as SASP in Japan, and this frequency of use is second to MTX. Its antirheumatic activity is slightly stronger, that is comparable to or higher than, that of SASP [41,42]. For this reason, BUC is used for treatment of mild to moderate RA. The pharmacologic actions that have been reported as likely to be involved in the drug's antirheumatic effects include suppression of cytokine production in the synoviocytes [43], suppression of antibody production from B-lymphocytes [44,45], and suppression of osteoclast differentiation [46]. According to a recent report, the effect of this drug in inhibiting Akt signals is involved in the suppression of antibody production from B-lymphocytes and the suppression of cytokine production by the synoviocytes [47,48]. Numerous adverse reactions including renal disorders and skin disorders are known, with serious adverse reactions including interstitial pneumonia and hematological disorders, and therefore patients must be watched closely. When used for the treatment of RA, BUC is administered at an initial dose of 100 mg/day, with a gradual increase up to 300 mg/day if efficacies are insufficient.

9. Tacrolimus (TAC)

TAC was initially sold as a drug for suppression host rejection of grafts. In 2005, its indication was expanded to encompass treatment of RA. The known effects of TAC include inhibition of the proliferation and differentiation of T lymphocytes involved in persistence of RA-associated inflammation and suppression of inflammatory cytokine production. The effect of this drug on RA is not strong when used as mono-therapy. It shows excellent efficacy when used as an additional drug in combination therapy for patients who have insufficient response to MTX alone [49]. In Western countries, this drug is not used frequently because the results of clinical trials of mono-therapy have been unsatisfactory, and the ACR has not advocated the use of TAC as a means of treating RA because of its insufficient efficacy [13]. Adverse reactions to TAC include headache, renal disorders, hyperglycemia, hyperuricemia, hypertension, and others. Since TAC is less likely to affect the respiratory system, it is occasionally used in patients who have respiratory complications. When used for the treatment of RA, this drug is usually administered at a dose of 3 mg/day, and at 1.5 mg/day in elderly patients.

10. Gold Compound

Two formulations of gold compound (injection and oral-dose preparations) are available. The efficacy and safety profiles partially differ between these 2 forms. Injection is performed intramuscularly once weekly at an initial dose of 50 mg/week, followed by maintenance dosing (once every 2 to 4 weeks). The response rate is relatively high, but effects are usually not evident until after 3 to 6 months. The frequency of discontinuation of treatment due to adverse reactions is high, with skin and mucosal disorders being the most frequent causes for discontinuation. Adequate monitoring for proteinuria and renal dysfunction is necessary, and care is also needed regarding hematological disorders, since leukopenia, thrombocytopenia, and hypoplastic anemia can develop following treatment with this drug. The oral-dose preparation is administered twice daily at a dose of 3 mg/dose. The efficacy of the oral-dose preparation is less than that of the injection and takes up to 9 months to appear. Adverse reactions to the oral-dose preparation are akin to those of the injection, although the incidence of renal and hematological disorders is slightly lower with the oral preparation.

11. Azathioprine

This drug is a purine analog and is shown to exert immunosuppressive effects by antimitotic action induced by inhibiting the synthesis of DNA and proteins. The efficacy of this drug against RA is comparable to that of other slow-acting drugs. Adverse reactions to azathioprine include gastrointestinal disorders, liver disease, leukopenia, and others.

12. Cyclosporine

Cyclosporine is an immune suppressor that is generally used as means of suppressing host rejection of grafts. This drug suppresses the production and physiological actions of interleukin-2 and lymphocyte growth factor, taking 6 to 12 weeks before manifestation of its efficacy against RA. Frequently observed adverse reactions to this drug include renal disorders, hypertension, gingival thickening, increased body hair, and others. Cyclosporine is recommended only for treatment of severe and advanced RA that has failed to respond to other drugs.

13. Cyclophosphamide

Cyclophosphamide is an alkylating agent with nonspecific cytotoxic activity. It suppresses the immune system by disturbing lymphocytes in a nonspecific manner. This dug has been positioned to play an important role in the treatment of SLE and vasculitis. It is rarely used for patients with RA because of strong adverse effects.

14. Changes in the position of small molecule DMARDs in the treatment of RA

According to the pyramid therapy [1] model that had been established by the beginning of the 1990s, RA treatment focused on alleviation of symptoms (pain, inflammation, etc.) with the use of NSAIDs and steroids at sufficiently high doses. Use of antirheumatic drugs was confined to cases with marked progression of bone erosion and other severe manifestations. It was noted that in cases requiring treatment by NSAIDs and steroids inflammation appeared to subside gradually by means of burnout over time. However, the RA itself remained unchanged and bone destruction continued to advance, accompanied by progression of joint dysfunction [50]. The primary drug therapy in those days played only the role of suppressing symptoms (i.e., pain and swelling), and it could not prevent progression of bone destruction, joint dysfunction, and other morbidity.

This situation changed dramatically during the period from the latter half of the 1990s to the 2000s. MTX had become clinically available for use in the treatment of RA in the 1980s to 1990s, and subsequently began to be used extensively as an anchor drug for the treatment of RA [2,3,4]. The term *anchor drug* refers to any drug used as a "protagonist" in the treatment of RA. In the management of RA, MTX was positioned as a drug whose necessity would be determined on the basis of the severity of the disease, and which would become indispensable in cases where the disease severity exceeded a certain level. After the mid-1990s, a series of data were published that provided new evidence of the efficacy of combined DMARD therapy (2 or 3 DMARDs) as compared to DMARD mono-therapy, stimulating active adoption of DMARD combination therapy. During this time, MTX also came to be positioned as a key drug in combination therapy, and to date, the prominence MTX as an anchor drug has not changed [5]. From the late 1990s to the 2000s, biologics, primarily TNF inhibitors, began to be introduced clinically as drugs expected to improve long-term prognosis and to maintain physical function [6,7,8], and by the 2000s, these events had led to an acceleration in some countries to revise existing treatment guidelines and diagnostic criteria for RA, which was accompanied by a shift of the focus of treatment from anti-inflammatory analgesia and delay of disease progression to achievement of disease remission and prevention of progression. The RA management guidelines that were published by the ACR in 2002 positioned DMARDs as first-line drugs for RA treatment, which were to be started within 3 months after disease onset, while positioning NSAIDs and steroids as auxiliary drugs for symptoms such as pain and inflammation [9]. These guidelines additionally recommended switching patients to different DMARDs if the initially prescribed DMARDs failed to exert sufficient efficacy within 3 months of the initiation of treatment. This guideline clearly positioned MTX as an anchor drug, allowing clinicians to acknowledge that a current framework of RA treatment had been decided at that time. It was also recommended by this guideline that biologics should be used in cases that were failing to respond well to treatment with DMARDs, including MTX. We may infer that in their early days, the clinical use of biologics was confined to intractable cases because this class of drug had not yet been evaluated in a sufficient number of cases (Figure 1).

During the period from the late 1990s to 2000s, as a series of new biologics were introduced and the clinical trial data on these drugs accumulated, it was suggested by some of these data that active use of biologics beginning soon after disease onset might be advantageous in some patients in terms of efficacy of long-term RA management, notably when focusing on the effects of biologics in suppressing progression of bone destruction and physical dysfunction, which were not seen with small molecule DMARDs [11,12]. In some patients, primarily those anticipated to have poor prognoses and those with rapidly progressive RA, biologics began to replace small molecule DMARDs. In 2008, noting this trend, the ACR made public a new recommendation on RA treatment that stated that the use of TNF inhibitors should be recommended as an option for first-line

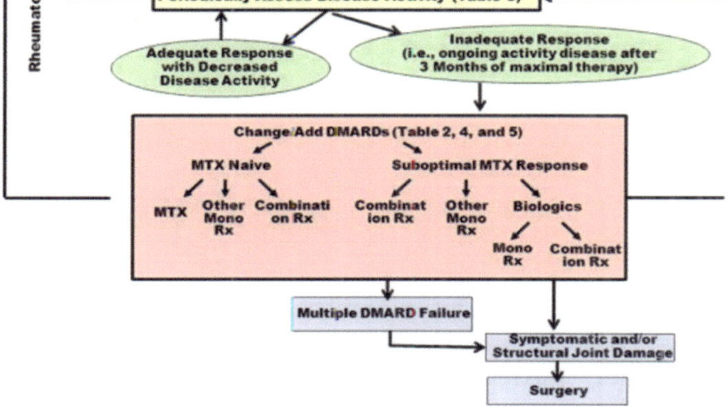

Figure 1. Guidelines for the management of rheumatoid arthritis: 2002 Update

medication for patients with high disease activity at 3 months to less than 6 months after disease onset, and patients with high disease activity and factors associated with poor prognosis at less than 3 months after disease onset [18] (Figure 2). Campaigns promoting a better long-term prognosis by earlier start of treatment with biologics based on these developments and bolstered by financial programs that assisted patients with out-of-pocket payments for biologics created stiff competition over biologics among manufacturers, and has reportedly promoted an increase in the quantity of biologics used for RA treatment. However, there are still many open issues surrounding biologics, including the high percentage of patients who fail to respond to biologics [14], the high price that causes large burdens on individuals and society [15], and the risk of serious adverse reactions such as infection [16,17]. The use of DMARDs, primarily in combination therapy, has also fallen under renewed scrutiny following publication of new studies. These events may stimulate further revision of the current guidelines/guidance on RA treatment.

Restriction of the use of biological preparations due to the necessity of out-of-pocket payment of their cost

Figure 3 illustrates the sales of 3 biological TNF antagonists per 100,000 populations in each country. It shows that biologics are used a lot in European countries such as Norway and Sweden. In these countries, patients are usually required to pay no money or only very small amounts (less than 1,000 yen) as out-of-pocket payment during each visit to a medical facility [10,51]. The consumption tax rate is high (about 20 to 30%) in these countries, and a large portion of the consumption tax collected is spent for social welfare, including medical expense. This is the reason why the out-of-pocket payment is small for patients in these countries.

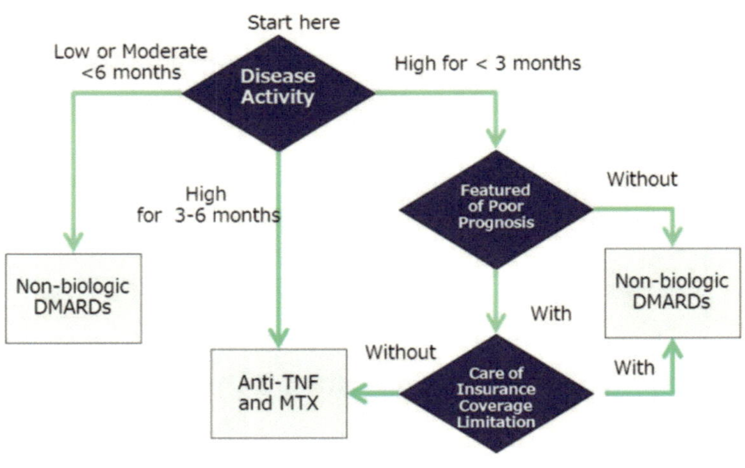

Figure 2. American College of Rheumatology 2008 recommendations on indications for the use of biologic Disease-modifying antirheumatic drugs in patients with RS <6 months

The United States, on the other hand, is the only developed country having no universal public health insurance. Excluding Medicare and Medicaid for elderly people, physically handicapped citizens and low-income families, healthcare in the United States depends on private sector insurance not mandatory for individual citizens. The premium for private health insurance is high, and a high percentage of uninsured people is often highlighted as a social problem in this country. For individuals covered by health insurance, the out-of pocket payment is not very large, although it varies depending on the insurance plan selected by individuals. Furthermore, unique campaigns by pharmaceutical companies are available in the United States, promoting the treatment with biologics. Under such campaigns, a majority of individual patient drug cost will be borne by the manufacturer to take over if the patients agree to treatment with specific drugs for a certain period of time and are registered with the treatment programs (RemiStart, Enbrel Support, My Humira, etc).

In Japan, however, annual out-of-pocket payment amounting to about 400,000 to 500,000 yen (about 5000 to 6500 dollars) is needed for many patients receiving treatment with biologics, excluding some patients covered by social welfare programs for reduction of out-of-pocket payment of healthcare expenses (specific physically handicapped individuals, individuals covered by poverty program, and so on). (Japan and Korea are the only countries belonging to the OECD where individuals covered by health insurance are required to make out-of-pocket payment to bear 30 % of health care costs.) This amount of out-of-pocket payment is about 25 times as large as the out-of-pocket payment needed for conventional DMARDs. There are patients who give up receiving treatment with biologics because they cannot afford to pay the expense [51].

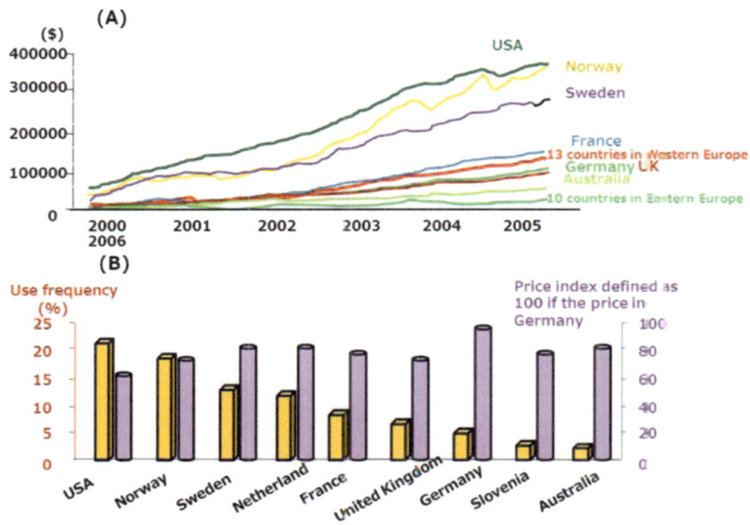

Figure 3. Sales of three biologics TNF antagonists per 100,000 population (A) and Price index and the percentage of patients using biologics TNF antagonist in the world in 2006 (B)

15. Current standard of care for RA

It has been shown that intervention with biologics at early stages of RA is expected to control the disease activity and suppress subsequent joint destruction, thus facilitating remission of RA, biologics free and cure [52]. However, according to the Best study [53], the long-term outcome of treatment differs little among different treatment strategies. It has thus been suggested to be more important to practice tight control through adjusting treatment flexibly depending on the disease activity in individual cases, instead of selecting biologics from the beginning (Figure 4).

In 2012, the ACR published the "2012 Update of the 2008 American College of Rheumatology Recommendations for the Use of Disease-Modifying Antirheumatic Drugs and Biologic Agents in the Treatment of Rheumatoid Arthritis," and recommended separate methods of treatment for patients at early stages of RA (less than 6 months after onset) and patients with established RA (6 months or more after onset) [18]. According to the revised guidelines, intervention with biologics is recommended for cases of established RA if the RA cannot be adequately controlled with recommended DMARD therapies (Figure 5). The guidelines also state that use of TNF inhibitors deserves to be considered even in patients with early stage RA if factors associated with poor prognosis are present and the disease activity is high, although it seems to be accepted that biologics have become a mode of treatment that is considered, as a rule, only in cases where the activity of RA cannot be controlled sufficiently by adequate treatment with small molecule DMARDs, including MTX.

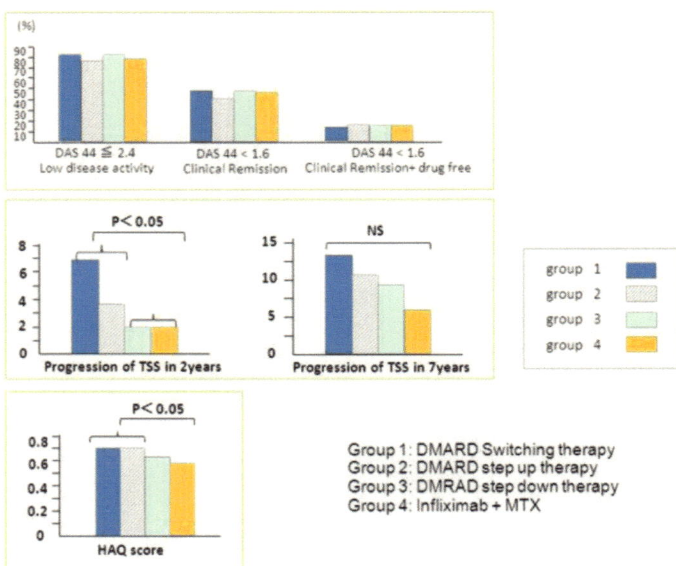

Figure 4. Seven year Results of DAS steered treatment in the BeSt Study: clinical and radiological outcome

http://dx.doi.org/10.5772/53320

Under the National Health Service (NHS) in the United Kingdom, in which prescription payments for individual patients are borne by the government, RA treatment is guided by the recommendations of the National Institute for Health and Clinical Excellence (NICE) [54]. The procedure for treatment under this system is more concrete than the ACR recommendations, and permits moving to therapy with biologics (anti-TNF preparations) or tocilizumab in cases that are poorly controlled despite attempts of treatment with DMARD combination therapy including MTX, even at the highest possible dose levels (Figure 6). However, permission for the use of these biologics under the British system requires that the manufactures bear any individual drug costs exceeding £9296 per year.

16. Comparison between small molecule DMARDs combination therapy and biologics plus MTX combination therapy

Regarding drug therapy at early stages of RA, the two-year data were recently reported on multicenter comparative clinical studies of three small molecule DMARDs combination therapy (MTX + SASP + HCQ) and biologics plus MTX combination therapy in the United States (TEAR study) [55] and Sweden (Swefot trial) [56]. In the TEAR study, the outcome as to DAS28-ESR did not differ between the oral triple therapy and the etanercept plus MTX combination therapy (first endpoint), and ACR20 and 50 was observed no difference between the two groups. The only significant difference was between two groups for ACR70 (Figure 7). In the

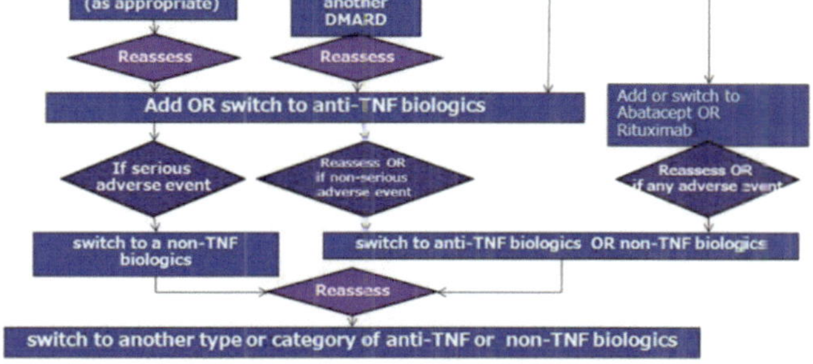

Figure 5. update of the 2008 American College of Rheumatology recommendations for the use of disease-modifying antirheumatic drugs and biologic agents in the treatment of rheumatoid arthritis.

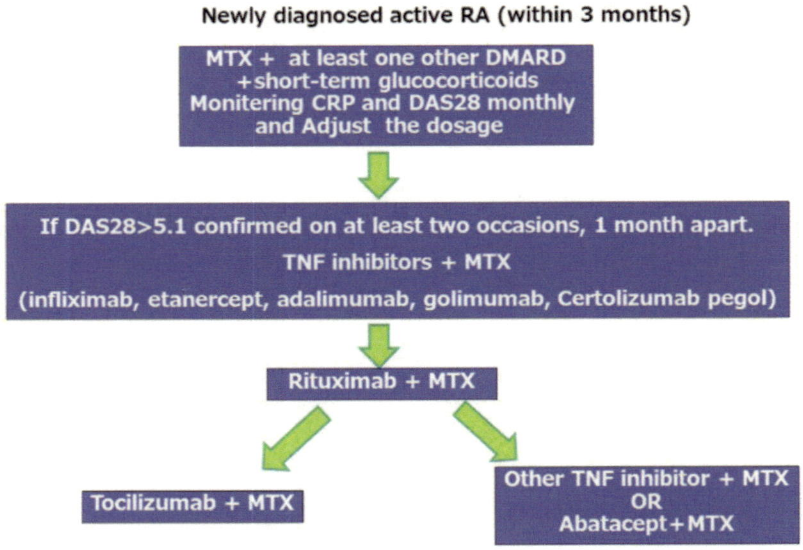

Figure 6. Summary of the management of rheumatoid arthritis in National Institute for Healt and Clinical Exellence guideline for rheumatoid arthritis

Swefot trial, there was no difference between the three small molecule DMARDs combination therapy group and the infliximab plus MTX combination therapy group in terms of ACR 20, 50 or 70 or EULAR good/moderate response. The TEAR study revealed no difference between the oral triple therapy group and the biologics plus MTX combination therapy group from the 12th month on after the start of treatment, while the Swefot trial disclosed higher efficacy of biologics plus MTX combination therapy during the first 6-12 months of treatment, followed by gradual disappearance of the inter-group difference during the two-year follow-up period. Also according to the long-term data from Best study conducted in the Netherlands [53], there was no significant difference in clinical improvement or the degree of bone/joint destruction on radiographic examination between Group 3 (treatment started with 3 drugs, MTX + SASP + steroid) and Group 4 (treatment started with biological preparations).

Regarding the degree of bone/joint destruction on radiographic examination, both TEAR study and Swefot trial demonstrated significant reduction in the biologics plus MTX combination therapy group, with the inter-group difference being 1-2 in terms of total Sharp Heijde score (full point: 448) of the mean progression of destruction per year relative to the baseline at the start of treatment. It might be thought that it is questionable to use the expensive biologics as the initial means of intervention into RA if only such slight suppression of bone/joint destruction on X-ray can be achieved.

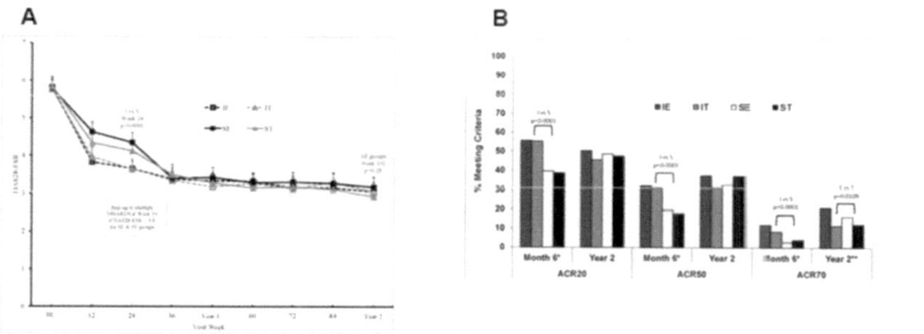

Figure 7. Results from the TEAR trial: oral triple Therapy vs. etanercept plus methotrexate in early RA (A): Observed DAS28-ESR,(B): Percentage of participants in TEAR achieving ACR20, 50, and 70 criteria at time of step-up at 6 months and at the 2 year conclusion of the study.

17. Three small molecule DMARD combination therapy in Japan (JaSTAR study)

The ACR recommendation and the NICE (U.K.) guidance state that the three DMARDs combination therapy should be applied before treatment with biologics [18,54]. In Japan, HCQ has not been approved for use in the treatment of RA because of adverse reactions. The three drug combined therapy (MRX + SASP + HCQ) is therefore not practically possible in Japan. We thus started a multicenter comparative clinical study on treatment of early stage RA with three small molecule DMARD combination therapy and biological TNF antagonists plus MTX combination therapy, involving nationwide 32 facilities of rheumatologist in Japan (JaSTAR study: Japan Strategic Treatment of Aggressive RA) [57].

The DMARDs used in the JaSTAR study were MTX, SASP and Bucillamine (Buc). Buc was used instead of HCQ for the following reasons:

1. Buc is a DMARD used frequently in Japan; and
2. this combination of three drugs with Recommendation Level "A" according to the Guidelines of the Ministry of Health, Labour and Welfare seemed to be appropriate for this study [41].

To date, case registration has been completed, achieving the targeting number (160 cases), and each patient enrolled to the study is now under follow-up. Interim analysis of the data during the first 6 months revealed a similar DAS28 remission rate between the three DMARDs combination therapy group and the biological TNF antagonists plus MTX combination therapy group (Figure 8). The treatment continuation rate among the 33 cases where one-year data have been analyzed was superior over the anti-TNF therapy continuation rate previously reported from the DANBIO registry [68] (Figure 9). We are looking forward to the results from final data analysis.

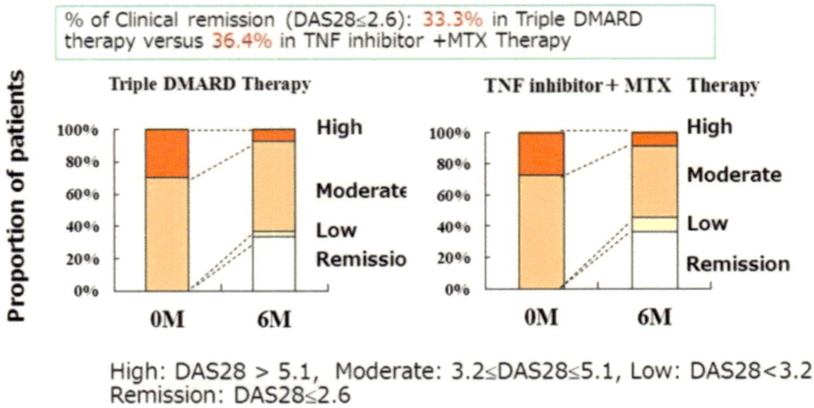

Figure 8. Distribution of disease activity of patients before and after treatment for 6 monts in JaSTAR Study

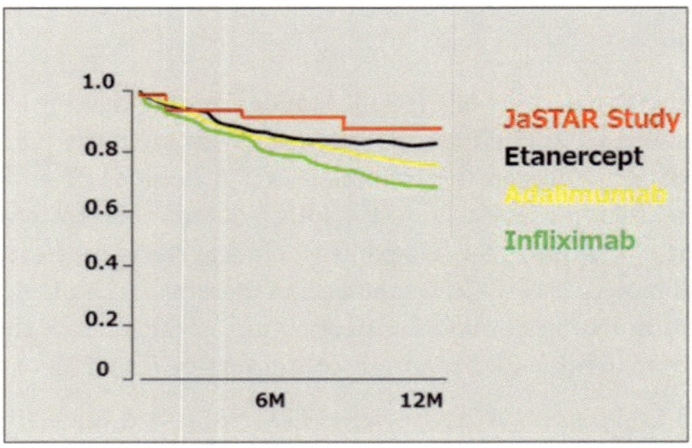

Figure 9. Cumulative continuation rate of triple DMARDs combination therapy in JaSTAR Stady, Cumulative continuation rate of TNF inhibitors in DANBIO study was superimposed.

18. Introduction of new small molecule DMARDs for RA treatment

It is known that among the drugs currently used for treatment of RA, those targeted at cytokines, all of which fall under the category of biologics, have yielded particularly favorable outcomes. However, unless the open issues mentioned above are resolved, it is unlikely that biologics will play a central role in the treatment of RA. In 2012 and 2013, there were 2 new DMARDs scheduled for introduction for RA treatment. One of them, tofacitinib, has been developed with attention focused on the role of cytokines in RA. If tofacitinib is shown in clinical practice to be a means of RA treatment possessing both the advantages of biologics and the advantages of small molecule DMARDs, it is expected that another paradigm shift will occur in RA management. The 2 new DMARDs are described in further detail below.

19. Tofacitinib

Tofacitinib has been developed as a drug for treatment of RA. It is shown to be an inhibitor of Janus kinase 3 (JAK3), an enzyme reported to be involved in cytokine receptor signal transduction. To date, tofacitinib has been experimentally shown to suppress all JAKs (1 through 3), rather than manifesting selective action against any particular JAK. Tofacitinib suppresses cytokines through inhibition of JAK-stat signals. In May 2012, the US FDA issued an approval recommendation for the use of this drug in adults with moderate or severe RA. According to the results of clinical trials, treatment with tofacitinib for 3 months achieved a semi-favorable (about 50%) ACR20 in patients who were responding poorly to TNF inhibitor treatment, with a placebo group achieving about 25%. Clinical trials have also been conducted for tofacitinib as a first-line drug, and in patients responding poorly to MTX, each yielding favorable outcomes. This drug is therefore reported to be promising not only as an additional option during biologic therapy but also as a first-line drug. Adverse reactions that require caution are elevations in blood cholesterol levels and neutrophilia.

20. Iguratimod

Iguratimod was formulated as a COX2 inhibitor and was later found to have immune modulating activity. It was thus developed as a DMARD. Iguratimod has been shown to be useful in combination with other drugs in patients failing to respond well to MTX. Elevation in liver enzymes is known as an adverse reaction.

21. Conclusion

As detailed herein, small molecule DMARDs have played a central role in treatment of RA since before the introduction of biologics, and it has been shown that modification of DMARD regimens (e.g., consideration of combination therapy beginning soon after disease onset) can improve the long-term prognosis, allowing small molecule DMARDs to serve as valid alternatives for biologics in RA treatment. While it is also known that treatment with biologics is useful in cases of high activity RA, even in these cases, there may be patients for whom combination therapy using existing DMARDs should be considered before introduction of biologics. Further changes in the paradigm of RA treatment are expected pending results of clinical use of new oral-dose small molecule DMARDs that have shown effects similar to both biologics and small molecule DMARDs.

Author details

Hiroaki Matsuno*

Address all correspondence to: info@toyama-ra.com

Matsuno Clinic for Rheumatic Diseases, USA

References

[1] Schenkier, S., & Golbus, J. (1992). Treatment of rheumatoid arthritis. New thoughts on the classic pyramid approach. Postgrad Med 289-92, 91(1), 285-6.

[2] Michael, E., Weinblatt, M. D., Jonathan, S., Coblyn, M. D., David, A., Fox, M. D., Patricia, A., Fraser, M. D., Donald, E., Holdsworth, M. D., David, N., Glass, M. B., Ch, B., David, E., & Trentham, M. D. (1985). Efficacy of Low-Dose Methotrexate in Rheumatoid Arthritis. *N Engl J Med*, 312, 818-822.

[3] Sokka, T., & Pincus, T. (2002). Contemporary disease modifying antirheumatic drugs (DMARD) in patients with recent onset rheumatoid arthritis in a US private practice: methotrexate as the anchor drug in 90% and new DMARD in 30% of patients. *Rheumatol*, 29(12), 2521-4.

[4] Pincus, T., Yazici, Y., Sokka, T., Aletaha, D., & Smolen, J. S. Methotrexate as the "anchor drug" for the treatment of early rheumatoid arthritis. *Clin Exp Rheumatol*, 21(5, 31), S179-85.

[5] O'Dell, J. R., Haire, C. E., Erikson, N., Drymalski, W., Palmer, W., Eckhoff, P. J., Garwood, V., Maloley, P., Klassen, L. W., Wees, S., Klein, H., & Moore, G. F. (1996). Treatment of rheumatoid arthritis with methotrexate alone, sulfasalazine and hydroxychloroquine, or a combination of all three medications. *N Engl J Med*, 334, 1287-91.

[6] Lipsky, P. E., van der Heijde, D. M., St, Clair. E. W., Furst, D. E., Breedveld, F. C., Kalden, J. R., Smolen, J. S., Weisman, M., Emery, P., Feldmann, M., Harriman, G. R., & Maini, RN. (2000). Anti-Tumor Necrosis Factor Trial in Rheumatoid Arthritis with Concomitant Therapy Study Group. Infliximab and methotrexate in the treatment of rheumatoid arthritis. Anti-Tumor Necrosis Factor Trial in Rheumatoid Arthritis with Concomitant Therapy Study Group. *N Engl J Med*, 343, 1594-602.

[7] Maini, R., St Clair, E. W., Breedveld, F., Furst, D., Kalden, J., Weisman, M., Smolen, J., Emery, P., Harriman, G., Feldmann, M., & Lipsky, P. (1999). Infliximab (chimeric anti-tumour necrosis factor alpha monoclonal antibody) versus placebo in rheumatoid arthritis patients receiving concomitant methotrexate: a randomised phase III trial. *ATTRACT Study Group. Lancet*, 354, 1932-9.

[8] Weinblatt, ME, Kremer, J. M., Bankhurst, A. D., Bulpitt, K. J., Fleischmann, R. M., Fox, R. I., Jackson, C. G., Lange, M., & Burge, D. J. (1999). A trial of etanercept, a recombinant tumor necrosis factor receptor:Fc fusion protein, in patients with rheumatoid arthritis receiving methotrexate. *N Engl J Med*, 340, 253-9.

[9] Guidelines for the management of rheumatoid arthritis:. American College of Rheumatology Subcommittee on Rheumatoid Arthritis Guidelines. Update., *Arthritis Rheum.*, 46(2), 328-46.

[10] Jönsson, B., Kobelt, G., & Smolen, J. (2008). The burden of rheumatoid arthritis and access to treatment: uptake of new therapies. *Eur J Health Econ*, 8(2), S61-86.

[11] van der Heijde, D., Klareskog, L., Rodriguez-Valverde, V., Codreanu, C., Bolosiu, H., Melo-Gomes, J., Tornero-Molina, J., Wajdula, J., Pedersen, R., Fatenejad, S., & TEMPO Study Investigators. Comparison of etanercept and methotrexate, alone and combined, in the treatment of rheumatoid arthritis: two-year clinical and radiographic results from the TEMPO study, a double-blind, randomized trial. 54, 1063-74.

[12] van der Heijde, D., Breedveld, F. C., Kavanaugh, A., Keystone, E. C., Landewé, R., Patra, K., & Pangan, A. L. (2010). Disease activity, physical function, and radiographic progression after longterm therapy with adalimumab plus methotrexate: 5-year results of PREMIER. *J Rheumatol*, 37, 2237-46.

[13] Saag, K. G., Teng, G. G., Patkar, N. M., Anuntiyo, J., Finney, C., Curtis, J. R., Paulus, H. E., Mudano, A., Pisu, M., Elkins-Melton, M., Outman, R., Allison, J. J., Suarez, Almazor. M., Bridges, S. L. Jr, Chatham, W. W., Hochberg, M., Mac Lean, C., Mikuls, T., Moreland, L. W., O'Dell, J., Turkiewicz, A. M., & Furst, D. E. (2008). American College of Rheumatology. American College of Rheumatology '08 recommendations for the use of nonbiologic and biologic disease-modifying antirheumatic drugs in rheumatoid arthritis. *Arthritis Rheum*, 59, 762-84.

[14] Finckh, A., Simard, J. F., Gabay, C., & Guerne, P.-A. (2012). for the SCQM physicians. Evidence for differential acquired drug resistance to anti-tumour necrosis factor agents in rheumatoid arthritis. *Rheumatology (Oxford)*, 51(5), 22-30.

[15] Michaud, K., Messer, J., Choi, H. K., & Wolfe, F. (2003). Direct medical costs and their predictors in patients with rheumatoid arthritis: a three-year study of 7,527 patients. *Arthritis Rheum*, 48, 2750-62.

[16] Dixon, W. G., Hyrich, K. L., Watson, K. D., Lunt, M., Galloway, J., & Ustianowski, A. (2010). BSRBR Control Centre Consortium, Symmons DP; BSR Biologics Register. Drug-specific risk of tuberculosis in patients with rheumatoid arthritis treated with anti-TNF therapy: results from the British Society for Rheumatology Biologics Register (BSRBR). *Ann Rheum Dis*, 69, 522-8.

[17] Furst, D. E. (2010). The risk of infections with biologic therapies for rheumatoid arthritis. *Semin Arthritis Rheum*, 39, 327-46.

[18] Singh, J. A., Furst, D. E., Bharat, A., Curtis, J. R., Kavanaugh, A. F., Kremer, J. M., Moreland, L. W., O'Dell, J., Winthrop, K. L., Beukelman, T., Bridges, S. L., Jr Chatham, W. W., Paulus, H. E., Suarez-Almazor, M., Bombardier, C., Dougados, M., Khanna, D., King, C. M., Leong, A. L., Matteson, E. L., Schousboe, J. T., Moynihan, E., Kolba, K. S., Jain, A., Volkmann, E. R., Agrawal, H., Bae, S., Mudano, AS, Patkar, N. M., & Saag, K. G. (2012). update of the 2008 American College of Rheumatology recommendations for the use of disease-modifying antirheumatic drugs and biologic agents in the treatment of rheumatoid arthritis. *Arthritis Care Res (Hoboken)*, 64, 625-39.

[19] Montesinos, M. C., Desai, A., & Cronstein, B. N. (2006). Suppression of inflammation by low-dose methotrexate is mediated by adenosine A2A receptor but not A3 receptor activation in thioglycollate-induced peritonitis. *Arthritis Res Ther*, 8, R53.

[20] Sharp, J. T., Strand, V., Leung, H., Hurley, F., & Loew-Friedrich, I. Treatment with leflunomide slows radiographic progression of rheumatoid arthritis: results from three randomized controlled trials of leflunomide in patients with active rheumatoid arthritis. *Leflunomide Rheumatoid Arthritis Investigators Group*, 43, 495-505.

[21] Kerstens, P. J., Boerbooms, A. M., Jeurissen de Graaf, ME R., Mulder, J., & van de Putte, L. B. (2000). Radiological and clinical results of longterm treatment of rheumatoid arthritis with methotrexate and azathioprine. *J Rheumatol*, 27, 1148-55.

[22] Kremer, J. M., Alarcón, G. S., Lightfoot, R. W., Jr Willkens, R. F., Furst, D. E., Williams, H. J., Dent, P. B., & Weinblatt, M. E. Methotrexate for rheumatoid arthritis. Suggested guidelines for monitoring liver toxicity. *American College of Rheumatology*, 37, 316-28.

[23] Morgan, S. L., Baggott, J. E., Vaughn, W. H., Austin, J. S., Veitch, T. A., Lee, J. Y., Koopman, W. J., Krumdieck, C. L., & Alarcón, G. S. (1994). Supplementation with folic acid during methotrexate therapy for rheumatoid arthritis. A double-blind, placebo-controlled trial. *Ann Intern Med*, 121, 833-41.

[24] Morgan, S. L., Baggott, J. E., Vaughn, W. H., Young, P. K., Austin, J. V., Krumdieck, C. L., & Alarcón, G. S. (1990). The effect of folic acid supplementation on the toxicity of low-dose methotrexate in patients with rheumatoid arthritis. *Arthritis Rheum*, 33, 9-18.

[25] Shiroky, J. B., Neville, C., Esdaile, J. M., Choquette, D., Zummer, M., Hazeltine, M., Bykerk, V., Kanji, M., St-Pierre, A., Robidoux, L., et al. (1993). Low-dose methotrexate with leucovorin (folinic acid) in the management of rheumatoid arthritis. Results of a multicenter randomized, double-blind, placebo-controlled trial. *Arthritis Rheum*, 36, 795-803.

[26] Alarcón, G. S., Kremer, J. M., Macaluso, M., Weinblatt, ME, Cannon, G. W., Palmer, W. R., St Clair, E. W., Sundy, J. S., Alexander, R. W., Smith, G. J., & Axiotis, CA. (1997). Risk factors for methotrexate-induced lung injury in patients with rheumatoid

arthritis. A multicenter, case-control study. Methotrexate-Lung Study Group. *Ann Intern Med*, 127, 356-64.

[27] Matsuno, H., Yoshida, K., Ochiai, A., & Okamoto, M. (2007). Requirement of methotrexate in combination with anti-tumor necrosis factor-alpha therapy for adequate suppression of osteoclastogenesis in rheumatoid arthritis. *Rheumatol*, 34, 2326-33.

[28] Morabito, L., Montesinos, M. C., Schreibman, D. M., Balter, L., Thompson, L. F., Resta, R., Carlin, G., Huie, MA, & Cronstein, B. N. (1998). Methotrexate and sulfasalazine promote adenosine release by a mechanism that requires ecto-5′-nucleotidase-mediated conversion of adenine nucleotides. *J Clin Invest*, 101, 295-300.

[29] Hirohata, S., Ohshima, N., Yanagida, T., & Aramaki, K. (2002). Regulation of human B cell function by sulfasalazine and its metabolites. *Int Immunopharmacol*, 2, 631-40.

[30] Chambers, C. D., Johnson, D. L., Robinson, L. K., Braddock, S. R., Xu, R., Lopez-Jimenez, J., Mirrasoul, N., Salas, E., Luo, Y. J., Jin, S., & Jones, K. L. (2010). Organization of Teratology Information Specialists Collaborative Research Group. Birth outcomes in women who have taken leflunomide during pregnancy. *Arthritis Rheum*, 62, 1494-503.

[31] Brent, R. L. Teratogen update: reproductive risks of leflunomide (Arava); a pyrimidine synthesis inhibitor: counseling women taking leflunomide before or during pregnancy and men taking leflunomide who are contemplating fathering a child. *Teratology*, 63(2), 106-12.

[32] Ben-Zvi, I., Kivity, S., Langevitz, P., & Shoenfeld, Y. (2012). Hydroxychloroquine: from malaria to autoimmunity. *Clin Rev Allergy Immunol*, 42, 145-53.

[33] Fox, R. I., & Kang, H. I. (1993). Mechanism of action of antimalarial drugs: inhibition of antigen processing and presentation. *Lupus*, 2(1), S9-12.

[34] Kyburz, D., Brentano, F., & Gay, S. (2006). Mode of action of hydroxychloroquine in RA-evidence of an inhibitory effect on toll-like receptor signaling. *Nat Clin Pract Rheumatol*, 2, 458-9.

[35] Tsakonas, E., Fitzgerald, A. A., Fitzcharles, M. A., Cividino, A., Thorne, J. C., M'Seffar, A., Joseph, L., Bombardier, C., & Esdaile, J. M. (2000). Consequences of delayed therapy with second-line agents in rheumatoid arthritis: a 3 year followup on the hydroxychloroquine in early rheumatoid arthritis (HERA) study. *J Rheumatol*, 27, 623-9.

[36] O'Dell, J. R., Blakely, K. W., Mallek, J. A., Eckhoff, P. J., Leff, R. D., Wees, S. J., Sems, K. M., Fernandez, A. M., Palmer, W. R., Klassen, L. W., Paulsen, G. A., Haire, C. E., & Moore, G. F. (2001). Treatment of early seropositive rheumatoid arthritis: a two-year, double-blind comparison of minocycline and hydroxychloroquine. *Arthritis Rheum*, 44, 235-41.

[37] O'Dell, J. R., Paulsen, G., Haire, CE, Blakely, K., Palmer, W., Wees, S., Eckhoff, P. J., Klassen, L. W., Churchill, M., Doud, D., Weaver, A., & Moore, G. F. (1999). Treatment

of early seropositive rheumatoid arthritis with minocycline: four-year followup of a double-blind, placebo-controlled trial. *Arthritis Rheum*, 42, 1691-5.

[38] Tilley, B. C., Alarcón, G. S., Heyse, S. P., Trentham, D. E., Neuner, R., Kaplan, D. A., Clegg, DO, Leisen, J. C., Buckley, L., Cooper, S. M., Duncan, H., Pillemer, S. R., Tuttleman, M., & Fowler, S. E. Minocycline in rheumatoid arthritis A 48-week, double-blind, placebo-controlled trial. *MIRA Trial Group*, 122, 81-9.

[39] Kloppenburg, M., Breedveld, F. C., Terwiel, J. P., Mallee, C., & Dijkmans, BA. (1994). Minocycline in active rheumatoid arthritis. A double-blind, placebo-controlled trial. *Arthritis Rheum*, 37, 629-36.

[40] Federici, T. J. (2011). The non-antibiotic properties of tetracyclines: clinical potential in ophthalmic disease. *Pharmacol Res*, 64, 614-23.

[41] Mimori, T. (2004). Anti-rheumatic drugs. *In: Ochi T, Yamamoto K, Ryuu. J, editors. Manual of diagnosis and guideline for treatment of RA. Tokyo: Japanese rheumatism foundation*, 84-98, in Japanese.

[42] Ichikawa, Y., Saito, T., Yamanaka, H., Akizuki, M., Kondo, H., Kobayashi, S., et al. (2005). Therapeutic effects of the combination of methotrexate and bucillamine in early rheumatoid arthritis: a multicenter, double-blind, randomized controlled study. *Mod Rheumatol*, 15, 323-8.

[43] Matsuno, H., Sugiyama, E., Muraguchi, A., Nezuka, T., Kubo, T., Matsuura, K., & Tsuji, H. (1998). Pharmacological effects of SA96 (bucillamine) and its metabolites as immunomodulating drugs--the disulfide structure of SA-96 metabolites plays a critical role in the pharmacological action of the drug. *Int J Immunopharmacol*, 20, 295-304.

[44] Hirohata, S., & Lipsky, P. E. (1994). Comparative inhibitory effects of bucillamine and D-penicillamine on the function of human B cells and T cells. *Arthritis Rheum*, 37, 942-50.

[45] Hirohata, S., & Lipsky, P. E. (1993). Regulation of B cell function by bucillamine, a novel disease-modifying antirheumatic drug. *Clin Immunol Immunopathol*, 66, 43-51.

[46] Suematsu, A., Tajiri, Y., Nakashima, T., Taka, J., Ochi, S., Oda, H., Nakamura, K., Tanaka, S., & Takayanagi, H. (2007). Scientific basis for the efficacy of combined use of antirheumatic drugs against bone destruction in rheumatoid arthritis. *Mod Rheumatol*, 17(1), 17-23.

[47] Tsuji, F., Seki, I., Aono, H., Odani, N., Mizutani, K., Okamoto, M., & Sasano, M. (2007). Bucillamine mechanism inhibiting IL-1beta-induced VEGF production from fibroblast-like synoviocytes. *Int Immunopharmacol*, 7, 1569-76.

[48] Tsuji, F., Setoguchi, C., Okamoto, M., Seki, I., Sasano, M., & Aono, H. (2012). Bucillamine inhibits CD40-mediated Akt activation and antibody production in mouse B-cell lymphoma. *Int Immunopharmacol*, 14, 47-53.

[49] Kawai, S., Takeuchi, T., Yamamoto, K., Tanaka, Y., & Miyasaka, N. (2011). Efficacy and safety of additional use of tacrolimus in patients with early rheumatoid arthritis

with inadequate response to DMARDs--a multicenter, double-blind, parallel-group trial. *Mod Rheumatol*, 21, 458-68.

[50] Kirwan, J. R. (1999). Conceptual issues in scoring radiographic progression in rheumatoid arthritis. *J Rheumatol*, 26, 720-5.

[51] Matsuno, H. (2010). Medical economy. *In:Abe C, Kondo M, Matsubara T, Yasaki K The manual of rheumatoid arthritis therapy with biologics. Tokyo:NIHON IGAKUKAN*, 200-209.

[52] van der Bijl, A.E., et al. (2007). Infliximab and methotrexate as induction therapy in patients with early rheumatoid arthritis. *Arthritis Rheum*, 56(7), 2129-34.

[53] van den Broek, M., Dirven, L., Klarenbeek, N. B., Molenaar, T. H., Han, K. H., Kerstens, P. J., Huizinga, T. W., Dijkmans, BA, & Allaart, C. F. (2012). The association of treatment response and joint damage with ACPA-status in recent-onset RA: a subanalysis of the 8-year follow-up of the BeSt study. *Ann Rheum Dis*, 71(2), 245-8.

[54] Chiu, Y., Ostor, A. J., Hammond, A., Sokoll, K., Anderson, M., Buch, M., Ehrenstein, M. R., Gordon, P., Steer, S., & Bruce, I. N. (2012). Access to the next wave of biologic therapies (Abatacept and Tocilizumab) for the treatment of rheumatoid arthritis in England and Wales : Addressing treatment outside the current NICE guidance. *Clin Rheumatol*, 10.1007/s10067-011-1936-6.

[55] Moreland, L. W., O'Dell, J. R., Paulus, H. E., Curtis, J. R., Bathon, J. M., William, St., Clair, E., Louis, Bridges. S., Jr Zhang, J., Mc Vie, T., Howard, G., van der Heijde, D., & Cofield, S. S. for the TEAR Investigators. A randomized comparative effectiveness study of oral triple therapy versus etanercept plus methotrexate in early, aggressive rheumatoid arthritis. *Arthritis Rheum*, 10.1002/art.34498.

[56] van Vollenhoven, R. F., Geborek, P., Forslind, K., Albertsson, K., Ernestam, S., Petersson, I. F., Chatzidionysiou, K., & Bratt, J. Swefot study group. Conventional combination treatment versus biological treatment in methotrexate-refractory early rheumatoid arthritis: 2 year follow-up of the randomised, non-blinded, parallel-group Swefot trial. *Lancet*, 379(9827), 1712-20.

[57] Matsuno, H. (2011). Directions in pharmacotherapy desired by patients with rheumatoid arthritis-When to use traditional disease modifying antirheumatic drugs versus biological agents-. *Clin Rheumatol*, 23(4), 356-364.

[58] Hetland, M. L., Christensen, I. J., Tarp, U., Dreyer, L., Hansen, A., Hansen, I. T., Kollerup, G., Linde, L., Lindegaard, H. M., Poulsen, U. E., Schlemmer, A., Jensen, D. V., Jensen, S., Hostenkamp, G., & Ostergaard, M. (2010). All Departments of Rheumatology in Denmark. Direct comparison of treatment responses, remission rates, and drug adherence in patients with rheumatoid arthritis treated with adalimumab, etanercept, or infliximab: results from eight years of surveillance of clinical practice in the nationwide Danish DANBIO registry. *Arthritis Rheum*, 62(1), 22-32.

Chapter 9

Gas-Therapy in Rheumatoid Arthritis Treatment: When West Meets East – Actual Medical Concepts with Ancient World Ideas

Michal Gajewski, Slawomir Maslinski,
Przemyslaw Rzodkiewicz and
Elzbieta Wojtecka-Lukasik

Additional information is available at the end of the chapter

http://dx.doi.org/10.5772/54506

1. Introduction

The significant number of rheumatoid arthritis (RA) patients do not respond to the typical treatment. To develop new anti-inflammatory therapies, studies on identification of new pathways involved in modulation of inflammation are still conducted. Inflammation is a local, protective response to injury and pathogen invasion. Following tissue damage manifests clinically by swelling, pain, redness and heat. Relations between the processes which enhance or suppress the inflammatory response are subject of precise regulation. Disorders of this delicate balance between proinflammatory and anti-inflammatory agents may even lead to necrosis or tissue damage. Too weak response to the agent that causes inflammation and may effect in immunodeficiency and on the other hand, too intense inflammatory response, causes the tissue damage such as occurs for example in RA. Regulation of inflammation by anti-inflammatory processes is an important condition for maintaining health and homeostasis [1,2].

The acute inflammatory process lasts from minutes to days. Its development depends on hemodynamic alterations, mechanisms of specific leukocyte-endothelial adhesive interactions, chemotaxis, and leukocyte activation and phagocytosis. These steps are regulated on humoral way by variety of soluble inflammatory mediators (eg. cytokines, histamine, NO, prostaglandins etc.) produced both by stationary cells (eg. fibroblasts, mast cells etc.) and circulating cells (lymphocytes, neutrophils etc.). Inflammatory reaction can be also regulated by neural signaling. In contrast to humoral regulation neural control is short-lived: after a brief refractory period, responding cells can resume function as required in the absence of further neural input. Recovery of immune function after transient inhibition enables necessary local inflammatory responses to be mobilized during persisting threat or infection [1,2]. Neural regulation of discrete, distributed, localized inflammatory sites provides a mechanism for integrating responses in real time. In RA patients imbalance between an overly active adrenergic nervous system (ANS) and reduced cholinergic neural system (CHNS) activity is observed [3]. ANS stimulation results in bringing the body to a state of raised activity and attention, usually called the *fight or flight* response. In contrast, stimulation of the cholinergic nervous system (CHNS) can be summarized as the *rest and digest* response, as this returns the body functions back to normal. Idea of manipulation of the autonomic nervous system (adrenergic and cholinergic) could be interesting approach in RA treatment [4].

2. Cholinergic neural system

The CHNS consists mainly (75%) of the vagus nerve, which is the largest nerve and owes its name because of the wandering course along the body [5]. CHNS, through the vagus nerve, plays an important role in regulation of inflammation. Main neurotransmitter of CHNS is acetylocholine (ACh). ACh acts through two, widely expressed types of receptors - the muscarinic (mAChR) and the nicotinic (nAChR) receptors. The ACh receptors are found not only on neurons, but also are widely expressed on other non-neural cells such as endothelial cells (EC), monocytes, macrophages, T and B lymphocytes, dendritic cells and neutrophils, which can act in an autocrine / paracrine way, modifying immune responses [1,2]. There is no neuroanatomical evidence for parasympathetic or vagal nerve innervations of any immune organs but ACh can be also locally expressed and released from splenic immune cells [6]. ACh is detectable in blood of several animal species [7]. In humans, the mean concentration of ACh in plasma is approximately 3 nmol L-1 (or 456 pg mL-1, range 151–1312 pg mL-1). Sixty per cent of the total ACh in human blood is contained in mononuclear leukocytes and the rest is found in plasma [8]. The nonneuronal cells that can produce ACh are for example: epithelial, endothelial, mesothelial, muscle cells and immune cells. Release of ACh from these sources is regarded as nerve-independent, which raises the possibility of immune cell-derived cholinergic activity that can modulate inflammation. These cells possess also all functional components of the cholinergic system and the cholinergic signaling in these cells is comparable to regular neurotransmission, this could be relevant in inflammatory conditions occurring with decreased activity of the vagus nerve [1,2,4].

3. Cholinergic anti-inflammatory pathway

Identification of 'cholinergic anti-inflammatory pathway' which is neural mechanism that deactivates macrophages through parasympathetic outflow changed our understanding of the mechanisms that regulate inflammation. It was shown that experimental activation of the cholinergic anti-inflammatory pathway by direct electrical stimulation of the efferent vagus nerve inhibits the synthesis of TNF in liver, spleen and heart, and attenuates serum concentrations of TNF during endotoxaemia [9,10]. Vagotomy significantly exacerbates TNF responses to inflammatory stimuli and sensitizes animals to the lethal effects of endotoxin. This connection between the nervous and immune systems functions as an anti-inflammatory mechanism and is observed also in other models of inflammation [1].

Human macrophages exposed to ACh inhibit release of TNF-α, IL-1β, IL-6, primarily through nAChRs; contrary to that, production of the anti-inflammatory cytokine IL-10 was unaffected [4]. It was observed that exposure of human macrophages, but not peripheral blood monocytes, to nicotine or ACh inhibits the release of TNF, IL-1 and IL-18 but not anti inflammatory IL-10, in response to endotoxin. Because tissue macrophages are responsible for production of most of the TNF that appears during an excessive inflammatory response, it may be concluded that a nicotinic, α-bungarotoxin sensitive macrophage ACh receptor is responsible for connection between the cholinergic nervous system and the innate immune system [11]. Because ACh is produced also by nonneural cells such as epithelial cells, T lymphocytes and EC, inflammatory response can be modulated by these cells [1,2,4].

4. Reflex inhibition of inflammation

The presence of pathogens in the body activates inflammatory response. Innate immune cells release number of cytokines regulating development of the process. Inflammatory process activates sensory fibres that ascend in the vagus nerve to synapse in the nucleus tractus solitaries [1]. Increased efferent signals in the vagus nerve suppress peripheral cytokine release through macrophage nicotinic receptors and the cholinergic anti-inflammatory pathway[1,2]. The inflammation-sensing and inflammation-suppressing functions provide the principal components of the inflammatory reflex. The 'inflammatory reflex' is described as localized, rapid and discrete response. It can also induce systemic humoral anti-inflammatory responses. This occurs because vagus nerve activity can be relayed to the medullary reticular formation, to the locus ceruleus and to the hypothalamus, leading to increased release of corticotrophin from the anterior pituitary gland [2,4].

Increased cytokine production in tissues causes pain, providing another mechanism for transferring information from the immune system[1]. Neural regulation of discrete, distributed, localized inflammatory sites provides a mechanism for integrating responses in real time, moreover, Tracey suggest that the cholinergic anti-inflammatory pathway might also modulate processing events that promote neural memory of the peri-inflammatory events (that is, the 'hissing snake' or 'charging lion' that caused the wound and/or infection) [1].

5. Dysregulation of autonomic nervous system in rheumatoid arthritis

Both ANS and CHNS are important actors in maintaining immune homeostasis. Inflammatory mediators signal to the brain via the circulation or via afferent fibers of the vagus nerve.

Result of this action is activation of the ANS and/or CHNS. Tracey suggested that the tonic activity of the vagus nerve is crutial to maintain immune homeostasis [2]. Efferent ANS and vagal nerve fibers induce local catecholamine and ACh production by neurons or nonneuronal cells. Impairment of this activity could lead to unrestrained cytokine responses and damage to the host [4].

The way in which autonomic nervous synthesis is dysregulated is still unknown. It seems likely that it may by result of increase in ANS activity (for example, stress). Pain and stress can activate the flight-or-fight responses. Because of resultant increase of adrenaline and noradrenaline, macrophages activation is inhibited and synthesis of TNF and other proinflammatory cytokines decreases [12]. Result of this response is also increased release of IL-10, which is an important anti-inflammatory cytokine from monocytes [13]. Flight-or-fight activation of sympathetic responses also stimulates increased vagus nerve output. The combined action of these neural systems is significantly anti-inflammatory through both local (neural) and systemic (humoral) anti-inflammatory mechanisms [1].

Usually actions of the sympathetic and parasympathetic nervous systems are in opposition. But in some situations the two systems function synergistically. For example, simultaneous stimulation of both sympathetic and vagus nerves produces a higher increase in cardiac output than does isolated stimulation of either nerve alone [14]. Similar situation is observed in RA - autonomic dysfunction in RA patients is characterized by an increased overall sympathetic tone and decreased activity of the vagus nerve [4]. It seems probable that the autonomic imbalance observed in experimental arthritis and RA patients is at least partially responsible for sustaining the inflammatory status [4]. Imbalance between ANS and CHNS observed in RA may effect in induction and/or persistence of the inflammation [3,15,16]. Low tone of the vagus nerve means low activity of the cholinergic anti-inflammatory pathway, which results in higher cytokine levels, thereby contributing to this proinflammatory status [4].

6. Cytokine disease theory

For nearly 1,500 years, the dominant medical doctrine of the occurrence of disease was the humoral theory of disease, whose founder was Galen. The theory assumed that disease was due to an imbalance of bodily fluids (called "humors"). Produced by internal organs, humors maintain health, until their level are properly regulated and balanced [17].

Contemporary cytokine theory of disease, similarly to humoral theory of disease assumes that cytokines produced by the immune system are somehow the equivalent of "humors," and may themselves cause not only symptoms of disease, but also the damage characteristic to diseases. For example, the presence of a single cytokine, TNF which is completely sufficient to cause lethal septic shock analogous to a serious infection caused by Gram-negative bacteria. Administration of TNF to healthy mammals makes exactly the same changes in metabolism, such as immune response or pathological manifestations of the disease, as in the case of bacterial infection [17]. It has been suggested that some diseases can be developed as a simple result of the presence of abnormal amounts of cytokines. This discovery opened a new field of research on the physiological control mechanisms that maintain health by restraining or counterregulating cytokine release. As was shown by Kokkonen [18] blood samples obtained from individuals before the onset of symptoms of RA have elevated concentrations of proinflammatory cytokines, cytokine-related factors and chemokines, indicating activation of the immune system. Observed in this study activation, occurred before any symptoms of joint involvement. These findings present an opportunity for better predicting the risk of developing RA and, therefore, possibly preventing disease progression [18]. In the case of RA, the typical symptoms may be caused merely by exposure to TNF or IL-1. The success of drug therapy specifically blocking TNF in patients with RA clearly show the fundamental role of this cytokine in the course of inflammation, validateing fundamental premise of the cytokine theory of disease. Anti-TNF and anti–IL-1–based therapeutics are currently widely used in doses that reduce cytokine activity to levels compatible with health without causing significant immunosuppression. Today, it seems that ancient Greek concepts were not far off, since our modern theories about disease causation implicate an imbalanced production of body substances [17].

7. Ancient medical concepts and modern clinical problem

The balance between the activity of the vagus nerve, and the cholinergic anti-inflammatory pathway in modulating the activity of the inflammatory response seems to be the guarantor of the proper course of inflammation. It is possible that a permanent dysfunction of the vagus nerve, and thus distortion of the inflammatory reflex may contribute to the emergence of diseases characterized by chronic inflammation such as RA. The therapeutic approach based on direct stimulation of the vagus nerve has already been used to treat epilepsy. Also, hypnosis or meditation can significantly affect the transmission of stimuli through the vagus nerve and inhibit immediate and delayed type hypersensitivity [19]. It should now be possible to determine clinically whether these or other approaches activate the cholinergic anti-inflammatory pathway [1,2,4].

Early clinical observations suggested that cigarette smoking might be beneficial to patients with ulcerative colitis. Randomized clinical trials of nicotine administration demonstrated significant benefit in a subset of patients [20]. Nicotine inhibits cytokine production via an nAChR-dependent mechanism makes it plausible to consider whether this pathway is activated in the subset of patients that derive benefit from nicotine. Cigarette smoking confers some increased risk of the development of RA but is protective against osteoarthritis [21]. Cholinergic deficiency and decreased vagus nerve activity characterize Alzheimer disease and other brain degenerative disorders. Peripheral immune responses can be modulated by cholinergic agonists used in treatment of Alzheimer disease through activation of the cholinergic anti-inflammatory pathway [1,17].

Physical exercises reduces synthesis of TNF and other cytokines. It is widely known that physical activity reduces risk of cardiovascular disease, type 2 diabetes and atherosclerosis

[22]. This observation is at least partially connected with increased vagus nerve activity and increased in cholinergic anti-inflammatory pathway activity. Obesity, on the other hand, is characterized by diminished vagus nerve output and elevated cytokine levels, which have been implicated in mediating insulin resistance and atherosclerosis [22]. Since weight loss and exercise are each associated with increasing vagus nerve activity. One can consider whether enhanced activity in the cholinergic anti-inflammatory pathway might decrease cytokine production and reduce the damage and metabolic derangements mediated by chronic, low-grade systemic inflammation that is characteristic of the metabolic syndrome [1].

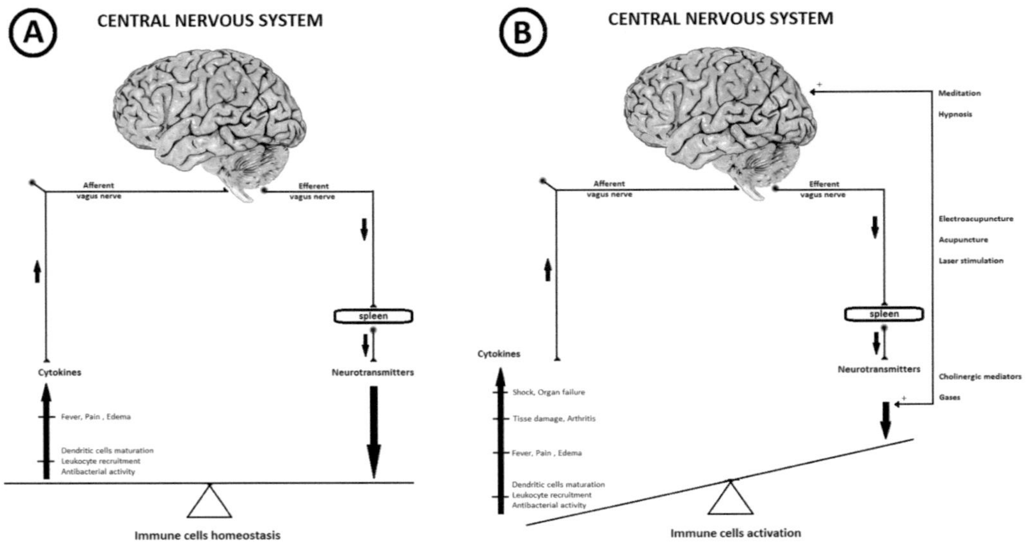

Figure 1. The therapeutic approach based on direct stimulation of the vagus nerve. A) At health cytokine production is balanced: low levels are required to maintain homeostasis. B) Overproduction of some cytokines causes diseases for example arthritis. Humoral and neural regulatory pathways regulate the magnitude of the inflammatory response. Cytokines released at the inflammatory site activate afferent fibres of the vagus nerve and reach the nucleus tractus solitarius in the brain stem. Compensatory signals are conveyed by the efferent vagus nerve and reach the site of inflammation where neurotransmitters act upon macrophages and other cells of the immune system to attenuate the inflammatory response. Hypnosis, meditation, acupuncture, electroacupncture or laser stimulation can affect the transmission of stimuli through the vagus nerve and inhibit immediate and delayed type hypersensitivity. Complex interactions between vagus nerve modulation, acupuncture, cholinergic neurotransmitters, "biological gases" and redox status of inflammatory cells, involved in joint tissue damage, might be useful for the development of novel therapeutic strategies for RA.

One of the fundamental premises of the ancient Greeks was that dietary manipulation controlled humoral balances. This concept is now, at least in principle, supported by new evidence of a direct link between dietary composition and the regulation of cytokines by the cholinergic anti-inflammatory pathway [1]. In the folk medicine we see examples of diet, modulating the immune system functioning. For example, a diet rich in fats derived from fish may increase parasympathetic activity affecting the inhibition of synthesis of proinflammatory cytokines such as TNF-α, IL-1β, IL-2, IL-6 and IL-18. At the same time increased production of antiinflammatory IL-10 is observed. It has long been suspected that the presence of large amounts of fatty acids derived from fish may explain the reduced incidence of heart disease in Eskimos and Japanese [23]. Now, we understand that this is due to the increased activity of the cholinergic system. Suggested mechanisms for this cardio-protective effect focused on the effects of n-3 fatty acids on eicosanoid metabolism or inflammation, beta oxidation; but, none of these mechanisms could adequately explain the beneficial actions of n-3 fatty acids [23].

Contemporary clinical studies recognize the validity of dietary supplementation with fish fats, oil or soy oil. These particular oils cause an increase in vagal activity and reduce severity of inflammation in chronic inflammatory bowel disease or RA [21,22]. These clinical antiinflammatory responses may be linked to the fat-induced stimulation of the cholinergic anti-inflammatory pathway, as observed in rats [24]. Main source of TNF which is a major factor determining the course of inflammatory pathway is the spleen, the source of Galen's black bile. As Tracey said, jokingly: "One can not help but wonder: How did the ancient Greeks know?" [17].

The physiology of the cholinergic anti-inflammatory pathway can also be used to consider the design of clinical experiments for anti-inflammatory therapies that were previously difficult to reconcile with classical mechanisms. Hypnosis and meditation can significantly affect the transmission of stimuli through the vagus nerve and inhibit immediate and delayed type hypersensitivity [1]. Acupuncture is used to modulate the activity of the vagus nerve to change the course of inflammatory bowel function and heart rate [1,17] Modulation of autonomic nervous system, especially the vagus nerve, by various means (including acupuncture) may be a breakthrough in the treatment of inflammatory diseases [1]. Because measurable increases in vagus nerve activity after acupuncture treatement was observed, it is theoretically possible that acupuncture can modulate the cytokine response via the cholinergic anti-inflammatory pathway [1]. High concentrations of neurotransmitters and hormones, including ACh and Norepinephrine were found within the boundary of most acupuncture points and meridian lines [25].

8. Acupuncture – Integrative functions of connective tissue

The ancient Chinese believed that there are two forces the Yang and the Yin. They are not two independent forces, as it is sometimes called, but they represent two extreme and opposite varieties of Chi energy, and thus - two opposing properties of the body, nature and the universe. Yang and Yin are defined opposites in nature, the cosmos and in man. As two opposite poles, Yin and Yang are represented in any substance at the same time, however, cannot exist alone, cannot be separated, exist in mutual relationship, in a constant balance and harmony. Imbalance between them leads to a disequilibrium in the world of phenomena, processes of change in charge of the life and phenomena of nature (homeostasis). Balance between Yin and Yang is basis of traditional Chinese medicine, which was created over 2500 years ago [26,27]. This concept is very similar to the pneuma of ancient Greek medicine. The great historian and biochemist Joseph Needham suggested that both Qi and pneuma are rarefied form of energy [28].

Acupuncture is an unconventional technique for treatment that came from the East but it seems that similar techniques were used in ancient Europe and America - ancient mummies (stone aged) that have tattoo lines partly overlapping meridians were discovered in Europe ("Ice Man") [29].

Acupuncture is used to reduce pain and maintain or restore the body's Qi energy balance, which is the condition for its effective functioning. The technique involves piercing the body with silver or gold needles in appropriate points, corresponding to the highest activity of internal organs. These points are located along the so-called meridians [30].

According to traditional Chinese medicine, the human body has designated pathways (meridians), which circulates in the Qi. The harmonious, stable and smooth flow of Qi through the meridians is health. While the symptoms appear when the energy flow stops (which does not mean that less and less Qi, only that it does not participate in the circulation) or is impaired. Each meridian is connected with region of cerebral cortex of specific internal organ [25]. It is believed that needling acupuncture point is the way to influence on flow of Qi and regulate homeostasis of the body. Significant correlation between the distribution of connective tissue and the meridians has been shown. Distribution of acupuncture points is consistent with the distribution of connective tissue, whats more acupuncture points are places with the largest grouping of connective tissue [30,31]. It was found an 80% correspondence between the sites of acupuncture points and the location of intermuscular or intramuscular connective tissue planes in postmortem tissue sections. Langevin et al. [30] hypothesized that the network of acupuncture points and meridians can be viewed as a representation of the network formed by interstitial connective tissue. Transmission of stimuli (mechanical, bioelectrical and biochemical) through connective tissue may have a powerful potential for integration across physiological systems (connective tissue surrounds all the organs, nerves, blood vessels and lymphatic) and between different parts of the body [31].

It was suggested by Fung [27] that the anatomical structure of meridian channels and acupoints are related not only to the connective tissues but also the connective tissue interstitial fluid (CTIF) system. This hypothesis, called CFMDD (Connective Fluid, Mechanotransduction, and Degranulation Durotaxis cells), postulated to be valid not only the connective tissue (hard part), but also liquids (soft part) is an integrated network to maintain the integrity of body shape against gravity [27]. Connective tissue consists of cells and extracellular material secreted by some of those cells. Ground substance consists largely of proteoglycans, hyaluronic acid, collagen fibers, proteins such as elastin, fibronectin, laminin. Various cell types were found in connective tissue interstitial fluid: macrophages, lymphocytes, T- and NK cells, eosinophils, adipocytes, plasma cells, fibroblasts, chondroblasts, osteoblasts, stem cells and mast cells [27]. Moreover, the CTIF system embeds a large numbers of nerve endings which contain receptors that are near mast cell migration tracks would have much better chances of interaction with the mast cells, leading to the degranulation of these cells. There is evidence that acupuncture could also cause degranulation of mast calls directly through mechanical stress [32].

http://dx.doi.org/10.5772/54506

Mast cells have a circular or oval shape (size ~10–20 μm) are produced in bone marrow BM arising from myeloid precursors (probably the same as basophils), to the final settlement they reach the bloodstream. Mast cells are important actors in inflammatory reaction. Their granules are rich in histamine and heparin. In addition, activated secrete prostaglandins and cytokines (eg IL-4 and TNF-α). They also contain proteases (eg tryptase and chymase). On the surface there is a receptor FcεRI IgE antibody binding. Mast cells are believed to interact with connective tissue matrix components through integrins. The interaction between mast cells and nerve cells would cause degranulation of the former leading to the release of said biomolecules as physiological or pathophysiological responses. In fact, the mast cell densities were found to be high around acupoints [33] and these cells could be mediators of the effector functions of acupuncture action. Fung [27] suggested that the solid substrate tissues can serve as the tracks of migration for the cells for physiological functions. He hypothesized that there are special migration tracks for fibroblasts and mast cells. The anatomical findings suggest that the densities of the collagen fibers plus some proteins are higher along certain tracks correlating with the Chinese medicine meridian channels. Mechanical properties of extracellular matrix not only affect the cell structure, but also cell locomotion. It was demonstrated that when cells are cultured on substrates of different rigidities (but with the same chemical properties), the morphology and motility rates of cells are different [27].

Manipulation of acupuncture needle may result in modification of extracellular matrix surrounding needle. Mechanical stimulus of the meridian can be transduced into bioelectrical and/or biochemical signals and can lead to downstream effects, including cellular actin polymerization, signaling pathway activation, changes in gene expression, protein synthesis, and extracellular matrix modification [30]. Actin polymerization in connective tissue fibroblasts may cause further pulling of collagen fibers and a "wave" of connective tissue contraction and cell activation spreading through connective tissue during acupuncture treatment [31].

Acupuncture meridians for more than 2500 years were believed to form a network throughout the body, connecting "via" connective tissue all internal tissues and organs. A form of signaling (biochemical, bioelectrical, or mechanical) transmitted through tissues or organs, therefore may have integrative functions. It is commonly known that connective tissue permeates all organs and surrounds all nerves, blood vessels, and lymphatics. Langevin et al. [30] propose that connective tissue plays a key role in the integration of several physiological functions with ambient levels of mechanical stress. Finally, as was concluded by E.S. Yang: "the ancient model appears to have withstood the test of time surprisingly well confirming the popular axiom that the old wine is better than the new" [26]

9. Intercellular communication or energetic modulation – Gasotransmitters as Qi equivalent?

As was suggested by Ralt [34] the transmission of Qi along the meridians is based on small molecules that travel *via* connective tissue. Acupuncture at specific points enhances the flow of these small signaling molecules. In this hypothesis the nitric oxide (NO) is a prime candidate to be a signaling molecule in the meridian system. The tight relations between NO and acupoint manipulation was observed [35]. NO has been shown to play a role in mediating the cardiovascular responses to electroacupuncture at point 36ST [35], moreover it was demonstrated that acupuncture increased the level of iNOS mRNA in macrophages [36]. It was also shown that NO contents and nNOS expression were consistently higher in the skin acupoints/ meridians associated with low electric resistance [36]. These data clearly show that NO is associated with the functions of acupoint/meridian including their low electric resistance. It is described that NO contents of peripheral blood increases significantly after acupuncture/moxibustion at point 36ST. Manipulating a distant point on the meridian and measure NO in another part of the body, demonstrate the meridian net via the NO biochemistry and the essentiality of NO in the control mechanisms of Chinese medicine. The similar results were obtained by blocking NO in one part of the body and measure inhibition of a distant meridian manipulation [36].

The three gases; CO, NO, and H_2S, are generated endogenously [37-39]. Cytochrome oxidase (COX), the terminal enzyme of mitochondrial complex is a mediator of mitochondrial respiration not only through its natural ligand, O_2, but also through the binding of CO, NO, and H_2S [37]. At physiological concentrations, all three gases act as anti-inflammatory and cytoprotective agents [37-39]. The inhibition of COX by CO, NO, and H_2S suppresses oxidative phosphorylation reduces energy production and decrease intensity of energy metabolism. Simultaneously, this down regulation of this phosphorylation changes the redox state of the electron transport chain and produces reactive oxygen species (ROS). In many cases, ROS function as signaling molecules, thereby controlling cell and tissue functions. This process is known as "mitochondrial redox signaling (MRS)". It is noting that near 1% of the O2 consumed is used for this reaction. The production of NO, H_2S, and CO is determined by stimulated NO synthase (eNOS), cystathionine γ-lyase, and heme oxygenase, respectively. All these enzymes are activated by Ca^{2+}-calmodulin, via stimulation of ACh receptors on EC. NO and CO diffuse into the adjacent smooth muscle cells and activate soluble guanylyl cyclase to produce cyclic GMP, being a functional part of cholinergic system. H_2S also diffuses into smooth muscle cells, where it likely activates K^+ channels, part of cholinergic system. These three gasotransmitters are known to inhibit O_2 consumption by inhibiting cytochrome oxidase, the terminal and crucial enzyme of the electron transport chain in mitochondria. In result, all these enzymes finally reduce energy production.

NO, similarly to CO and H_2S is known to inhibit O_2 consumption by inhibiting COX, the terminal electron acceptor of the electron transport chain. NO binds COX both reversibly and irreversibly. The tissue levels of NO is in a range between 10 and 450 nM, and NO can bind to COX in vivo. It was suggested that the effect of NO inhibition of COX may be the induction of MRS, which secondarily regulates many cellular responses, including, O2 redistribution, and regulation of energy metabolism [37]. NO also has a vasodilatory effect through the GMP pathway, which can increase the blood flow to the tissue. Thus, both the classic cGMP pathway and the MRS pathway seem to cooperate [37].

The tissue CO concentrations are in the micromolar range, and it may be assumed that CO inhibits COX in cells and tissues. CO is known to produce antiinflammatory and antiapoptotic effects, what seems to be regulated at the level of COX blocking and mediated by MRS. Furthermore, CO upregulates superoxide dismutase 2 (SOD) expression and because SOD converts O_2 to the signaling molecule H_2O_2, this effect may also enhance the MRS [37,38].

H_2S is an additional competitive inhibitor of COX [37], in a range of H_2S tissue concentration between 1 to 10mM. H_2S can also induce this phenomenon of "suspended animation" which is a physiologic response to anoxia in which all life processes reversibly arrest the most of physiological functions. This phenomenon completely returns to normal without any damage when animals are released from stress. In experiments of Blackstone et al. [40] inhalation of a nontoxic level (80 ppm) of H_2S in awake self-breathing mice could reversibly reduce the metabolic rate to as low as 10% of the normal state. Similar results were obtained in experiments with CO and NO. It seems, although these gases may have different pathways to induce the suspended phenomenon, COX inhibition is the common characteristic [40].

O_2 stimulation metabolism factor, may be recognized as yang (hot, light), contrary to CO, NO, and H_2S, inhibiting metabolism factors, which may be recognized as yin (cold, dark). It was also proposed that yin-yang balance may be an antioxidation-oxidation balance with yin representing antioxidation and yang as oxidation. These hypothesis opens an avenue to systematicall study the yin-yang balance and its health implications with the use of modern biochemical tools [41].

10. Qi as a modulator of redox imbalance?

In modern western medicine, the balance between antioxidation and oxidation is believed to be a critical concept for maintaining health. Very similar concept of balance called yin-yang has existed in Traditional Chinese medicine for more than 2000 years. As was suggested by Ou [41] the yin-yang balance may be compared to the antioxidation-oxidation balance with yin representing antioxidation and yang as oxidation. This hypothesis is supported by the fact that the "yin-tonic" traditional Chinese herbs have high efficiency in detoxification of ROS. They show about six times more antioxidant activity and polyphenolic contents than the "yang-tonic" herbs [41].

ROS are produced during normal aerobic cell metabolism, mainly during oxidative phosphorylation and by activated phagocytic cells during oxidative burst. Many studies have demonstrated a role of ROS and oxidative stress in the pathogenesis of RA. Oxidative stress is defined as an imbalance between oxidants and anti-oxidants in favour of the oxidants, leading to a disruption of redox signalling and control and/or molecular damage [42]. The living cells possess antioxidant molecules, including thiols- mainly glutathione (GSH) for defense. The major barrier against oxidative stress is the redox equilibrium of sulfhydryl/disulfides [43]. It is commonly accepted that ROS and the resulting redox imbalance play an important role in chronic inflammatory states like RA [43].

As was shown by Crapo [44] this stress may be a potent initiator of cytokine release. The redox conditions may be important factor in determining the reactivity of the innate immune cells. In the tissues an extremely high level of extracellular antioxidants activity to maintain extracellular spaces in a highly reduced state to keep the tissue and extracellular fluids in a highly reduced state is necessary to normal physiological functions was observed [44]. Immune system activation is regulated by oxidation and reduction balance and thus the responsiveness of the immune system is influenced by the general tissue redox state, moreover, it was suggested that the imbalance in redox equilibrium may be associated with hyperresponsiveness of innate immune system [44].

11. Redox regulation of endothelial progenitor cells

The pathogenesis of RA is critically dependent on neovascularization of the synovium. It is important to note, that this microvascular expansion is occurring before clinical symptoms appear. Synovial neovascularization creates a direct conduit for the entry into the joint of circulating leukocytes that exacerbate inflammation, and provides nutrients to the hyperproliferative synovium [45].

The discovery of endothelial progenitor cells (EPC) indicated the contribution of circulating bone marrow-derived (BM) progenitor cells to new blood vessel formation, rather than migration and replication of local adult EC. Recently it was shown that EPC are not only restricted to the BM, but could also be detected in the peripheral circulation of adults. It was indicated the inverse correlation of circulating EPC numbers with cardiovascular risk factor. Moreover that conditions, which reduce the cardiovascular risk increase the levels of EPC [46].

It was observed by Paleolog [47] that the EPC cells were generated at a higher rate from BM samples taken from RA patients compared with normal subjects. The capacity of BM-derived EPC from RA patients to progress into mature EC positively correlates with the synovial microvessel density [47]. It was also shown that, in patients with active RA, EPC levels in peripheral blood, contrary to BM, were significantly lower than in healthy control. The presence of EPC in RA synovium could result from their enhanced recruitment from peripheral blood. This might then lead to increased RA synovial blood vessel formation in pannus, perpetuating chronic inflammatory disease [47]. In collagen induced arthritis Silverman et al. [45] observed EPC cells in the inflammatory infiltrate of arthritis joins, whereas they did not detect these cells in the joint lining form control animals. This correlates well with observations that the number of EPC in human RA synovial tissue samples was elevated 25-fold over the number of EPCs localized in normal synovial tissue [45]. Regulation of EPC function may have to important clinical beneficient effects. In RA the inhibition of neovacularization and in consequence inhibition of expansion of invasive tissue of pannus may be very positive clinically effect [45].

Actually it is commonly accepted that blood vessels in adult can arise not only during angiogenesis (formation of new capillaries from preexisting vessels), but also be result of vasculogenesis (de novo new vessel formation from BM-derived progenitor cells after recruitment of a progenitor subpopulation into blood vessels) [45]. Dernbach et al [48] examined whether EPCs are equipped with an antioxidative defence to provide resistance against oxidative stress occurring in chronic inflamed joints. It was shown that the expression of the intracellular antioxidative enzymes catalase, and superoxidase dismutase was significantly higher in EPCs than EC. They are excellently equipped to be protected against redox imbalance, consistent with their progenitor cell character in chronic inflamed environment [48].

It is known that many progenitor cells functions are under redox regulation [49]. Factors promoting self-renewal cause the reduction of the redox state, whereas molecules promoting differentiation lead to excess oxidation in neural progenitor cells [50]. ROS, in non-toxic amounts, seem to be involved in the balance between self-renewal and differentiation of progenitor cells. ROS are involved in normal progenitor cells functions, such as proliferation, differentiation, apoptosis and survival. Although excess amounts of ROS are toxic, they are balanced by ROS-generating and antioxidant enzymes [50]. The stem cells are embedded in a local BM environment (so-called stem cells "niche") and are maintained to be quiescent with low oxygen and ROS level. The increased ROS in BM facilitates stem cells to exit from the quiescent state, thereby stimulating proliferation and differentiation [50].

ROS at low levels function as signaling molecules to mediate cell proliferation, migration, differentiation, and survival. ROS regulated both angiogenic gene expression in ECs and vasculogenic gene expression in EPC [51]. Understanding these mechanisms may provide insight into NADPH oxidase and its mediators as potential therapeutic targets for chronic inflammatory disease.

It was suggest that essential attribute of the "stemness" is high resistance to stress. It was observed that the ROS levels in EPC are lower than those in mature ECs. Moreover, the higher expression of antioxidant enzymes (SOD, CAT, GPx) in EPC than in EC was shown. It seems that this is required for preserving stemness, such as undifferentiated, self-renewal state [49]. It seems that oxidative stress increases circulating cytokine levels, thereby stimulating NADPH oxidase dependent ROS production in BM, which may promote reparative mobilization of EPC from BM and the resulting revascularization of synovial tissue [50,51].

In summary, the ROS are involved in BM stem cells proliferation, differentiation, and migration, moreover, the NADPH oxidase-dependent ROS play an important role in redox signaling involved in the mobilization of BM progenitor cells [49]. Moreover there is strong evidence that EPC express eNOS- enzyme generating NO. The activity of this enzyme is regulated under inflamed conditions [51]. Compounds or molecules that increase eNOS expression improve EPC function, contrary to that the eNOS inhibitory substances have deleterious effects on EPC activity. Besides overexpression of eNOS, carbon monoxide (CO) also enhanced EPC proliferation [52]. Since NO serves as an important factor for mobilization of EPC use of organic nitrates, which are powerful NO donators, should enhance the number and function of circulating EPC. In general, low levels of ROS may activate EPC, whereas higher ROS levels significantly impair EPC function. In diseases, which result in increased ROS levels such as RA, EPC numbers and function may be modificated be redox potential in environment [52].

12. Regulation of endothelial progenitor cells by low density granulocytes

The presence of low density granulocytes (LDGs) in mononuclear cell fractions from patients with lupus or RA was observed by Denny [53]. It was shown that mature neutrophils are capable of producing many factors in response to certain stimuli, including the proinflammatory cytokines TNF-α and IL-1β or IFN-γ. Inhibition of neutrophil-derived cytokines is viewed as a potentially useful strategy for therapeutic in chronic diseases as was suggested by Denny [53]. LDGs induce significant EC cytotoxicity and synthesize sufficient levels of type I IFNs to disrupt the capacity of EPC to differentiate into mature EC. Moreover LDG depletion restores the functional capacity of EPC. As was concluded by Denny [53] LDGs may play an important dual role by simultaneously mediating enhanced vascular damage while inhibiting vascular repair. Patients with systemic lupus erythematosus SLE and RA have a strikingly higher risk of developing cardiovascular complications when compared to age- and gender-matched controls. It was proposed that this is due to a strong imbalance between vascular damage (EC apoptosis) and repair (by EPCs,) [53].

Further, IFN-α is cytotoxic to EPCs. This suggests that this neutrophil subset may play an important role in the induction of premature vascular damage in SLE and RA. Therefore, future strategies aimed at characterizing the origin of these cells and therapeutic mechanisms to deplete them or replenish are warranted [53].

13. Redox regulation of circulating inflammatory cells

The functioning of cells infiltrating inflamed joints is markedly influenced by alterations in the intracellular redox balance. The study of Biagioni et al. [54] clearly demonstrated a markedly decreased GSH/GSSG ratio index of an increased redox imbalance in neutrophils from patients with chronic inflammation.

Neutrophils from synovial fluid (SF) of patients with RA undergo transdifferentiation to cells with dendritic-like characteristics [55] and start to express MHC class II molecules [56]. Because MHC class II positive PMN activate T cells, the activation of neutrophils and T cells might contribute to the perpetuation of the local inflammatory process, and consequently to the enhanced of destructive process in RA [55]. Transdifferentiated into dendritic like cells neutrophils might be responsible for controlling migration and activation of lymphocytes

In T lymphocytes, intracellular GSH/GSSG levels seem to be a critical for their functions. However T lymphocytes require exogenous thiols for activation and function, therefore to sustain lymphocytes activation exogenous thiols can be generated in the microenvironment of an immune response. Angelini et al. [57] have shown that human dendritic cells (DCs) release cysteine in the extracellular space thus providing a reducing microenvironment that facilitates immune response. On the other hand, the migration of monocytes in inflamed joint is depended upon neutrophils activity. The two subpopulations of monocytes "resident" monocytes and "inflammatory" monocytes have been identified [58]. Extravasation of inflammatory monocytes, but not resident monocytes, may be enhanced by local treatment with secretion of activated neutrophils. Lysates of neutrophils were shown to exert chemotactic activity on monocytes suggesting an important role for the neutrophils-monocyte axis in the physiology of the onset, intensity and resolution of inflammatory process. Components of the neutrophils secretion were found to directly activate inflammatory monocytes and further enhanced of redox imbalance [58]. The hyporesponsiveness state observed in SF T lymphocytes from patients with RA strictly correlates with markers of oxidative stress and redox imbalance. Decreased of intracellular levels of antioxidant GSH and increased of GSSG in circulating cells was observed [59]. The redox balance alterations play a critical role in the abrogation of the cellular activation of the SF T lymphocytes from patients with RA [59]. Similar conclusion was performed by Cemersky et al. [60]. Oxidative stress and redox potential imbalance plays an important role in the induction of T lymphocyte hyporesponsiveness observed in RA.

The results obtained by Remans [61] show that chronic oxidative stress observed in synovial T lymphocytes is not secondary to exposure to extracellular ROS, but originates from intracellularly produced ROS. Chronic redox imbalance in SF T lymphocytes inhibits T cell receptor-dependent activation of signaling molecules required for efficient T cell proliferation, thus contributing to severe hyporesponsiveness of these cells to antigenic stimulation [61].

It seems that modification of the inflammatory environment by neutrophils and their granule proteins creates a milieu favoring further extravasation of inflammatory subtypes of monocytes. The targeting neutrophils without causing serious side effects seems futile, it may be more very promising to aim at interfering with subsequent neutrophils-driven proinflammatory events [58]. On the other hand, accumulating evidence suggests that intracellular redox status regulates many cellular function in macrophages [66].

Two classes of macrophages, ie. reductive macrophages (RMF), with a high intracellular content of glutathione, and oxidative macrophages (OMF) with a reducent content of glutathione were described by Murata et al.[66]. Moreover, it was observed that the Th1/Th2 balance is regulated by the balance between RMF and OMF. Type 1 helper T cells (Th1) are characterized by the production of pro-inflammatory cytokines like IFN-γ, IL-2, and TNF-β. These cells are involved in cell-mediated immunity. RA have been described as Th1 dominant disease. Type 2 helper T cells (Th2) are characterized by the production of IL-4, IL-5, IL-9, IL-10, and IL-13, and these cells are thought to play a role in humoral-mediated immunity. The balance Th1/Th2 was due to the disparate production of Il-12 vs IL-6 and 10. The OMF showed an elevated IL-6 and IL-10 production, and reduced NO and IL-12 production. Contrary to that RMF elicited a elevated IL-12 and NO production and reduced IL-6 and IL-10 production [66].

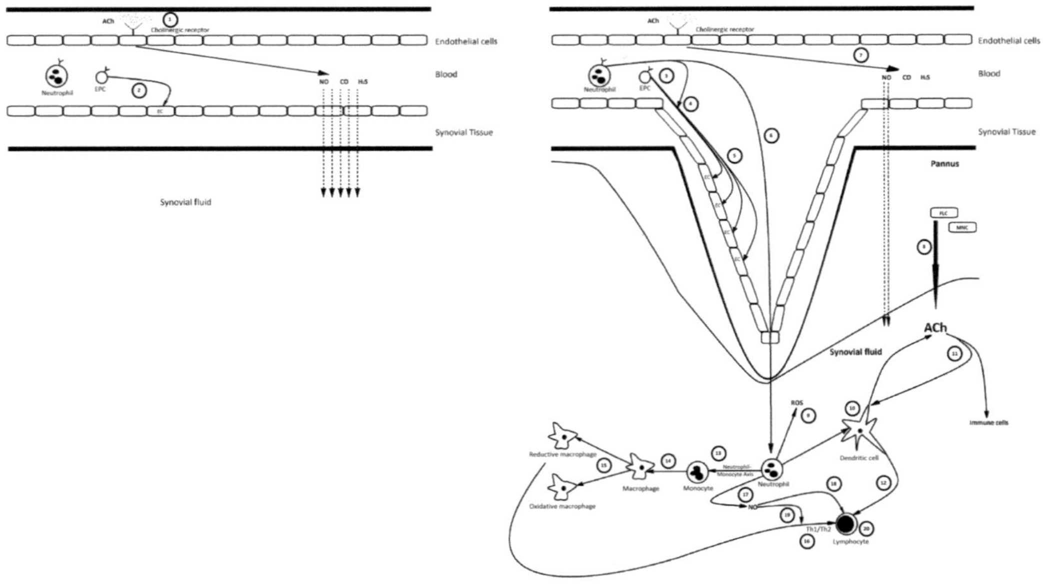

Figure 2. The role of neutrophils and importance of cholinergic anti-inflammatory pathway in interactions netrophils-cells in RA. 1. Stimulation of ACh receptors on EC cells results in release of gases which may regulate function of neutrophils and EPC. 2. EPC have ability to differentiate into EC. 3. Acetylcholine by its receptor on EPC improves the functional activity of EPC [62]. 4. The low density granulocytes (LDGs) partially disrupt the capacity of EPC to differentiate into mature EC. 5. Increased vasculature of ST in RA is a result of intensified processes of angiogenesis and neovascularisation. 6. Raised neutrophil migration into the articular cavity in RA patients is observed. 7. Decreased activity of the vagus nerve results in inhibited production of biologic gases. 8. In RA tissue in which cholinergic innervation is not proven to exist is supplied with ACh via production in non-neural cells within the tissue. Fibroblast-like cells and mononuclear-like cells may produce ACh [63]. 9. Reactive Oxygen Species released by neutrophils cause toxic effects. 10.The neutrophils are capable to transdifferentiate into dendritic like cells (DC). 11. DC expresss the muscarinic receptors and enzymes for production of ACh. ACh modulates the function of DC through autocrine/paracrine loop [64]. 12. DC are responsible for controlling migration and activation of lymphocytes. 13. The neutrophils activate inflammatory monocytes. 14. Monocytes transform to macrophages. 15. There are two classes of macrophages- reductive macrophages (RMF) and oxidative macrophages (OMF) with a reducent content of glutathione. 16. The Th1/Th2 balance is regulated by the balance between RMF and OMF. 17. The neutrophils are capable of generating NO in the inflamed synovium. 18. The NO regulate T cell functions under physiological conditions, but overproduction of NO may contribute to T lymphocyte dysfunction [65]. 19. The NO profoundly alters T cell activation and Th1/Th2 balance. 20. Chronic redox imbalance in SF contribute T lymphocytes hyporesponsiveness to antigenic stimulation.

The cytokines propensities of OMF and RMF were intercoverted to each other. Taken together RMF induction may generate the amplification loop of a RMF/Th1 circuit and OMF that of OMF/Th2. The findings implicate that the alteration in MF functions because altered intracellular glutathione may play a relevant role in the pathological progression of inflammation, as was suggested [66]. IL-12 is secreted physiologically by MF and plays a pivotal role in regulating cell-mediated immunity. Moreover, IL-12 also plays an important role in maintaining the in vivo balance between TH1 and Th2 responses. The development of Th1 cells from TH0 cells requires IL-12 and is prevent by prostaglandin E2 and IL-10. The differentiation TH0 into TH2 cells requires IL-4 and IL-6. It was proven that the Th1/Th2 balance is certainly regulated by the balance between RMF and OMF [66]. Moreover, the lymphocytes functions may be regulated by biological gases, it is commonly accepted that NO regulate T cell functions under physiological conditions, but overproduction of NO may contribute to T lymphocyte dysfunction [65].

Several different cell types are capable of generating NO in the inflamed synovium, including neutrophils and other circulating and stationary cells [67]. NO-dependent tissue injury has been implicated in RA. It was shown that NO serves as a potent immune-regulatory factor by influenceing the cytoplasmic redox balance and may inhibit cytochrome c oxidase, leading to cell death through ATP depletion. It seems that T cell activation is associated with NO production [13]. Several studies have documented evidence for increased endogenous NO synthesis, suggesting that overproduction of NO may be important in the pathogenesis of RA [67].

It seems that the NO profoundly alters T cell activation and Th1/Th2 balance. Because NO may plays an important role in the pathogenesis of RA, it seems reasonably that "biologic gases" may represent a novel therapeutic approach in the treatment of chronic autoimmune diseases like RA.

14. Conclusions – Proposed therapies

The parasympathetic nervous system, through the vagus nerve down-regulate inflammation. The vagus nerve exert anti-inflammatory effect via a ACh, primary on the nicotinic receptor on macrophages. As was shown by Maanen et al.[68], experimental arthritis may be ameliorated by cholinergic agonist, nicotine. Bruchfeld et al. [69] showed that addition of nicotine to the blood cultures, from patients with RA, significantly suppressed cytokine production. These experiments showed that it is possible to therapeutically target the ACh receptors dependent control of cytokine release in RA patients with suppressed vagus nerve activity.

Strong expression of nicotinic receptor in the synovium of RA patients was detected by Das [70]. Both peripheral macrophages and synovial fibroblasts respond to specific cholinergic stimulation with potent inhibition of proinflammatory cytokines. It was proposed by Das [70] that vagal nerve stimulation, or nicotinic agonists may augment the formation of anti-inflammatory lipid molecules: lipoxins, resolvins, protectins and maresins. This implies that new therapies focused on directed regulation of the cholinergic mediated mechanisms and enhancing the formation of lipoxins, resolvins, protectins and maresins may halt and/or ameliorate RA [70]. It is very important to note, that electrical stimulation of the vagus nerve, ie. activating antiinflamatory pathway, attenuates inflammatory injury without unwanted secondary effects on organ and tissue functions, such as heart rate or gut motility [11].

It is commonly accepted that, similarly to vagus nerve stimulation, acupuncture may activate the cholinergic anti-inflammatory pathway in treatment of inflammatory diseases [12]. Moreover, stimulation of auricular afferents excites vagal efferents [14] and may modulate the cholinergic anti-inflammatory pathway activity [71]. Aricular acupuncture (AA) has been used for a wide varieties of pain conditions but unlike body acupuncture, the mechanism of AA remains largely uninvestigated. Since the auricle is innervated by a mix of V, VII, IX and X cranial sensory nerves and has central connections distinct from those of body acupoints, the physiological responses produced by AA may be substantially different from those produced by body acupuncture.

AA is a method based on normalizing the body's dysfunction through stimulation of some definite points on the ears [72]. AA, a distinct form of acupuncture. It is based on a somatotopic relation of the external ear to other body regions. It as was shown that ear acupressure is effective in increasing oxygen uptake and lowering lactic acid following exercise. Lin et al. [72] shown that AA enhance the physiological abilities by lowering athletes' heart rates at rest, decreasing oxygen intake, and expediting excretion of post-exercise blood lactic acids. Electroacupunture, another form of acupuncture increases the cannabinoid receptor expression not only on "stationary" keratinocytes but also on "circulating" infiltrating inflammatory cells, like macrophages or T-lymphocytes [73].

Acupressure or physical exercise has been also proposed to be a physiological way to modulate immunity and inflammation. These processes are controlled mainly by alterations in ROS level and redox balanced [74]. Moreover it was observed that acute severe exercise (ASE) usually impedes immunity, contrary to chronic moderate exercise (CME) which improves it [74]. It was shown that ASE stimulates the secretion of many pro-inflammatory cytokines, such as TNF-α, IL-6, and IL-1β. Nevertheless, CME potently elevates the an anti-inflammatory cytokine like IL-10. Since ASE and CME have opposite effects on inflammatory cytokines, they differentially regulate ROS level as well as redox balance [74].

A number of drugs or drug candidates (in clinical trials) exert their effects via donation of "biological gases", on redox balance, such as NO, CO and H_2S [39,75]. Szabo [39] suggested that the endogenous generated molecules may have a distinct advantage when applied as therapeutics, because the body 'already knows' how to 'deal with them'. Moreover, the cellular responses are predictable, and specific elimination pathways are present. It seems that gaseotransmitter therapy may be viewed as 'hormone replacement therapy' [38]. Many therapeutic approaches (in clinical or preclinical stages) are based on various aspects of gaseotransmitter pharmacology, for example as the therapeutic administration of these gases in inhaled gaseous form [39].

The main anti-inflammatory effects of NO, CO and H_2S involve multiple more complex pathways, but at high local concentrations, the cytotoxic effects of NO, CO and H_2S cause a direct inhibition of mitochondrial respiration [76]. It was demonstrated that the inhibition of cytochrome c oxidase (followed by inhibition of mitochondrial respiration, and generation of ROS) is responsible for both the toxic effects of this gases and for the therapeutic modulation of anti- inflammatory phenomenon [76]. It may be assumed that the direction of the net biological effect (protection or toxicity) is a function of the degree of cytochrome c inhibition by "biological gases", and in consequence modulation of redox homeostasis. Since NO, CO and H_2S are produced in human body, there are basal levels of these gases in many cells and tissues. Szabo postulated that endogenous levels of all three gaseotransmitters may increase or decrease in various disease conditions, moreover, it may be interesting for diagnostic purposes [77]. The beneficial anti-inflammatory effects of these gases typically occur at low (near-physiological) concentrations, while at higher concentrations the effects diminish, and toxicity may ensue, according to Paracelsus (1493-1541) definition that "all drugs are poisons; the benefit depends on the dosage".

Taken together, understanding of the complex interactions between vagus nerve modulation, acupuncture, cholinergic neurotransmitters, "biological gases" and redox status of inflammatory cells, involved in joint tissue damage, might be useful for the development of novel therapeutic strategies for RA. The significant number of RA patients do not respond to the typical treatment. To develop new anti-inflammatory treatments, studies on identification of new pathways involved in modulation of inflammation are still conducted. One of interesting approaches could be idea of manipulation of the autonomic nervous system. In conclusion, it may be posited that the combined medical knowledge of the East and the West, the ancient and the actual concepts may offer new possibilities to the modern medicine.

Author details

Michal Gajewski[1], Slawomir Maslinski[2], Przemyslaw Rzodkiewicz[1,2] and
Elzbieta Wojtecka-Lukasik[1]

1 Department of Biochemistry, Institute of Rheumatology, Warsaw, Poland

2 Department of General and Experimental Pathology, Medical University of Warsaw, Warsaw, Poland

References

[1] Tracey KJ. The inflammatory reflex. Nature. 2002;420(6917):853-9.

[2] Tracey KJ. Reflex control of immunity. Nat Rev Immunol. 2009;9(6):418-28.

[3] Evrengul H, Dursunoglu D, Cobankara V, Polat B, Seleci D, Kabukcu S, Kaftan A, Semiz E, Kilic M. Heart rate variability in patients with rheumatoid arthritis. Rheumatol Int. 2004;24(4):198-202.

[4] Koopman FA, Stoof SP, Straub RH, Van Maanen MA, Vervoordeldonk MJ, Tak PP. Restoring the balance of the autonomic nervous system as an innovative approach to the treatment of rheumatoid arthritis. Mol Med. 2011;17(9-10):937-48.

[5] Berthoud HR, Neuhuber WL. Functional and chemical anatomy of the afferent vagal system. Auton Neurosci. 2000;85(1-3):1-17.

[6] Wess J. Molecular biology of muscarinic acetylcholine receptors. Crit Rev Neurobiol. 1996;10(1):69-99.

[7] Fujii T, Yamada S, Yamaguchi N, Fujimoto K, Suzuki T, Kawashima K. Species differences in the concentration of acetylcholine, a neurotransmitter, in whole blood and plasma. Neurosci Lett. 1995;201(3):207-10.

[8] Kawashima K, Fujii T. Extraneuronal cholinergic system in lymphocytes. Pharmacol Ther. 2000;86(1):29-48.

[9] Borovikova LV, Ivanova S, Zhang M, Yang H, Botchkina GI, Watkins LR, Wang H, Abumrad N, Eaton JW, Tracey KJ. Vagus nerve stimulation attenuates the systemic inflammatory response to endotoxin. Nature. 2000;405(6785):458-62.

[10] Bernik TR, Friedman SG, Ochani M, DiRaimo R, Ulloa L, Yang H, Sudan S, Czura CJ, Ivanova SM, Tracey KJ. Pharmacological stimulation of the cholinergic antiinflammatory pathway. J Exp Med. 2002;195(6):781-8.

[11] Rosas-Ballina M, Tracey KJ. Cholinergic control of inflammation. J Intern Med. 2009;265(6):663-79.

[12] Molina PE, Zambell KL, Zhang P, Vande Stouwe C, Carnal J. Hemodynamic and immune consequences of opiate analgesia after trauma/hemorrhage. Shock. 2004;21(6): 526-34.

[13] Woiciechowsky C, Asadullah K, Nestler D, Eberhardt B, Platzer C, Schöning B, Glöckner F, Lanksch WR, Volk HD, Döcke WD. Sympathetic activation triggers systemic IL-10 release in immunodepression induced by brain injury. Nat Med. 1998;4(7):808-13.

[14] Koizumi K, Terui N, Kollai M, Brooks CM. Functional significance of coactivation of vagal and sympathetic cardiac nerves. Proc Natl Acad Sci U S A. 1982 Mar;79(6): 2116-20.

[15] Dekkers JC, Geenen R, Godaert GL, Bijlsma JW, van Doornen LJ. Elevated sympathetic nervous system activity in patients with recently diagnosed rheumatoid arthritis with active disease. Clin Exp Rheumatol. 2004;22(1):63-70.

[16] Stojanovich L, Milovanovich B, de Luka SR, Popovich-Kuzmanovich D, Bisenich V, Djukanovich B, Randjelovich T, Krotin M. Cardiovascular autonomic dysfunction in systemic lupus, rheumatoid arthritis, primary Sjögren syndrome and other autoimmune diseases. Lupus. 2007;16(3):181-5.

[17] Tracey KJ. Physiology and immunology of the cholinergic antiinflammatory pathway. J Clin Invest. 2007;117(2):289-96.

[18] Kokkonen H, Söderström I, Rocklöv J, Hallmans G, Lejon K, Rantapää Dahlqvist S. Up-regulation of cytokines and chemokines predates the onset of rheumatoid arthritis. Arthritis Rheum. 2010;62(2):383-91.

[19] Peng CK, Henry IC, Mietus JE, Hausdorff JM, Khalsa G, Benson H, Goldberger AL. Heart rate dynamics during three forms of meditation. Int J Cardiol. 2004;95(1):19-27.

[20] Pullan RD, Rhodes J, Ganesh S, Mani V, Morris JS, Williams GT, Newcombe RG, Russell MA, Feyerabend C, Thomas GA, et al. Transdermal nicotine for active ulcerative colitis. N Engl J Med. 1994;330(12):811-5.

[21] Felson DT, Anderson JJ, Naimark A, Hannan MT, Kannel WB, Meenan RF. Does smoking protect against osteoarthritis? Arthritis Rheum. 1989;32(2):166-72.

[22] Facchini M, Malfatto G, Sala L, Silvestri G, Fontana P, Lafortuna C, Sartorio A. Changes of autonomic cardiac profile after a 3-week integrated body weight reduction program in severely obese patients. J Endocrinol Invest. 2003;26(2):138-42.

[23] Das UN. Beneficial effect(s) of n-3 fatty acids in cardiovascular diseases: but, why and how? Prostaglandins Leukot Essent Fatty Acids. 2000;63(6):351-62.

[24] Luyer MD, Greve JW, Hadfoune M, Jacobs JA, Dejong CH, Buurman WA. Nutritional stimulation of cholecystokinin receptors inhibits inflammation via the vagus nerve. J Exp Med. 2005;202(8):1023-9.

[25] Omura Y. Connections found between each meridian (heart, stomach, triple burner, etc.) & organ representation area of corresponding internal organs in each side of the cerebral cortex; release of common neurotransmitters and hormones unique to each meridian and corresponding acupuncture point & internal organ after acupuncture, electrical stimulation, mechanical stimulation (including shiatsu), soft laser stimulation or QI Gong. Acupunct Electrother Res.1989;14(2):155-86.

[26] Yang ES, Li PW, Nilius B, Li G. Ancient Chinese medicine and mechanistic evidence of acupuncture physiology. Pflugers Arch. 2011;462(5):645-53.

[27] Fung PC. Probing the mystery of Chinese medicine meridian channels with special emphasis on the connective tissue interstitial fluid system, mechanotransduction, cells durotaxis and mast cell degranulation. Chin Med. 2009;4:10

[28] Temple R (1986) The genius of China: 3,000 years of science, discovery and invention. Simon and Schuster, New York

[29] Dorfer L, Moser M, Spinder K, Bahr F, Egarter-Vigl E, Dohr G. 5200-year-old acupuncture in central Europe? Science. 1998;282(5387) :242-3.

[30] Langevin HM, Yandow JA. Relationship of acupuncture points and meridians to connective tissue planes. Anat Rec. 2002;269(6):257-65.

[31] Langevin HM, Churchill DL, Cipolla MJ. Mechanical signaling through connective tissue: a mechanism for the therapeutic effect of acupuncture. FASEB J. 2001;15(12): 2275-82.

[32] Yu XJ, Ding GH, Yao W, Zhan R, Huang M. [The role of collagen fiber in "Zusanli" (ST 36) in acupuncture analgesia in the rat]. Zhongguo Zhen Jiu. 2008;28(3):207-13. Chinese.

[33] Zhang D, Ding G, Shen X, Yao W, Zhang Z, Zhang Y, Lin J, Gu Q. Role of mast cells in acupuncture effect: a pilot study. Explore (NY). 2008;4(3):170-7.

[34] Ralt D. Intercellular communication, NO and the biology of Chinese medicine. Cell Commun Signal. 2005;3(1):8.

[35] Chen S, Ma SX. Nitric oxide in the gracile nucleus mediates depressor response to acupuncture (ST36). J Neurophysiol. 2003;90(2):780-5.

[36] Ma SX. Enhanced nitric oxide concentrations and expression of nitric oxide synthase in acupuncture points/meridians. J Altern Complement Med. 2003;9(2):207-15.

[37] Kajimura M, Fukuda R, Bateman RM, Yamamoto T, Suematsu M. Interactions of multiple gas-transducing systems: hallmarks and uncertainties of CO, NO, and H_2S gas biology. Antioxid Redox Signal. 2010;13(2):157-92.

[38] Mustafa AK, Gadalla MM, Snyder SH. Signaling by gasotransmitters. Sci Signal. 2009;2(68):re2.

[39] Szabo C. Gaseotransmitters: new frontiers for translational science. Sci Transl Med. 2010;2(59):59ps54.

[40] Blackstone E, Morrison M, Roth MB. H2S induces a suspended animation-like state in mice. Science. 2005;308(5721):518.

[41] Ou B, Huang D, Hampsch-Woodill M, Flanagan JA. When east meets west: the relationship between yin-yang and antioxidation-oxidation. FASEB J. 2003;17(2):127-9.

[42] Filippin LI, Vercelino R, Marroni NP, Xavier RM. Redox signalling and the inflammatory response in rheumatoid arthritis. Clin Exp Immunol. 2008;152(3):415-22.

[43] Pedersen-Lane JH, Zurier RB, Lawrence DA. Analysis of the thiol status of peripheral blood leukocytes in rheumatoid arthritis patients. J Leukoc Biol. 2007;81(4):934-41.

[44] Crapo JD. Oxidative stress as an initiator of cytokine release and cell damage. Eur Respir J Suppl. 2003;44:4s-6s.

[45] Silverman MD, Haas CS, Rad AM, Arbab AS, Koch AE. The role of vascular cell adhesion molecule 1/ very late activation antigen 4 in endothelial progenitor cell recruitment to rheumatoid arthritis synovium. Arthritis Rheum. 2007;56(6):1817-26.

[46] Distler JH, Beyer C, Schett G, Lüscher TF, Gay S, Distler O. Endothelial progenitor cells: novel players in the pathogenesis of rheumatic diseases. Arthritis Rheum. 2009;60(11):3168-79.

[47] Paleolog E. It's all in the blood: circulating endothelial progenitor cells link synovial vascularity with cardiovascular mortality in rheumatoid arthritis? Arthritis Res Ther. 2005;7(6):270-2.

[48] Dernbach E, Urbich C, Brandes RP, Hofmann WK, Zeiher AM, Dimmeler S.Antioxidative stress-associated genes in circulating progenitor cells: evidence for enhanced resistance against oxidative stress. Blood. 2004;104(12):3591-7.

[49] Haneline LS. Redox regulation of stem and progenitor cells. Antioxid Redox Signal. 2008;10(11):1849-52.

[50] Ushio-Fukai M, Urao N. Novel role of NADPH oxidase in angiogenesis and stem/progenitor cell function. Antioxid Redox Signal. 2009;11(10):2517-33.

[51] Schröder K, Kohnen A, Aicher A, Liehn EA, Büchse T, Stein S, Weber C, Dimmeler S, Brandes RP. NADPH oxidase Nox2 is required for hypoxia-induced mobilization of endothelial progenitor cells. Circ Res. 2009;105(6):537-44.

[52] Fleissner F, Thum T. Critical role of the nitric oxide/reactive oxygen species balance in endothelial progenitor dysfunction. Antioxid Redox Signal. 2011;15(4):933-48.

[53] Denny MF, Yalavarthi S, Zhao W, Thacker SG, Anderson M, Sandy AR, McCune WJ,Kaplan MJ. A distinct subset of proinflammatory neutrophils isolated from patients with systemic lupus erythematosus induces vascular damage and synthesizes type I IFNs. J Immunol. 2010;184(6):3284-97.

[54] Biagioni C, Favilli F, Catarzi S, Marcucci T, Fazi M, Tonelli F, Vincenzini MT, Iantomasi T. Redox state and O2*- production in neutrophils of Crohn's disease patients. Exp Biol Med (Maywood). 2006;231(2):186-95.

[55] Iking-Konert C, Ostendorf B, Sander O, Jost M, Wagner C, Joosten L, Schneider M, Hänsch GM. Transdifferentiation of polymorphonuclear neutrophils to dendritic-like cells at the site of inflammation in rheumatoid arthritis: evidence for activation by T cells. Ann Rheum Dis. 2005;64(10):1436-42.

[56] Cross A, Bucknall RC, Cassatella MA, Edwards SW, Moots RJ. Synovial fluid neutrophils transcribe and express class II major histocompatibility complex molecules in rheumatoid arthritis. Arthritis Rheum. 2003;48(10):2796-806.

[57] Angelini G, Gardella S, Ardy M, Ciriolo MR, Filomeni G, Di Trapani G, Clarke F, Sitia R, Rubartelli A. Antigen-presenting dendritic cells provide the reducing extracellular microenvironment required for T lymphocyte activation. Proc Natl Acad Sci U S A. 2002;5;99(3):1491-6.

[58] Soehnlein O, Lindbom L, Weber C. Mechanisms underlying neutrophil-mediate monocyte recruitment. Blood. 2009;114(21):4613-23.

[59] Gringhuis SI, Leow A, Papendrecht-Van Der Voort EA, Remans PH, Breedveld FC, Verweij CL. Displacement of linker for activation of T cells from the plasma membrane due to redox balance alterations results in hyporesponsiveness of synovial fluid T lymphocytes in rheumatoid arthritis. J Immunol. 2000;164(4):2170-9.

[60] Cemerski S, Cantagrel A, Van Meerwijk JP, Romagnoli P. Reactive oxygen species differentially affect T cell receptor-signaling pathways. J Biol Chem. 2002;277(22): 19585-93.

[61] Remans PH, van Oosterhout M, Smeets TJ, Sanders M, Frederiks WM, Reedquist KA,Tak PP, Breedveld FC, van Laar JM. Intracellular free radical production in syno-

vial T lymphocytes from patients with rheumatoid arthritis. Arthritis Rheum. 2005;52(7):2003-9.

[62] Yu M, Liu Q, Sun J, Yi K, Wu L, Tan X. Nicotine improves the functional activity of late endothelial progenitor cells via nicotinic acetylcholine receptors. Biochem Cell Biol. 2011;89(4):405-10.

[63] Grimsholm O, Rantapää-Dahlqvist S, Dalén T, Forsgren S. Unexpected finding of a marked non-neuronal cholinergic system in human knee joint synovial tissue. Neurosci Lett. 2008;442(2):128-33.

[64] Salamone G, Lombardi G, Gori S, Nahmod K, Jancic C, Amaral MM, Vermeulen M, Español A, Sales ME, Geffner J. Cholinergic modulation of dendritic cell function. J Neuroimmunol. 2011;236(1-2):47-56.

[65] Nagy G, Koncz A, Telarico T, Fernandez D, Ersek B, Buzás E, Perl A. Central role of nitric oxide in the pathogenesis of rheumatoid arthritis and systemic lupus erythematosus. Arthritis Res Ther. 2010;12(3):210.

[66] Murata Y, Shimamura T, Hamuro J. The polarization of T(h)1/T(h)2 balance is dependent on the intracellular thiol redox status of macrophages due to the distinctive cytokine production. Int Immunol. 2002;14(2):201-12.

[67] Nagy G, Clark JM, Buzás EI, Gorman CL, Cope AP. Nitric oxide, chronic inflammation and autoimmunity. Immunol Lett. 2007;111(1):1-5.

[68] Maanen van MA, Vervoordeldonk MJ, Tak PP. The cholinergic anti-inflammatory pathway: towards innovative treatment of rheumatoid arthritis. Nat Rev Rheumatol. 2009;5(4):229-32.

[69] Bruchfeld A, Goldstein RS, Chavan S, Patel NB, Rosas-Ballina M, Kohn N, Qureshi AR, Tracey KJ. Whole blood cytokine attenuation by cholinergic agonist sex vivo and relationship to vagus nerve activity in rheumatoid arthritis. J Intern Med. 2010;268(1): 94-101.

[70] Das UN. Can vagus nerve stimulation halt or ameliorate rheumatoid arthritis and lupus? Lipids Health Dis. 2011;10:19.

[71] Chung WY, Zhang HQ, Zhang SP. Peripheral muscarinic receptors mediate the anti-inflammatory effects of auricular acupuncture. Chin Med. 2011;6(1):3.

[72] Lin ZP, Wang CY, Jang TR, Ma TC, Chia F, Lin JG, Hsu JJ, Ho TJ. Effect of auricular acupuncture on oxygen consumption of boxing athletes. Chin Med J (Engl). 2009;122(13):1587-90.

[73] Zhang J, Chen L, Su T, Cao F, Meng X, Pei L, Shi J, Pan HL, Li M. Electroacupuncture increases CB2 receptor expression on keratinocytes and infiltrating inflammatory cells in inflamed skin tissues of rats. J Pain. 2010;11(12):1250-8.

[74] Syu GD, Chen HI, Jen CJ. Severe exercise and exercise training exert opposite effects on human neutrophil apoptosis via altering the redox status. PLoS One. 2011;6(9):e24385.

[75] Chen JX, Ibe BO, Ma SX. Nitric oxide modulation of norepinephrine production in acupuncture points. Life Sci. 2006;79(23):2157-64.

[76] Zuckerbraun BS, Chin BY, Bilban M, d'Avila JC, Rao J, Billiar TR, Otterbein LE. Carbon monoxide signals via inhibition of cytochrome c oxidase and generation of mitochondrial reactive oxygen species. FASEB J. 2007;21(4):1099-106.

[77] Papapetropoulos A, Pyriochou A, Altaany Z, Yang G, Marazioti A, Zhou Z,Jeschke MG, Branski LK, Herndon DN, Wang R, Szabó C. Hydrogen sulfide is an endogenous stimulator of angiogenesis. Proc Natl Acad Sci U S A. 2009;106(51):21972-7.

Chapter 10

Laryngeal Manifestations of Rheumatoid Arthritis

Stevan Stojanović and Branislav Belić

Additional information is available at the end of the chapter

http://dx.doi.org/10.5772/51730

1. Introduction

Rheumatoid arthritis is the most common inflammatory disease of joints. It is described as symmetric, persistent and destructive polyarthritis which is often followed by positive rheumatoid factor and/or positive results on anticyclic citrulined peptide immunoglobulins. The larynx is rarely considered affected, and the patients come at terminal phase of rheumatoid arthritis when the changes are so progressive and irreversible and the treatment is very difficult. The larynx is a part of upper respiratory system and an aerodigestive crossroads and is, therefore, often affected by pathological changes specific for rheumatoid arthritis. Damage of its anatomical structures and physiological functions happens in the early phases of rheumatoid arthritis, as many authors have written about it (Hart, 1966), which is manifested by different pathoanatomical and pathophysiological changes. Sequence and intensity of the symptoms' appearance depend on the size, localization, spread and duration of pathological changes in rheumatoid arthritis. Clinical picture of laryngeal manifestations of rheumatoid arthritis is characterized by numerous and various symptoms.Because of the perplexity and length of the symptoms' manifestations of this disease on other localizations of a human body, it is rarely thought about the laryngeal symptoms and signs when they are in the initial phase and of weak intensity. Patients with progressive symptoms and signs of rheumatoid arthritis in the larynx do not get routine examination by otorhinolaryngologists, but this disease is usually diagnosed only when breathing and/or swallowing are very compromised.One patient with rheumatoid arthritis in its terminal phase was treated at the ORL Clinic of the Clinical Center in Kragujevac. The disease was diagnosed by techniques of indirect laryngoscopy, microlaryngoscopy with the use of laryngoscopic claws, computered endovideostroboscopy and multislice scanner larynx examination. Previously, the patient underwent surgical tracheotomy because of asphyxia and very reduced breathing space. Modern diagnostics recommended by other authors include electromyography of the larynx with the aim of differential diagnostics of cricoarytenoid joint immobility because of the paralysis of nervus reccurens of other etiology.With the aim of timely diagnostics of pathological changes in the larynx in the patients with the rheumatoid arthritis, a routine indirect laryngoscopy is necessary to be carried out. When otorhinolaryngologists notice reduced mobility of one half of the larynx, laryngomicroscopy, electromyography of the larynx, multislice scanner neck examination are recommended in these patients. In diagnosed laryngeal changes, the therapy of intra-articular injection of corticosteroids in every affected cricoarytenoid joint should be considered as a possibility.

2. Larynx and rheumatoid arthritis

Rheumatoid arthritis is a generalized disease, but because of anatomical, physiological and pathoanatomial characteristics of the larynx, this disease has its manifestations in the larynx. Clinical picture, diagnostics and therapy of rheumatoid changes in the larynx have their characteristics to which every clinician must pay attention when treating clinical manifestations of this disease on other localizations and organs. In RA, the larynx is affected in 25% of the patients (Dockery, 1991). Symptoms and signs of rheumatoid arthritis in the larynx must be noticed and treated adequately in its earliest phase. This is necessary for preventing the progress of the disease and manifestation of the symptoms and signs that are life threatening, while the ultimate effect would be bringing back the quality of life to a satisfying level.

2.1. Anatomy and embryology of the larynx

The larynx or voice box is located in the median line of the anterior neck. It is placed at the aerodigestive crossroads and is the beginning of lower respiratory system. It is a fibroelastic tube between the hyoid bone and trachea, whose external layer is made of cartilage and muscles, and internal layer is mucous. The larynx is tied by ligaments and muscles to the hyoid bone and, therefore, it follows its movements. The larynx extends from the third to the fourth cervical vertebrae. From its aperture on the front wall of the inferior pharynx, the larynx comes down through the anterior neck and continues its way through the trachea. Upper larynx border is presented by a free edge of epiglottis and aryepiglottic plicae. Lower edge of the cricoid cartilage makes the lower larynx border, Figure 1.

Topographically, hypopharynx with very mobile musculature is between the larynx and vertebral column at the back, while at the front, there is a gland thyroid on both sides of the larynx. Its anterior is covered with thin infrahyoid muscles.Voice box is tied and strained to scull base and lower jaw indirectly over the hyoid bone, suprahyoid muscles and fibroelastic connections. It follows the head and neck movements and it rises and descends while swallowing. Its angular prominence on the anterior neck is known as Adam's apple in men, and is more prominent than in women. Structure of the larynx is such that firm part is made of cartilages connected mutually as well as with other organs by fibrillar connections-membranes and joints-ligaments. Muscles move cartilages one to another. Submucous layer is made of fibroelastic membrane and the interior is encased by mucosa with blood vessels and nerves. Epiglottis bends backwards and closes the opening of the larynx while swallowing. Cavity of the larynx

http://dx.doi.org/10.5772/51730

or cavum laryngis at its frontal section reminds of a sandglass or two vertical funnels connected with their narrow ends, Figure 2. Upper floor or vestibule of the larynx is vestibulum laryngis that extends from the larynx aperture to upper plicae, so called false vocal cords – plicae vestibulares s. plicae vocales spuriae. Inferior mucous plicae or true vocal cords or plicae s. chordae vocales close the vocal gap or rima glottidis and it presents the entrance into the lower, subglottic floor of the larynx called cavum infraglotticum. Vocal cord is in its anterior, longer part, membranous and that part is called pars intermembranacea s. ligamentum vocale and in its posterior, shorter part it is cartilagenous and that part is called pars intercartilaginea s. processus vocalis. Rima glottidis or just glottis consists of vocal cords and vocal extention of arytenoid cartilage. The median floor consists of a mucous recessus or invagination which arises between the true and false vocal cords and it is larynx ventricle or sinus s. ventriculus laryngis Morgagni. That recessus between the plicae ventricularis and vocal cords has a role of resonator and its length is approximately 20mm in men and 15mm in women. Mucosa of the larynx ventricle external wall is full of glands or glandulae laryngis.

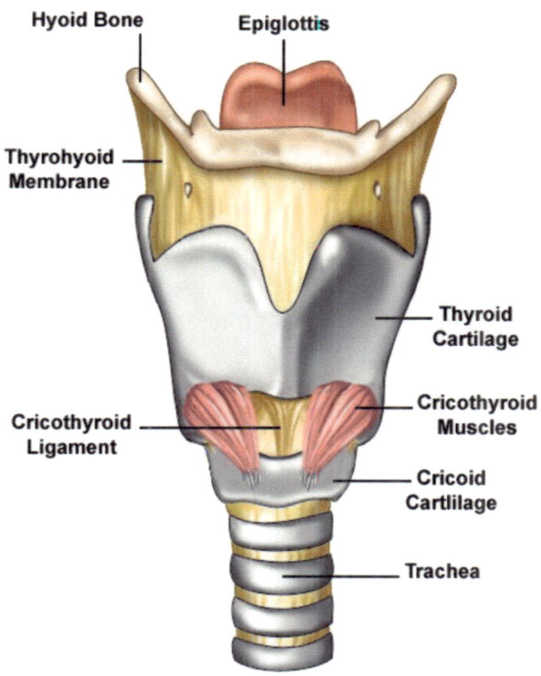

Figure 1. Anterior view of larynx.

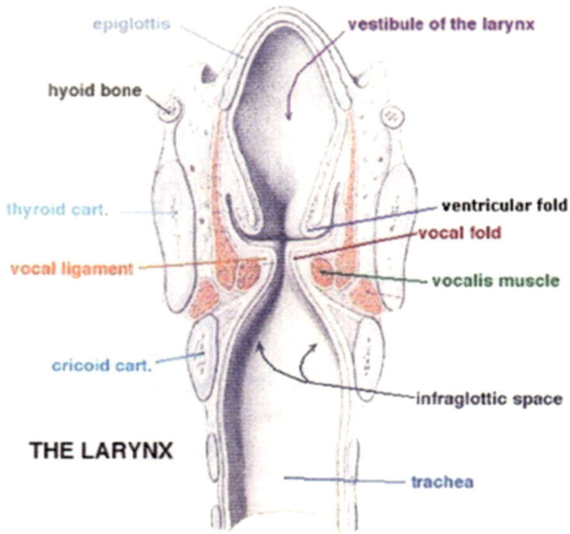

Figure 2. Coronal section of larynx.

2.1.1. Epiglottis, plicae ventricularis and glottis

The anterior side of epiglottis or pars lingulais is free and covered with weakly adhered mucosa, which allows easy stretchening around edema. Its posterior side called pars laryngis completely belongs to the larynx and is bent above the larynx aperture. Pedicle of epiglottis or petiolus is tied along the posterior side of the thyroid angle. Petiolus makes a bump on its mucosa, which covers the anterior commissure and, therefore, it can hardly be seen by indirect laryngoscopy. Mucosa of the epiglottic laryngeal side is tightly connected with its base. Vocal cords stretch from the back side of the thyroid angle and backwards to the vocal ending of the arytenoid cartilage, Figure 3.

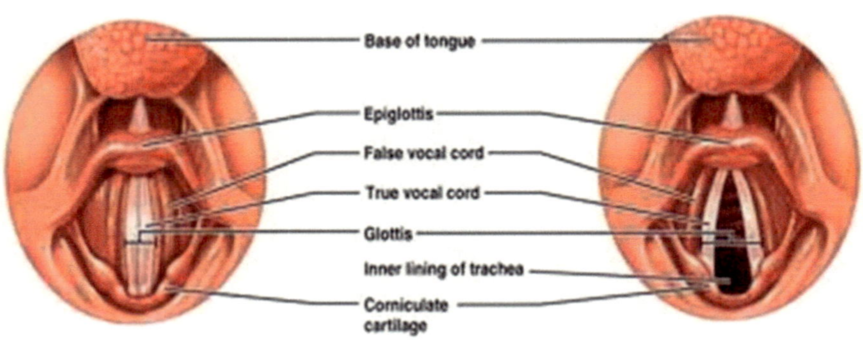

Figure 3. Internal view of larynx.

They present triangular prismatic plicae. Their upper side is turned upwards and outside and continues its way laterally on the base of the ventriculus Morgagni, while their inferior side is turned downwards and inside and continues its way slopingly into the subglottic space. When seen microscopically, they are whitish with vertical capillaries. Vocal ligament makes elastic skeleton of the vocal cord. Length of the vocal cord is changeable and it depends on its position and tighteness. When calm, it is about 30mm in men and 20mm in women. Subglottic space extends from the vocal cords down to the inferior edge of the cricoid cartilage and it has a conical shape. Its mucosa is tightly connected to the cartilage and they are separated only by elastic membrane.

2.1.2. Laryngeal cartilages

Skeleton of the larynx consists of 16 cartilages: 6 paired and 4 unpaired. There are four large cartilages: thyroid or cartilago thyreoidea, cricoid or anular or cartilago cricoidea, paired arytenoid or cartilago arytenoidea and epiglottic or cartilago epiglottica. The first three are hyaline and the fourth one is fibrocartilagenous. The thyroid cartilage is the gratest cartilage of the larynx. It has a shape of a shield or a shape of a book opened backwards, Figure 4.

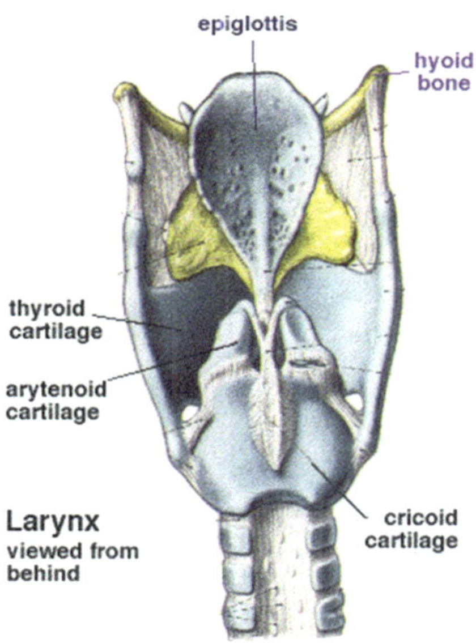

Figure 4. Lateral view of laryngeal cartilages.

Two thyroid quandrangle plates (lamine s. alae) are connected in their anterior middle part under the right angle in men and under 120 degrees in women. Plates become ossified around the age of 25 and the process ends around the age of 65. Its posterior edge extends upwards with the greater horn or cornu superior towards the hyoid bone and downwards with its interior side, little horn or cornu inferior is joined with the cricoid cartilage. The epiglottic cartilage is located in the anterior wall of the larynx and has a shape of a rose leaf. Its superior, wider part is the larynx lid, and lower narrower part is pedicle or petiolus. There are many concaves on the epiglottic cartilage that are filled with lymph tissue. The epiglottic cartilage is elastic and never ossifies in contrast to others that are hyaline and therefore start to ossify right after the puberty. Cricoid or anular cartilage is placed in the inferior part of the larynx. It has a shape of a ring which is narrow in front and wider in the back. Ossifying of this cartilage begins around the age of 65. There are two small smooth surfaces for joining with arytenoid cartilages on both sides on the superior edges of cricoid lamina. The anterior cartilage is made of an arch or arcus. There are round surfaces for joining with inferior horns of the thyroid cartilage on the joining of the arch and lamina. Arytenoid cartilages are paired and they are placed in the posterior wall of the larynx. They have a shape of a triangular pyramid. The base of the pyramid is turned downwards and is located on the superior edge of the anular cartilage plate. On the inferior part, near the base of this cartilage, there are two extensions and one of them is turned medially or processus vocalis and the other one is turned laterally or processus muscularis. Musculus vocalis (m. thyroarytenoideus) attaches on vocal extension. Glottis adductors and abductors attach on the muscular extension. The main extension of the arytenoid cartilage extends with an elastic connection (ligamentum vocale) which extends forward and ends on the interior side of the thyroid cartilage under its superior incesure. Right above the anterior joint of this connection, another connection or ligamentum vestibulare begins, and it continues backwards and ends on the anterior edge of the arytenoid cartilage on one small protuberance or colliculus.

2.1.3. Joints of the larynx

There are two important joints on every side. They are synovial and enforced by a capsule. Articulatio cricothyreoidea is located between cornu inferior of the thyroid cartilage and cricoid cartilage on the joint of the arcus and lamina.

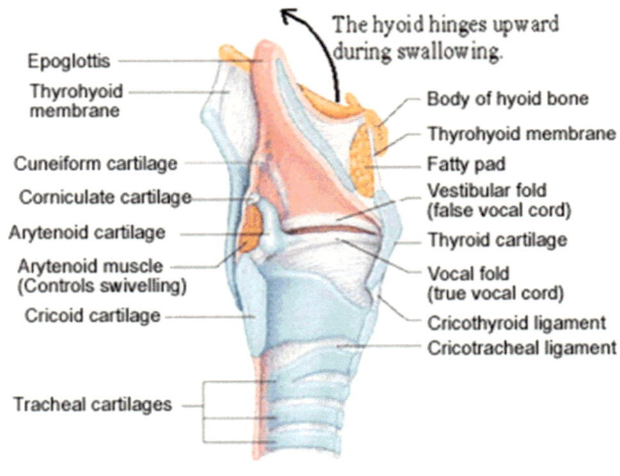

Figure 5. Joints of the larynx.

Movements in this joint are rotation around the horizontal arytenoid axis and very restricted movements of sliding. Articulatio crycoarytenoidea is located between the arytenoid base and joint surfaces on superior edge of the cricoid cartilage. Movements in the joint are rotation around the vertical arytenoid axis and movements of sliding when arytenoids adduct or abduct, Figure 5.

2.1.4. Fibrous links of the larynx – membranes and ligaments

Membranes and ligaments of the larynx are divided into three groups. The first group consists of ligaments of joints' capsules, cricothyroid and cricoarytenoid. The second group consists of interior fibrous tissue made of memrane elastica laryngis. Superior membrane supports aryepiglottic and plicae ventricularis, while inferior membrane or conus elasticus goes between the superior edge of the cricoid and inferior edge of the thyroid cartilage up to behind the vocal extension. Ligamentum vocale presents superior, free edge of conus elasticus. The anterior part of the conus elasticus is tightly thickened in the middle and it makes ligamentum thyreoepiglotticum, which links epiglottis and thyroid cartilage. The third group consists of: membrane thyrohyoidea with the aperture for upper laryngeal artery and vein and internal branch of superior laryngeal nerve, cricotrachealis membrane lies between the inferior edge of the cricoid cartilage and the first tracheal ring and ligamentum hyoepiglotticum, which attaches epiglottis to hyoid bone, Figure 6.

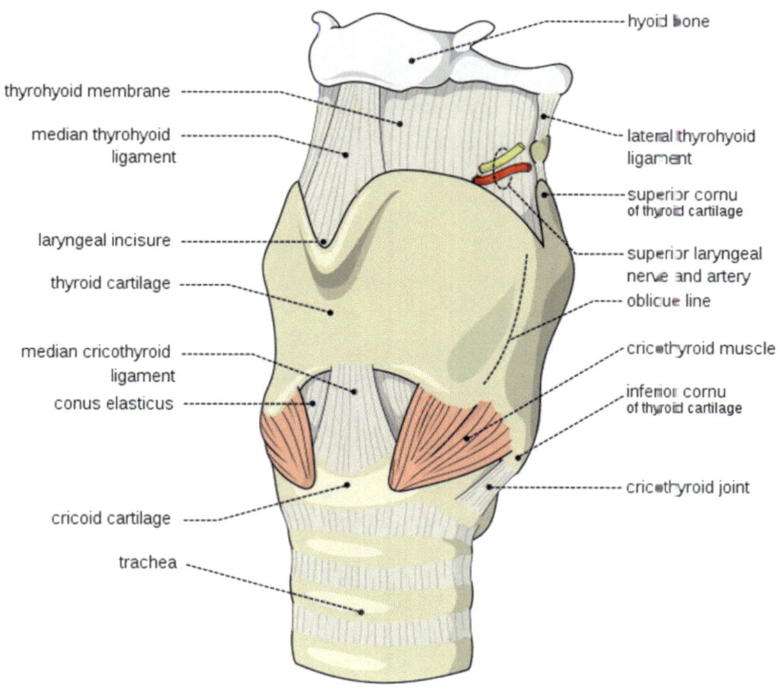

Figure 6. Membranes and ligaments of the larynx.

2.1.5. Muscles of the larynx

Muscles of the larynx are divided into A. internal and B. external. A. Internal muscles (Figure 7) are placed between some of the cartilages and are divided into 1. abductors, 2. adductors, 3. tensors and 4. covers of the larynx lumen. 1. Laryngeal abductors are two muscles on each side of the larynx, m. cricoarytenoideus posterior s. posticus. Its function is to abduct vocal cords from the middle line and thus to open glottis. 2. Adductors adduct vocal cords to the middle line and close glottis. These are: a) m. cricoarytenoideus lateralis s. lateralis b) m. interarytenoideus s. transversus c) m. thyroarytenoideus or pars externa s. externus. 3. Laryngeal tensors are: a) m. cricothyreoideus s. anterior is external laryngeal tensor. It adducts the thyroid cartilage to the cricoid cartilage from the anterior side, and thus tights the vocal cords intermediately. b) m. thyroarytenoideus or pars interna s. internus s. vocalis is known as internal larynx tensor and forms a vocal cord. 4) covers of the larynx lumen: a) m. interarytenoideus – pars obliqua has a role of glottic sphincter, b) m. aryepiglotticus represents an extension of pars transversa muscles interarytenoidus into aryepiglottic plicae and has a function of a supraglottic sphincter. B. External laryngeal muscles: a) m. sternothyroideus is pulling the larynx downwards, b) m. thyrohyoideus is raising the larynx if hyoid is fixed, in other words, lowering hyoid bone if the larynx is fixed.

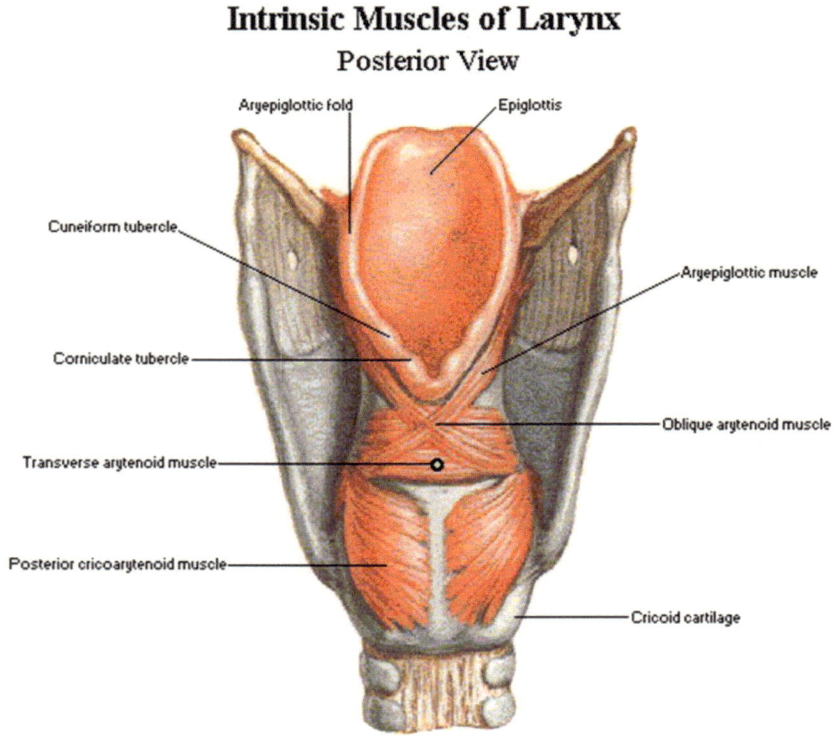

Figure 7. Internal laryngeal muscles.

2.1.6. Laryngeal mucosa

Laryngeal mucosa encases the whole of its cavity. It is separated from cartilage and muscles by submucosa and elastic membrane. On the superior larynx aperture, mucosa continues its way forward across the superior edge and anterior side of epiglottis into the mucosa of the root of the tongue, laterally and backwards into the pharynx mucosa, then it encases the external surface of the anterior wall of the larynx and it continues downwards into the trachea. Laryngeal mucosa is tightened very loosely to submucosa and elastic aperture, except at the front on the epiglottic cartilage and at the back on Santorini cartilages and superior ends of the arytenoid cartilages. There are many tubuloalveolar glands of serous or seromucous nature. Apart from tiny glands that can be found almost everywhere in laryngeal mucosa, three main groups of glands are placed :a) on the top of laryngeal epiglottic side and in the root of the lingual side, b) in the wall of ventriculus Morgagni and c) in the plicae ventricularis. Otherwise, there aren't mucous glands on the free edges of the vocal cords. Larynx mucosa epithelium can be: 1) placoid-layered; 2) cylindrical-ciliary, respiratory type and 3) transitory pseudo-layered cylindrical epithelium (transitory type). Placoid-layered epithelium encases the vocal cords, superior larynx aperture and it goes downwards into the vestibulum, free epiglottic edge, epiglottic plicae, internal side of the arytenoid and interarytenoid space. This epithelium covers the whole glottis from the anterior commissure at the front and back to processus vocalis and interior side of arytenoid. It goes under the free edge of glottis and laterally towards the plicae ventricularis for 6 to 8mm. There are 20 to 30 rows of cells in that region. Under normal conditions, the isles of placoid epithelium can be found scattered in the zones of cylindrical-ciliary epithelium and in the larynx vestibulum. The passage between placoid-layered and ciliar epithelium in the level of the vocal cords and free edges of the larynx is manifested as transformation of superficial planocells into cylindrical cells. And opposite, in the level of placoid cells isle, these variations can continue one to another without the passage. The most important of all the layers is the superficial layer which is made of more planocells that desquamate but don't keratinize. Under the ifluence of toxins, chronic irritation and inflammation, this epithelium can show similar characteristics as horny layer and epithelium extensions go into the derm so that papillae become higher. Cylindrical-ciliary epithelium of respiratory type covers the remaining, largest part of the larynx surface.

In 20 % of the cases, the anterior ends of the vocal cords are characterized by a narrow band of epithelium of transitory type. This epithelium is sometimes present in subglottis. Mucosa of the vocal cords has one macroscopic characteristic of a special importance like Reink spaces which goes along the whole length of the vocal cords between mucosa and vocal ligament. Macroscopically, there isn't a point of joining mucosa with a vocal ligament.

2.1.7. Blood vessels, nerves and lymph vessels of the larynx

Arterial vascularization of the larynx comes from: a) a. thyreoidea superior (branch a. carotis externa) via its branches aa. thyreoidea superior et media. These arteries go into the larynx on the posterior part of the thyrohyoid membrane, b) a. thyreoidea inferior (branch arteria subclavia) that follows n. recurrens on its way into the larynx. Veins of the larynx follow arteries of the same name. The larynx is innervated by the branch n. vagus: 1) n. laryngeus superior which has two laryngeal branches, internal and external (Figure 8). The internal branch is often sensitive and gives sensory innervation for the whole larynx lumen till the vocal cords height. It goes through the thyrohyoid membrane with superior laryngeal artery and vein. The external branch is motor and innervates the anterior cricothyroid muscle and goes along the inferior edge of superior pharynx constrictor; 2) n. laryngeus inferior s. recurrens which is on the left side much longer than on the right side. Left recurrens goes round the aortic arch and the right recurrens goes round the artery subclavia and then goes upwards in the gutter between the trachea and esophagus. It enters the larynx right behind the lower cricothyroid muscle and then divides into two branches: motor or anaetreolateral branch which innervates all internal muscles of the larynx, except the front cricothyroid muscle; and sensitive or postmedial branch for subglottic space. Nerve fibres n. recurrens that are on one side don't go on the opposite side. Lymph vessels of the larynx are divided into two parts, superior that are above the vocal cords or supraglottic and inferior, below the vocal cords or subglottic. Lymph vessels of the superior part flow into preepiglottic lymph nodes and superior deep neck lymph nodes. Lymph vessels of the inferior part flow into prelaryngeal lymph nodes and inferior deep neck lymph nodes. The vocal cords practically don't have their lymph vessels.

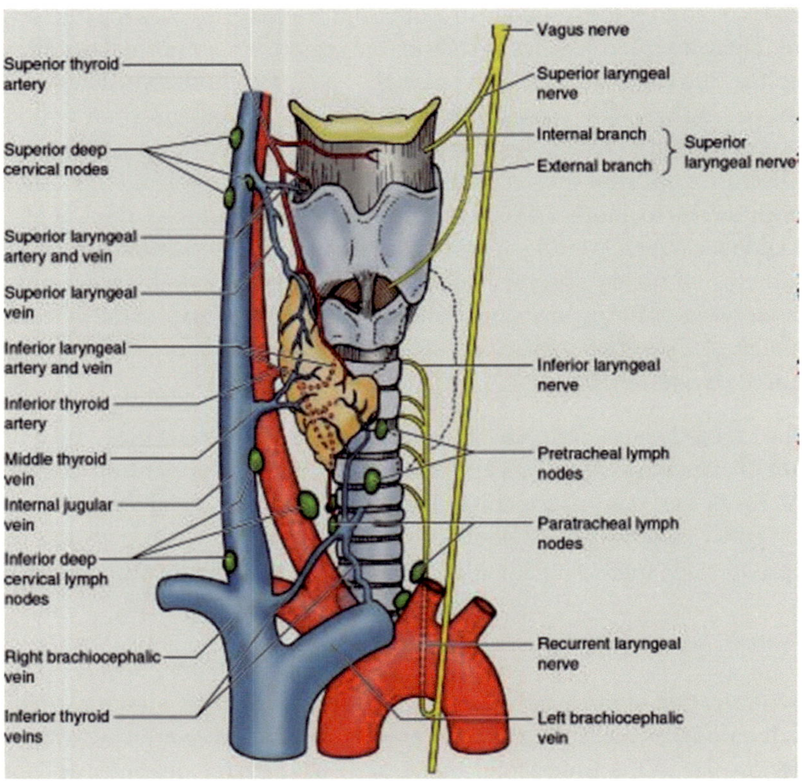

Figure 8. Blood vessels, nerves and lymph vessels of the larynx.

2.2. Physiology of the larynx

Functions of the larynx can be primary and secondary. Primary functions are phylogenetically the oldest and they contain the following functions: respirations, protection of airways, swallowing, thorax fixation. Secondary functions are adapted to breathing and swallowing organs, ant the most important of them is phonation.

2.2.1. Respiratory function of the larynx

Glottis opens one second before the air comes into it by lowering diaphragm. This opening is a consequence of cricoarytenoid muscle contraction which is innervated by nerve recurrens and it begins right before the motor activity of n. frenicus. It is led across the respiratory centre as the activity of n. frenicus, it increases with hypercapnia and ventilatory obstruction, and it decreases with artery hyperoxygenation and hyperventilation. This activity is deleted by tracheotomy, as a result of lowered ventilation resistence. Hemoreceptor corpusculs are identified in supraglottic mucosa, so their stimulation during hypercapnia decreases laryngeal resistence during the inspiration and expiration. Inspiratory dilation of the larynx isn't distributed to glottis and it doesn't depend on muscle activity. With inspiratory lowering of the larynx from hyoid downwards, true and false vocal cords contract, arytenoid cartilages go laterally and glottis opens. Passive opening of the larynx is still intensified also by the inspiratory phase, in other words activity of external laryngeal muscles. The result of glottis opening size variation during respiration allows the larynx to contribute significantly to internal air resistance during the respiration time, so abduction of the vocal cords produces glottis dilatation and reduction of opening during the inspiration time, and adduction of the vocal cords with glottis constriction produces greater resistence to expiratory air, which influences the depth and level of respiration. These reflex changes are a consequence of reaction on presoreceptors in lungs and subglottic part of the trachea and can help in mixing the air in the lungs. After vagus deafferention, neither inflation nor deflation influence respiratory activity in posterior cricoarytenoid. Corrections of glottis opening compensate changes in total air resistance which increased in the nose and bronchi.

2.2.2. Circulatory function of the larynx

Normal respiration, in other words normal air circulation through the larynx, allows normal functioning of the circulatory system, heart and blood vessels. Arrhytmia, bradycardia and periodical cardiac arrest, can result in stimulation of the larynx. The mechanism is connected to the nerve fibres stimulation that comes from aortal baroreceptors and goes to the central nervous system across n. laryngeus recurrens, ramus communicans and n. laryngeus superior. These fibres go through the larynx into the deep tissue near thyroid plates and they are stimulated when the larynx is dilated.

2.2.3. Protective function of the larynx

Almost at the same time with respiration, mechanism of protection of the inferior airways developed, protecting them from entering foreign bodies, and this protection is guided by following mechanisms: 1. Sphincter mechanism. There are three sphincters in the larynx and they are the vocal cords, ventriculous and aryepiglottic plicae so it comes to: adduction of the true vocal cords one to another, closing of the false vocal cords one to another and to the base of epiglottis, posterior commissure of the vocal cords is closed by rotation and adduction of the arytenoid cartilages, constriction of the false vocal cords by activity of internal laryngeal muscles, lifting and moving the larynx to the front, moving the base of epiglottis backwards and covering aditus, moving tyreoepiglottic ligamentum to the front. The previous movements, first of all the tongue base and aryepiglottic plicae, lead to direction of food bolus to peripheral sinus and thus allows the function of the larynx while swallowing; 2. Reflex inhibition mechanism of respiration starts when food bolus touches the posterior wall of the pharynx and because of that, breathing stops immediately. Respiration ceases while swallowing. This is a reflex which results from stimuli coming from the pharynx when food enters, and they transfer via n. glossopharyngeus and n. vagus. Receptors are the richest in mucosa of the laryngeal side of epiglottis, aryepiglottic and plicae ventricularis and interarytenoid area; 3. Cough reflex is weak or it doesn't exist in newborn children. Reflex centre is in medulla oblongata, and n. vagus is both afferent and efferent part of the reflex arch. Closing of the false vocal cords is an important moment for this reflex, because adduction of the true vocal cords one to another can bring by itself to preventing the air to come out of the lungs. When high subglottic pressure is reached, sphincter mechanism suddenly relaxes and the air under the accumulated pressure comes out. In this way, matters that initiated this reflex also go out. 4. Phonatory function is secondary adapted to respiratory and swallowing organs. It developed later in phylogenetic development thanks to high differentiation of the central nervous system. For proper accomplishment of all the activities that the larynx carries out, there has to be full coordination of both synergistic and antagonistic groups of muscles. During phonation, the vocal cords are in adduction near medial line by the action of cricothyroid muscles that present the vocal cords tensors. More subtle changes are a consequence of thyroarytenoid muscles action. Medial movement of the vocal cords towards the false ones are caused by: a) tension in the vocal cords, b) lowering of subglottic air pressure with every vibrating aperture of glottis and c) aspirating the air that ran away which is known as Bernuli phenomenon. The result of such repeated cycles of glottis opening and closing is freeing of small clouds from subglottic air column which forms sound waves.

2.2.4. Function of thorax fixation

When the larynx is closed, thorax is fixed and serves as adminiculum when some activities connected to the effort are held out: climbing, lifting burden, defaecation, delivery.

2.2.5. Function of emotions

Different mental conditions are expressed over the voice or they cause disorder in it.

2.2.6. Phonation function

This function of the larynx is philogenetically the youngest function which was adapted to breathing and swallowing organs and it developed thanks to high diferentiation of the central nervous system. Production of voice is a very complex process and it depends on compliance in the body. It presents integral function in which peripheral and central phonatory organs take part in. Peripheral organs are: voice activator (lungs, diaphragm), voice generator (larynx) and resonator (pharynx, mouth, nose and paranasal cavities). Central organs for voice and speech are located in the central nervous system (cortex, lower centres, reticular substance, cerebellum and others). Voice and speech of the humans are under the influence of psyche, neurovegetative system and endocrine system. One of the most important preconditions for normal development of speech is preserved hearing. A system called "feed back" participates in forming and maintaining voice and speech. Besides hearing, its main elements are eyesight and sensibility, and main activities in the sense of creating voice and speech happen in the central nervous system. Three-dimensional analysis of movements in cricoarytenoid joint shows that vocal ligaments, cricothyroid ligament and conus elasticus are the most important in the control of abduction, while posterior cricoarytenoid muscle and conus elasticus take part in restriction of adduction. Vocal ligament makes moving of the vocal arytenoid cartilage extension backwards impossible, while cricoarytenoid and posterior capsular ligament restrict movement of vocal extension forward. Anterior capsular ligament restricts slanting of the arytenoid cartilage posteriorly and moving of the arytenoid cartilage laterally across joint surface of the cricoid cartilage (Wang, 1998).

2.3. Etiology of rheumatoid arthritis and laryngeal rheumatoid arthritis

Rheumatoid arthritis (RA) is an inflammatory chronic systemic disease of unknown cause that affects peripheral joints symmetrically and permanently and is often connected to positive rheumatoid factor and/or positive results on anticyclic citrulined peptide immunoglobulins.. Annual incidence of RA in the world is 3 patients out of 1000 people, and the prevalence is from 0,5 – 5%. The disease is mainly present in some groups of population like North American natives, while it is less present in some other groups like black people in Carribean region. When gender is taken into consideration, the disease is three times more frequent in women than men. It can start at any age but its greatest frequency is in the fourth and fifth decade and it grows in the old age so it is the highest in people at the age of 25 to 50. Arthritis rate is from 5-6% in the Americans from Asian/Pacific islands, to 12% in Afro-Americans to 16% in white people. Etiology of rheumatoid arthritis includes more assumed theories. One of them says that obesity, weakness and morning rigidity are important in appearing of this disease. Apart from joints, RA can also have extra-articular localizations such as skin, heart, lungs and eyes. Another etiological theory implies presence of infectious cause of rheumatoid arthritis (Mycoplasma, Epstein-Bar virus, parvovirus, rubella) but none of the mentioned micro-organisms has been proved. Some of the medications from the group of medications that modify the disease also have antimicrobical activity and they are gold salts, antimalarial medications and minocyclin. In the joints of rheumatoid arthritis patients, bacterial DNA is found, which is also an indirect proof of the bacterial etiology. Autoimmune processes, as one more theory out of the assumed etiological theories, are tightly connected to RA but it isn't known if they appear as a primary or secondary process. In the RA patients, autoantibodies aren't directed towards one immunoglobulin G but also towards other different antigens, such as nuclear antigens (RA 33, EBNA), citrulined proteins (anti-CCP antibodies), collagen and glucose-6-isomarase phosphate. RA has an important genetic predisposition and that is one more theory about RA. About 60% of patients in the USA has a common epitope HLA-DR4 claster which consists of peptide connected place of the adequate HLA-DR molecule and it is joined with RA. As women suffer from RA about three times more often than men, sexual hormones explain one more etiological theory of RA. Complaints almost completely disappear during pregnancy, but in the postmenopause period, recurrences of the disease appear. RA rarely appears in women who use oral contraceptives. It is also described that hyperprolactinemia can be a risk factor for RA. Hyperplasia of synovial cells and activation of endothelial cells are early occurences in the pathological process that lead to uncontrolable inflammatory process and consequent cartilage and bone damage. Pathological production and regulation of both pro-inflammatory and anti-inflammatory cytokines are found in RA. In tissue immunity, the most important are Th1 CD4 cells, mononuclear phagocytes, fibroblasts, osteoclasts and neutrophils. B lymphocytes can serve as an antigen of the presenting cell and they create autoantibodies (for example rheumatoid factor – RF). One of the therapeutic possibilities is, therefore, the elimination of B lymphocytes population by mononuclear antibodies (for example rituximab^R which is often used in combination with methrotrexate). In RA patients, many other changed cells are found, such as numerous cytokines, hemokines. Other mediators of inflammation are also described: tumor necrosis factor-alpha, interleucins 1 and 6, transforming growth factor – beta, interleucin 8, fibroblast growth factor, growth factor received from thrombocytes. Finally, inflammation and uncontrolable synovial proliferation lead to damage of certain tissues, mostly cartilages, bones, strings, ligaments and blood vessels. Other predisposing factors are psychological stress and smoking. The so far known risk factors in RA are: female gender, positive family history, older age, exposure to silicates and smoking (Kuder, 2002). Drinking more than two cups of coffee a day, high intake of vitamin D, consuming of tea and oral contraceptives reduce risk for RA (Mikuls, 2002; Merlino, 2004).

2.4. Pathoanatomy of rheumatoid arthritis and laryngeal rheumatoid arthritis

Damage of joints in RA is caused by proliferation of synovial macrophages and fibroblasts, probably as a response to possible autoimmune and infectious triggers. Therefore, it comes to lymphocyte proliferation of perivascular region and proliferation of endothelial cells which cause new blood vessels to multiply and ingrow. In damaged joints, blood vessels become clogged by small clots or inflammatory cells. Furthermore, the progress of process leads to irregular growth (Firestein, 2005; Goldring, 2000). RA in the larynx can manifest in the following forms: 1) Arthritis of cricothyroid and/or cricoarytenoid joint (Ferdynus-Chromy, 1977; Gotze, 1973; Kubiak-Socha, 1973; Woldorf, 1971; De Gandt, 1969; Copeman, 1968), 2) Rheumatoid nodules (Bridger, 1980; Bonner, 1977; Abadir, 1974), 3) Laryngeal myositis, 4) Neuropathy of laryngeal nervus recurrens and 5) Postcricoid granulomas (Bienenstock H, 1963). Histological examinations of cricoarytenoid joints in RA have shown synovitis as the earliest change that leads to synovial proliferation, fibrinous deposit, forming of pannus on joint surfaces, erosion of the joint cartilage and finally obliteration and ankylosis of joints. Cricoid necrosis as the last phase of pathological changes on the cricoid cartilage can cause serious pathophysiological disturbances (Gatland, 1988). Neural atrophy of laryngeal muscles and degenerative changes in laryngeal nerves caused by vasculitis, can follow the degree of affection of cricoarytenoid joint (Voulgari PV, 2005; Lofgren RH, 1962). Rheumatoid nodules of different size in the larynx are mainly found with seropositive RA. Methotrexate can raise the development of nodules (Kerstens, 1992). Microtrauma, especially a repeated one, can create predisposition for RA. In the largest number of cases, nodules are found subcutaneously. A few small nodules can be noticed microscopically in submucous layer, and each of them consists of fibrinous necrosis focus surrounded by histiocytes arranged like palisades. There is a progressive proliferation of endothelial cells and fibroblasts as well as the infiltration of plasma cells and lymphocytes in fibrous supporting tissue that surrounds nodules (Webb J, 1972).

2.5. Pathophysiology of rheumathoid arthritis and laryngeal rheumatoid arthritis

Factors joined with RA include the possibility of infectious trigger, genetic predispositions and autoimmune response. $CD4^{+}T$ cells lead to immunological cascade reaction which causes secretion of cytokines such as tumor necrosis alpha and interleucin 1. Increased formation and expression of TNF-alpha cause inflammation of synovial membranes and joint destruction. Inflammation, proliferation and degeneration are typical for affected synovial membranes. Joint deformations and working inability happen because of erosion and destroying of synovial membranes and joint surfaces. Acute obstruction of the superior airways leads to inspiratory stridor, the use of subsidiary respiratory musculature which is manifested by entrainment in jugulum, intercostal spaces, supraclavicular pits and in epigastrium, respiratory weaknesses, peripheral cyanosis, state of shock and coma (Lehmann, 1997). Chronic obstruction of the superior airways can lead to hypoxia, hypercapnia and respiratory acidosis which cause pulmonary hypertension and cor pulmonale (McGeehan, 1989).

2.6. Clinical picture of rheumatoid arthritis and laryngeal rheumatoid arthritis

Clinical picture of RA can be divided into several groups of clinical manifestations of the disease, depending on the affected organs/systems: 1) Pulmonary, 2) Cardiovascular, 3) Constitutional, 4) Manifestations from rheumatoid nodules, 5) Eye manifestations, 6) Neurological, 7) Cutaneous, 8) Hematological, 9) Renal and 10) Hepatic manifestations. 1) Pulmonary manifestations of RA are pleuritic effusion, pulmonary nodules, interstitial fibrosis, pneumonitis and arteritis. 2) Cardiovascular manifestations are coronary disease, inflammatory pericarditis and pericarditis with effusion, myocarditis, mitral valves disease, disorder in conducting. 3) Constitutional manifestations of RA can be high body temperature, asthenia, weight loss, exhaustion and loss of appetite. 4) Rheumatoid nodules can manifest subcutaneously or in pulmonary parenchyma. 5) Eye manifestations are kretoconjuctivitis, episcleritis, scleritis and conjuctivitis. 6) Neurological manifestations of RA can be neuropathies such as carpal tunnel syndrome, multiple mononeuritis, cervical myelopathy, central nervous system diseases (stroke, hemorrhage, encephalopathy, meningitis). 7) Cutaneous manifestations in RA can appear as ulcus cruris, palmar erythema and skin vasculitis. 8) Hematological manifestations of RA appear as anemia, thrombocytosis, granulocytopenia, eosinophilia, cryglobunemia and hypertreaclines. 9) Renal manifestations can appear as glomerulonephritis, vasculitis and secondary amyloidosis. 10) Hepatic manifestations of RA are characterized by high level of liver enzymes. American association of rheumatologists has set up the following criteria for RA clasification: 1. Rigidity in and around joints that lasts at least one hour before maximum improvement in the morning hours. 2. Arthritis of three or more joint regions. At least three joint regions have soft tissue swellings or liquid which was diagnosed by a clinician. Fourteen possible regions include left and right superior interphalangeal (GIF) joint, metacarpophalangeal (MCF) joint, wrist joint, elbow joint, knee joint, ankle and metatarsophalangeal (MTF) joints; 3. Arthritis of wrist joints; at least one region of carpus, GIF and MCF are swollen; 4. Symmetric arthritis, in other words simultaneous affection of the same joint region on both sides of the body. Mutual affection of GIF, MCF and MTF without absolute proportion is also accepted; 5. Rheumatoid nodules are subcutaneous nodules that are present above the osseus bumps or extensory surfaces or surfaces around the regions that are close to joints; 6. Serum RF; 7. Radiographic changes typical for RA on postero-anterior radiographies of hand and carpus, that have to enclose erosions or disproportional decalcification of bones localized in or on the rims of the most common affected joints. Independent osteoarthritic changes are not a criterion for RA. Presence of four out of seven criteria are enough for diagnosis. Criteria from 1 to 4 have to be present at least 6 weeks, and the physician has to establish criteria from 2 to 5. RA is often manifested with constitutional symptoms such as myelalgia, weight loss, high body temperature, weight loss and exhaustion. Patients can have difficulties with every day activities (dressing up, getting up, walking, personal hygiene, the use of arms). In most of the patients, RA has a perfidious start. It can start with systemic manifestations such as high body temperature, exhaustion, arthralgia and weakness before the appearance of swelling joints and inflammation. In the lower percentage, the patients have abrupt start with acute development of synovitis and extra-articular manifestations. Laryngeal manifestations of rheumatoid arthritis were described for the first time in 1880. by Mackenzie M. and later, 1894. Mackenzie GH. (Mackenzie, 1880; Mackenzie, 1894). Cricoarytenoid arthritis can be divided into two phases, acute and chronic, and it appears in 27-78% of RA patients (Tarnowska, 2004), and according to some authors in 17-70% when the research is done laryngoscopically, by computered larynx tomography and histopathological cadaveric examinations (Voulgari, 2005). In 55% of patients, cricoarytenoid arthritis is asymptomatic (Jurik, 1984). At the beginning of the disease, symptoms are mild but usually subclinical. Acute cricoarytenoid arthritis is manifested by feeling of a foreign body in the throat or a feeling of tension in neck or even feeling of burning , hoarseness, odynophonia, voice weakness, changes in voice tone, odynophagia or dysphagia, pain or the feeling of hardness that becomes worse while speaking, spreading of pain to ear, feeling of suffocating, coughing, dyspnea or the feeling of rigidity. In the chronic phase of cricoarytenoid arthritis, patients often complain of hoarse speech, stridor that appears while making an effort, dyspnea, pain while speaking, neck swelling, hoarseness and these symptoms appear during an infection or during a dream (Braverman, 2007). Laryngeal symptoms during RA vary in their manifestations from 31-75%, while histopathological changes in the larynx are presented postmortem in 90% (Pearson, 1957; Copeman, 1957). According to some authors, stridor appears during exercising in 75% of the cases (Charlin, 1985) and can be the result of inflammation and swelling of arytenoid and posterior commissure during an acute affection of joint or because of joint ankylosis in the chronic RA phase. The most frequent symptoms are the feeling of a foreign body in the throat (51%), hoarseness (47%) and voice weakness (29%) (Amernik, 2007). Hoarseness appears only in 5% of RA patients (Fisher, 2008), while some other researches have shown that it appears in 30% of RA patients (Segebarth, 2007). Hard RA can be manifested by laryngeal obstruction and can lead to heart, pulmonary and fatal complications. Rheumatoid nodules of the larynx are often manifested by hoarseness and coughing.

2.7. Diagnosis of rheumatoid arthritis and laryngeal rheumatoid arthritis

Thorough anamnesis, careful examination of joints and periarticular soft tissue structures, as well as laboratory and imaging results are necessary for right diagnosis of RA. None laboratory test is specific for RA, so its diagnosis is primary clinical. A clinical examination can establish that mostly small wrists and ankles are affected relatively symmetrically. The most frequently affected joints, with decreasing frequency, are MCF, wrist joint, GIF, knee joint, MTF, shoulder joint, ankle, cervical spine, hip and temporomandibular joints. The patient whom we treated, had prominent changes on the wrists which can be clearly seen in the Figure 9.

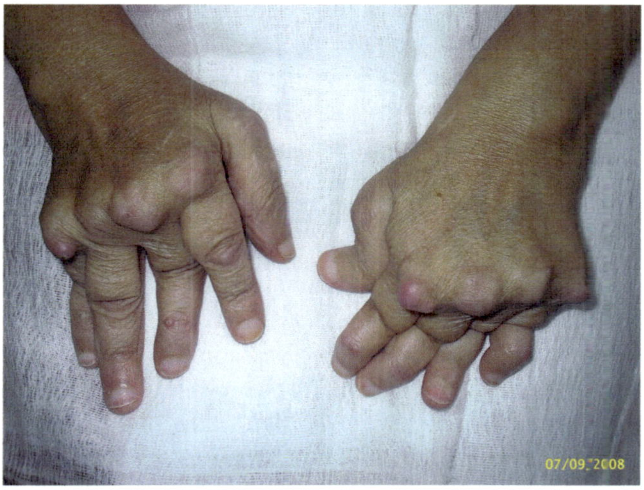

Figure 9. Hand changes of reumatoid arthritis.

Joints show inflammation with swelling, painfulness, locally high temperature and restricted movement. Atrophy of interosseus muscles of hands is a typical early sign. Joints and chordae damage can lead to deformities such as ulnar deviation, hammer like fingers and occasionally joint rigidity. Other muscle-skeletal manifestations that are usually found during the examination are tendosynovitis and joined chordae rupture during the ligament and chordae affection, the most often affected are chordae of the fourth and fifth finger extensor, periarticular osteoporosis during the localized inflammation, generalized osteoporosis during systemic chronic inflammation, changes connected to immobilization, or corticosteroid therapy and syndrom of carpal tunnel. Cutaneous changes in RA appear like subcutaneous nodules, often along the pressure points (for example olecranon), ulceration of feet cutis, rashes in vasculitis, palmar erythema, gangrenous pyodermia. Vascular lesions of cutis can be manifested as palpable purpura or cutis ulceration. Cardial changes in RA lead to increased cardiovascular morbidity and mortality. Myocardial infarction, myocardial disfunction and constrictive pericarditis are rare. Affection of lungs in RA can have several forms like pleural effusion, interstitial fibrosis, nodules (Caplan syndrom) and bronchiolitis obliterans, in other words ogranized pneumonia. In gastrointestinal tract, the affection of intestines is a side effect of medication action, inflammation and other diseases. Kidneys are usually intact by direct action of RA. Secondary kidney damage often happens during medicamentous therapy (nonsteroidal anti-inflammatory drugs, gold salt, cyclosporin), inflammation (amyloidosis) and joined diseases (Sjögren syndrom with kidney tubular disorders). Vascular lesions can affect any organ, but are often found on cutis where they can be manifested as palpable purpura, cutis ulcerations or digital infarcts. Hematological disorders are often manifested by secondary anemia which is normochromic-normocytic type, thrombocytosis and eosinophilia. Affection of nerves is often as in nervus medianus syndrom in the carpal tunnel. Vascular lesions, mononeuritis multiplex and cervical myelopathy can cause serious neurological prolapses. RA is manifested on eyes like keratoconjuctivitis sicca, as well as episcleritis, uveitis and nodular scleritis which can lead to scleromalacia. American college for rheumatology has determined criteria for progression, remission and functional state of RA patient. A) RA progression (clinical and radiological stages): Stage 1 (early RA) is characterized by: a) absence of destructive changes during the roentgenography examinations and b) possible radiography presence of osteoporosis; Stage 2 (advanced progression): a) radiography evidence of periarticular osteoporosis with or without light subchondral destruction of bones, b) possible light destruction of cartilage, c) possible restriction of joint movements, without joint deformities, d) joined myatrophy, e) possible soft tissue extra-articular lesions (for example nodules, tenosynovitis). Stage 3 (very advanced progression): a) radiographic evidence of cartilage and bone destruction followed by periarticular osteoporosis, b) joint deformities (for example subluxation, ulnar deviation, hyperextension) without fibrous or osseus ankylosis, c) massive myatrophy, d) possible extra-articular lesions of soft tissue (for example nodules, tenosynovitis); Stage 4: a) fibrous or osseus ankylosis and b) criteria for stage 3. B) RA remission (≥ 5 below induced states that last at least two months constantly): a) morning rigidity that doesn't stop for 15 minutes, b) without weakness, c) without pain in joints, d) without cracking in joints or pain while moving, e) without soft tissue swelling in joints or chorda wraping, f) erythrocyte sedimentation lower than 30 mm/h in women or lower than 20mm/h in men. C) Functional status of RA patients: a) Category I – completely able to fullfil everyday activities, b) Category II – able to fullfil regular personal hygiene and activities connected to their profession but limited in other activities, c) Category III – able to fullfil the activities of regular personal hygiene but limited in activities connected to their proffession and other activities that aren't connected to their profession, d) Category IV – limited to fulfill regular activities for personal hygiene, profession and activities that aren't connected to their profession. American College of Rheumatologists (ACR) and European League Against Rheumatism (EULAR) have regulated new criteria for classification of early RA, which include joint affection, autoantibodies status, answer to acute phase and symptoms duration (Aletaha, 2010). ACR/EULAR 2010 criteria: A) Joint affection (0-5): one median to large joint (0), two to ten median to large joints (1), one to three small joints (large joints aren't included) (2), four to ten small joints (small joints aren't included) (3), more than ten joints (at least one small joint) (5); B) Serology (0-3): negative RF and negative cell-Purkinje antibodies (APCA) (0), Light positive RF or light positive APCA (2), high positive RF or high positive APCA (3); C) Reactants of acute phase (0-1); normal CRP and normal percentage of erythrocyte sedimentation (ESR) (0), Abnormal CRP or abnormal ESR (1); D) Symptoms duration: a) shorter than 6 weeks (0), 6 weeks and more (1). Cut point for RA is 6 weeks or more. RA can be diagnosed in patients if they have: a) atypical erosions or b) long lasting disease which fullfils the previous classification criteria. Large joints are defined as: shoulder joints, elbow joints, hip joints, knee joints and ankles. Small joints are defined as: MCF, PIF, from the second to fifth MTF and interphalangeal thumb joints and carpus joints. Course of disease can be short and limited or progressive and hard. The following laboratory tests are necessary to be carried out: complete blood count with differential count, rheumatoid factor, erythrocyte sedimentation, C-reactive proteins, fibrinogen, haptoglobin, alpha-1-acid glycoprotein, alpha-1-trypsin, S-amyloid-A protein and hematocrit (Guerra, 1992). Erythrocyte sedimentation and C-reactive protein give the best information about the presence of acute phase of RA, but thrombocytosis, low level of iron in the serum and low values of hemoglobin also point to active disease (Crassi, 1998). It is also important to examine the function of liver and kidneys because of further choice of medicaments, which shows that it is necessary to carry out a complete biochemical blood analysis. Diagnosis of rheumatoid changes in the larynx includes anamnesis, clinical examination, videolaryngoscopy, computered tomography and electromyography (Amernik, 2007) Indirect laryngoscopy shows changes in the larynx in 32% of RA patients, unlike computered tomography where the changes are found in 54%, so indirect laryngoscopy reveals mucous and great pathoanatomical changes, and computered larynx tomography reveals structural lesions (Lawry, 1984). Cricoarytenoid arthritis can be asymptomatic because many RA patients have pathological changes in cricoarytenoid joint, proved by computered tomography, but they don't have laryngeal difficulties (Brazeau-Lamontagne, 1986). Laryngoscopy in acute cricoarytenoid arthritis shows light red medially expressed swellings in the region of arytenoid, epiglottis, cricoarytenoid arthritis and vocal cords nodules that can look normal or very edematous. In chronic cricoarytenoid arthritis, we can find thickened mucosa in the region of arytenoid, interarytenoid pachydermia, uneven rima glottidis, called "bamboo nodules" because of their appearance that reminds of knots on the bamboo branch. During laryngoscopy of bamboo nodules, subepithelial sallow mass on upper surface of glottis is noticed, often mushroomlike shape and directed by its longer axis transversely to the vocal cords, and they are usually surrounded by hyperemic mucosa (Immerman, 2007; Hilgert, 2008). Direct fiber laryngoscopy can establish pathological changes in the larynx in 75% of RA patients (Brazeau-Lamontagne, 2005). The most frequent rheumatoid changes in the larynx are hyperemia of the mucosa in arytenoid subregion in 41% of the patients and edema of the same region in 28% of the patients (Amernik, 2007). Safe diagnosis of laryngeal RA is set in direct laryngoscopy by arytenoid palpation when mechanical restriction of movements in cricoarytenoid joint can be proved (Woods, 2007). Computered endovideostroboscopy allows examination of the way mucosa vibrates on the affected side, determination of lesion depth in mucous layer, confirming the unique characteristics of these lesions. In this way, we can diagnose disorders of adduction and lateral torsion of the vocal cords when they are present. During the palpation of these lesions in general anesthesia, we can find tough fibroid masses tightened on the deep vocal cords structures. Radiographic manifestations of the disease on wrists are characterised by swelling and mild juxta-articular osteoporosis. Radiographic indicators of cricoarytenoid joint affection are cricoarytenoid prominention (46%), changes in thickness and volume of joint (46%), as well as cricoarytenoid subluxation (39,9%). Radiographic signs of erosive arthritis of cricoarytenoid joint are present in 45% of patients (Jurik 1984). Computered tomography of the larynx is a method of choice in diagnosing cricoarytenoid thickness, erosions, arytenoid subluxations, glottic or aryepiglottic nodules asymmetry and by using this method, changes are found in 72% of RA patients (Brazeau-Lamontagne, 2005). Deviation of the larynx in three surfaces is a characteristic finding for RA in the advanced stage and it includes: 1) moving of the larynx anterio-laterally, 2) rotation of the vocal cords clockwise and 3) slantedness of the larynx forward while its front aspect is lowered caudally in relation to its front part (Keenan, 1983). Similar changes on multislice scanner larynx examination in the woman patient treated at our clinic and triploid deviation of the larynx can clearly be seen in Figure 10.

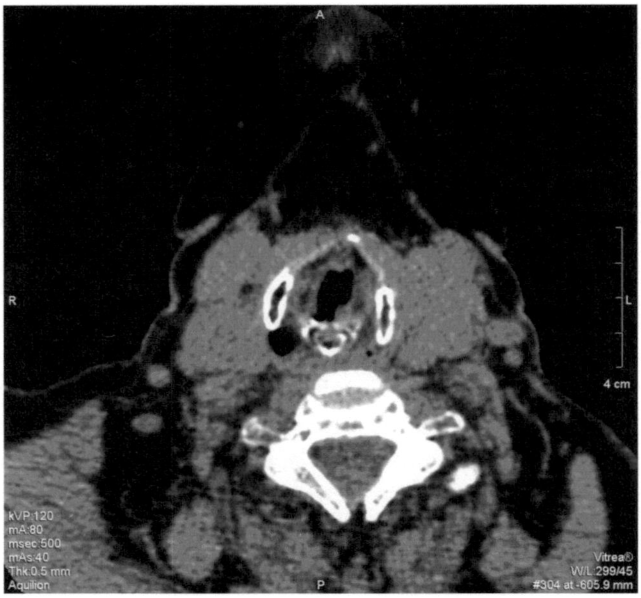

Figure 10. Sclerosis of the right arytenoid due the cricoarythenoid rheumatoid involvement. Also triplanar laryngeal deviation.

Nuclear magnetic resonance, computered tomography and scintigraphy can give useful information about pathological changes and their extension in RA. Ultrasonography is accepted for examination of joints, chordae and bursa affection in RA and it can advance early clinical diagnosis and following of patients, showing details such as synovial thicknesses in finger joints (Grassi W, 1998). In RA patients, electromyographic examinations of internal thyroarytenoid muscles show mutually normal bioelectric stimulation of thyroarytenoid muscles during phonation, while at rest there is no denervation activity (Tarnowska, 2004).

2.8. Complications of laryngeal rheumatoid arthritis

Complications of RA can begin to develop within several months since the appearance of clinical symptoms, so timely refering to a rheumatologist or his consultation are necessary for the beginning of treatment with DMARD (disease-modifying antireumatic drugs). A great number of acute respiratory insufficiency cases caused by rheumatoid arthritis in the larynx have been described (Chalmers, 1979; McGeehan, 1989). Acute respiratory insufficiency in RA patients can be provoked by bacterial infections of the larynx, mechanical larynx lesions or acute exacerbation of cricoarytenoid arthritis (Bolten, 1991; Geterud, 1986). Laryngeal obstruction required surgical tracheotomy of RA patients (Takakura, 2005; Jol, 1997; Daver, 1994; Ten Holter, 1988; Peters, 2011; Bossingham, 1996; Funk, 1975). Tracheotomy is necessary in 10-25% of patients with chronic cricoarytenoiditis (Tarnowska, 2004). Acute obstruction of airways is often connected to cervical spine ankylosis and impossibility of its extension (Miller, 1994). Cervical spine ankylosis was also present with the patient that we treated, it can easily be seen in Figure 6. and it can threaten surgical tracheotomy (Yonemoto, 2005).

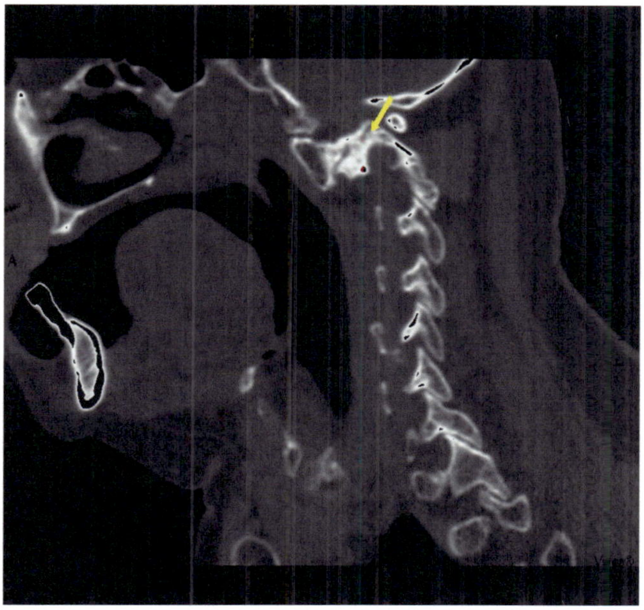

Figure 11. Atalantoccipital joint ankylosis. Arrow indicates patological process of cervical spine.

Vertical penetration of cerebral vertebra cusp was the most important manifestation of cervical spine disease, and one of the laryngeal deviation causes is the scoliotic trachea and the larynx deformation because of neck shortening as a consequence of the second cervical vertebra cusp penetration. Another machanism is rotational deformity of cervical vertebra caused by asymmetric osseous erosions (Keenan, 1983). Besides cricoarytenoid and cervical vertebra ankylosis, treatment of RA patients is also difficult because of temporomandibular joint ankylosis (Okuda, 1992; McGeehan, 1989). These pathological changes of RA patients can make endotracheal intubation very difficult and dangerous, especially if there is a triploid deviation of the larynx on computered tomography (Bamshad, 1989). Rheumatoid cricoarytenoid arthritis was complicated by ulcerous necrosis of cricoid esophagostenosis and therefore the patient underwent total laryngectomy (Montgomery, 1980).

2.9. Differential diagnosis of rheumatoid arthritis and laryngeal rheumatoid arthritis

Differential diagnosis is directed to artropathies caused by infection, seronegative spondyloartropathies and other connective tissue diseases such as systemic lupus eritematodes (Harris, 2005; Akil, 1995; Nanke, 2001).

RA should be distinguished from a wide range of diseases that are characterized by clinically prominent synovitis, such as viral, reactive and psoriatic arthritis as well as enteroarthritis and we can come to differential diagnosis by eliminating, because there isn't a specific test for RA (Grassi, 1998). Arthritis of cricoarytenoid joint is also caused by gout, mumps, tuberculosis, syphilis, gonorrhea, Tietz syndrom, lupus eritematodes and injuries (Fried, 1991). Rheumatoid nodules of the larynx as initial signs of systemic lupus eritematodes are described in the literature (Schwartz, 1980). Rheumatoid nodules of the larynx can be differentially diagnostic problem if they are mixed up with vascular lesions (Friedman, 1975). It is often important to distinguish by differential diagnosis asthma and psychoneurosis from cricoarytenoid joint arthritis which is rarely manifested by acute laryngeal obstruction and colapse (Leicht 1987; Absalom 1998). Secondary amyloidosis during rheumatoid arthritis or secondary Sjögren syndrom are rarely causes for laryngeal symptoms (Bayar, 2003). The case of RA and systemic sclerosis union is also described, which led to mutual immobility of the vocal cords and was manifested by dysphonia and dyspnea as main symptoms and treatment by sphygmic doses of methylprednisolone led to slow improvement (Ingegnoli, 2007). With other autoimmune diseases, transversal, white-yellow, striped lesions can be found, in the median part of membranous link of the vocal cords, mostly bilateral, but they aren't symmetrical (Ylitalo, 2003). Rheumatoid cricoarytenoid arthritis should be distinguished from neurogenic disorders, traumatic changes, infections, neoplastic processes and psychosomatic illnesses (Bolten, 1991; Chen, 2005). The most difficult differential diagnosis is in cricoarytenoid ankylosis and bilateral paresis/paralysis of recurrent laryngeal nerves. Mutual immobility of cricoarytenoid joint and Hashimoto thyroiditis are next differentially diagnostic problem which requires multidiscipline approach (Stojanovic, 2010). Then normal electromyogram of vocal muscles and fixation of cricoarytenoid joints during laryngoscopy set by application of laryngoscopic claws, confirm the diagnosis of ankylosis. Differential diagnosis of these two conditions is possible by using electromyography and laryngoscopy, and mutual fixation of the arytenoid cartilages is confirmed with long-term endotracheal intubation (in 68,8% of patients), short-term endotracheal intubation (in 9,4%), Wegener granulomatosis (in 9,4%) of rheumatoid arthritis (in 6,3%) of previous surgery in the larynx (in 3,1%) and caustic ingestion (in 3,1%) (Eckel, 2003).

2.10. Treatment of rheumatoid arthritis and laryngeal rheumatoid arthritis

The aims of early prevention and early treatment of RA are to reduce pain, inflammation and inability, to prevent radiologically found damages and progression and to reduce the development of comorbidity. Joint damage in rheumatoid arthritis begins a few weeks since the begining of the disease symptoms and that's why the early treatment reduces the disease progression rate (Emery, 2002). Pharmacotherapy generally includes several groups of medications: nonsteroidal anti-inflammatory drugs (NSAID) for pain control, oral or intra-articular glucocorticoids in low doses and start with DMARD. "Reverse pyramid" approach is required in RA treatment today, when DMARD are started immediately in order to slow down the disease progression as soon as possible (Rindfleisch, 2005). This approach is accepted on the basis of several facts: joint damages start in the early phase of the disease (Emery, 2002), DMARD have a significant use when they are used in the early phase of the disease, the uses of DMARD can be helped when the medications are used in the combination (Pincus, 1999; Lipsky, 2000; Weinblatt, 2004), a great number of medications from this group with positive evidence of useful effects are accessible. RA patients of medium stage and normal radiographic results should start the treatment with hydroxychloroquine, sulphasalazine or minocycline, although methotrexate is also a possibility. Patients with heavier stage of disease or radiographic changes should start treatment with methotrexate. If the disease symptoms aren't controlled well by mentioned medications, leflunomid or combined therapy should be taken into consideration (methotrexate together with one medication of newer generation). For initial RA treatment for reducing pain and joint swelling together with the combination of the mentioned medications, NSAID, salicylate or ciclooxygenease-2 inhibitors should be used. These medications can't be used independently because they don't change clinical course of RA. Glucocorticoids, usually in the dose that is equivalent to 10 mg of prednisone a day are highly important for freeing from RA symptoms and they can slow down joint damage (Kirwan, 1995). Their dosing should be kept at minimum because of a great risk of unwanted effects, which include osteoporosis, cataract, hyperadrenocorticism and altered glycemia levels. American college for rheumatology has recommended the intake of 1500mg of calcium and 400-800 IU of vitamin D a day. The most often used medications for RA treatment are methotrexate, hydroxychloroquine, sulphasalazine, leflunomide, infliximab and etanercept. Newer DMARD are leflunomide, antagonists tumor necrosis factor (TNF) and anakinra. Pharmacotherapeutic approaches for RA are very different depending on certain studies. One of such approaches is a combination of these two medications from the DMARD group, mainly methotrexate and sulphasalazine or methotrexate and cyclosporine (Dougados, 1999; Tugwell, 1995). Combination of methotrexate, sulphasalazine and high doses of corticosteroids has brought up to prolonged effects on radiographic progression in comparison to monotherapy by sulphasalazine (Landewe, 2002). In the two-year study, 197 RA patients were chosen by coincidence to take therapeutic protocol with four medications, methotrexate, sulphasalazine, hydroxychloroquine and prednisolone (5mg/a day) or individual medication from DMARD where it has been noticed that greater number of patients in remission got combined therapy, while fewer number of patients in remission were in the group of monotherapy by some other medication from DMARD group (Korpela, 2004). In some studies, cricoarytenoid arthritis treatment in a 65-

year-old male patient and 56-year-old female patient was carried out by local, intra-articular injections of triamcinolone combined with prednisolone (Jol, 1997; Simpson, 1980; Habib, 1977). Systemic application of corticosteroids brought up to significant mobility of the arytenoid cartilages in a 63-year-old patient (Jurik, 1985). Beclomethasone diproprionat in the treatment of rheumatoid changes in the larynx was useful (Sladek, 1983). Surgical approach to immobility of the vocal cords from paramedial position, in other words rheumatoid ankylosis of cricoarytenoid joints implies mobilizational and laterofixational techniques (Ejnell, 1985). Arytenoid adduction surgery was carried out successfully in a 57-year-old female patient who didn't have dyspnea year and a half after the surgery (Kumai, 2007). Endoscopic arytenoidectomy is usually a surgery of choice (Koufman, 2003).

3. Conclusion

Rheumatoid arthritis is a disease of unknown cause with several assumed etiological theories, but pathoanatomical and pathophysiological changes are mostly familiar. It is manifested on different organs and tissues and about 25% of all patients have clinical manifestations in the larynx. Patients with RA manifested on more than one joint, must be sent to and examined by a rheumatologist 6 weeks since the beginning of the disease symptoms. Joint and bones swelling points to early arthritis especially if at least two joints are involved and/or morning rigidity lasts longer than 30 minutes and/or if there is an affection of metacarpophalangeal and/or metatarsophalangeal joints (Emery, 2002). Following the disease course includes counting of painful and swollen joints, complete cooperation between the patient and the physician, determining erythrocyte sedimentation and C - reactive protein. Disease activities should be followed in the intervals from 1 to 3 months until the remission period is reached. Structural damages must be followed rardiographically every 6 to 12 months during the first several years. Family doctor must think about the structural damage of the larynx in the patients with advanced arthritis and he must send these patients to periodical otorhinolaryngological examinations every 1 to 3 months. At that time, it is necessary to carry out indirect laryngoscopy and graphic flow/volume which is enough for the initial screening. Forced inspiratory/expiratory relationship between the flow and volume provide a simple non-invasive test for revealing stenosis in upper airways. Pathological results of screening cause additional examinations by fiberoptical laryngoscopy, laryngomicroscopy with the examination of the arytenoid cartilages fixation, helped by multislice scanner larynx examination every six months to a year, computered stroboscopy and electromyography of the larynx. This is important because laryngoscopy provides better view of the mucous and functional integrity preservation, and multislice scanner larynx examination offers more precise visualisation of the structural changes. Periodical otorhinolaryngological examinations should be routine when treating patients with rheumatoid arthritis and they are always undertaken when family doctor and/or the rheumatologist of the clinic find the smallest disease progression on laryngeal and/or extralaryngeal localizations. Then, together with basic rheumatological therapy, intra-articular application of corticosteroid medications needs to be applied into every sick cricoarytenoid joint. When conservative treatment fails, after providing airways by tracheostomy, it is indicated to carry out endoscopic arytenoidectomy which presents a surgery of choice. For patients of extremely bad state to bear laryngeal surgery, or with those patients where surgical procedures failed to provide adequate airway, permanent tracheostomy is the final therapeutic possibility. In RA patients where a surgery in general endotracheal anesthesia is indicated, the otorhinolaryngologists inform the anesthesiologist after every examination about every laryngeal disorder. Anesthesiological risk is always present in the patients with rheumatoid arthritis in the larynx during endotracheal intubation and immediately after the extubation (Segebarth, 2007). In these patients, a careful search for cricoarytenoid arthritis is the basic thing, especially in those with laryngeal stridor which can be inforced after general anesthesia.

Acknowledgements

I would like to give credit to my wife Tatjana, my daughter Nina and my son Luka for their support and immense patience during elaboration of this chapter, as well as for their recognition of the importance of this work in diagnosis and treatment of all rheumatoid arthritis patients.

Author details

Stevan Stojanović* and Branislav Belić

*Address all correspondence to: stevan67@gmail.com

Faculty of Medical Sciences, University of Kragujevac, Republic of Serbia

References

[1] Firestein, G. S. (2005). Etiology and pathogenesis of rheumatoid arthritis. *Kelley's Textbook of rheumatology, Ruddy, S, Harris, E.D, Sledge, C.B. et al, (Ed.)*, 996-1042, 7th ed, W.B. Saunders, 0721601413, Philadelphia, USA.

[2] Aletaha, D., Neogi, T., Silman, A. J., Funovits, J., Felson, D. T., & Bingham, C. O. (2010). Rheumatoid arthritis classification criteria: an American College of Rheumatology/European League Against Rheumatism collaborative initiative. *Arthritis Rheum*, 62(9), 2569-81.

[3] Goldring, S. R. (2000). A 55-year-old woman with rheumatoid arthritis. *JAMA*, 283, 524-31.

[4] Kuder, S. A., Peshimam, A. Z., & Agraharam, S. (2002). Environmental risk factors for rheumatoid arthritis. *Rev Environ Health*, 17, 307-15.

[5] Merlino, L. A., Curtis, J., Mikuls, T. R., et al. (2004). Vitamin D intake is inversely associated with rheumatoid arthritis: results from the Iowa Women's Health Study. *Arthritis Rheum*, 50, 72-7.

[6] Emery, P., Breedveld, F. C., Dougados, M., et al. (2002). Early referral recommendation for newly diagnosed rheumatoid arthritis: evidence based development of a clinical guide. *Ann Rheum Dis*, 61, 290-7.

[7] Harris, E. D. (2005). Clinical features of rheumatoid arthritis. *In: Kelley's Textbook of rheumatology Ruddy, S, Harris, ED, Sledge, C.B, et al, (Ed.)*, 1043-78, 7th ed, W.B. Saunders, 0721601413, Philadelphia, USA.

[8] Akil, M., & Amos, R. S. (1995). ABC of rheumatology. Rheumatoid arthritis-I: clinical features and diagnosis. *BMJ, Review*, 310, 587-90, 0959-8138.

[9] Bridger, M. W., Jahn, A. F., & van Nostrand, A. W. (1980). Laryngeal rheumatoid arthritis. *Laryngoscope*, 90(2), 296-303, 0023-852X.

[10] Lofgren, R. H., & Montgomery, W. W. (1962). Incidence of Laryngeal Involvement in Rheumatoid Arthritis. *N Engl J Med*, 267, 193-5.

[11] Bonner, F. M. 3rd. (1977). Rheumatoid nodule. Pathological quiz case 1. *Arch Otolaryngol*, 103(2), 112-4.

[12] Ferdynus-Chromy, J., & Wagner, T. (1977). Comparative studies of synovial membranes of cricoarytenoid and knee joints in rheumatoid arthritis. *Reumatologia*, 15(1), 13-21.

[13] Grassi, W., De Angelis, R., Lamanna, G., & Cervini, C. (1998). The clinical features of rheumatoid arthritis. *Eur J Radiol*, 27(1), 18-24, 0720-048X.

[14] Mackenzie, M. (1880). *Diseases of the pharynx, larynx and trachea*, William Wood & Co., New York.

[15] Mackenzie, G. H. (1894). Rheumatism of the larynx. *Edin Med J*, 40, 507-9.

[16] Voulgari, P. V., Papazisi, D., Bai, M., et al. (2005). Laryngeal involvement in rheumatoid arthritis. *Rheumatol Int*, 25(5), 321-5.

[17] Kerstens, P. J., Boerbooms, A. M., Jeurissen, M. E., et al. (1992). Accelerated nodulosis during low dose methotrexate therapy for rheumatoid arthritis. An analysis of ten cases. *J Rheumatol*, 19, 867-71, 0315-162X.

[18] Fried, M.P., & Shapiro, J. (1991). Acute and chronic laryngeal infections. *Otolaryngology*, edn 3, Paperella, M.M., Shumrick, D.A., Gluckman, J. I., Meyerhoff, W.L., (Ed), W. B. Saunders, Philadelphia, USA. 0721615074 9780721615073, 2245-56.

[19] Webb, J., & Payne, W. H. (1972). Rheumatoid nodules of the vocal folds. *Ann Rheum Dis*, 31, 122-5.

[20] Bienenstock, H., Ehrlich, G. E., & Breyberg, R. H. (1963). Rheumatoid arthritis of the cricoarytenoid joints: a clinicopathologic study. *Arthritis Rheum*, 6, 48-63.

[21] Pearson, J. E. (1957). Rheumatoid arthritis of the larynx. *Br Med J*, 2, 1047, 0007-1447.

[22] Copeman, W. S. (1957). Rheumatoid arthritis of the cricoarytenoid joints. *Br Med J*, 1(5032), 1398-9.

[23] Bayar, N., Kara, S. A., Keles, I., et al. (2003). Cricoarytenoid in rheumatoid arthritis: Radiologic and clinical study. *J Otolaryngol*, 32(6), 373-8.

[24] Charlin, B., Brazeau-Lamontagne, L., Levesque, Ry., et al. (1985). Cricoarytenoiditis in rheumatoid arthritis: Comparision of fibrolaryngoscopic and high resolution computerized tomographic findings. *J Otolaryngol*, 14, 381-6.

[25] Hamdan, A. L., El -Khatib, M., Dagher, W., et al. (2007). Laryngeal involvement in rheumatoid arthritis. *M E J Anesth*, 19(2), 335-46.

[26] Chen, J. J., Branstetter, B. F., & Myers, E. N. (2005). Cricoarytenoid rheumatoid arthritis: an important consideration in aggressive lesions of the larynx. *Am J Neuroradiol*, 26(4), 970-2.

[27] Lawry, G. V., Finerman, M. L., Hanafee, W. N., Mancuso, A. A., Fan, P. T., & Bluestone, R. (1984). Laryngeal involvement in rheumatoid arthritis A clinical, laryngoscopic, and computerized tomographic study. *Arthritis Rheum*, 27(8), 873-82.

[28] Jurik, A. G., & Pedersen, U. (1984). Rheumatoid arthritis of the crico-arytenoid and crico-thyroid joints: a radiological and clinical study. *Clin Radiol*, 35(3), 233-6.

[29] Ingegnoli, F., Galbiati, V., Bacciu, A., Zeni, S., & Fantini, F. (2007). Bilateral vocal fold immobility in a patient with overlap syndrome rheumatoid arthritis/systemic sclerosis. *Clin Rheumatol*, 26(10), 1765-7.

[30] Leicht, M. J., Harrington, M. H., & Davis, D. E. (1987). Cricoarytenoid arthritis: A cause of laryngeal obstruction. *Annals of Emergency Medicine*, 16(8), 885-8.

[31] Amernik, K. (2007). Glottis morphology and perceptive-acoustic characteristics of voice and speech in patients with rheumatoid arthritis. *Ann Acad Med Stetin*, 53(3), 55-65, 1427-440X.

[32] Amernik, K., Tarnowska, C., Brzosko, I., Grzelec, H., & Burakl, M. (2007). Glottis morphology in rheumatoid arthritis. *Otolaryngol Pol*, 61(1), 85-90

[33] Immerman, S., Sulica, L., & Bamboo, Nodes. (2007). *Otolaryngol Head Neck Surg*, 137(1), 162-3.

[34] Braverman, I., Malatskey, S., & Avior, G. (2007). Bilateral vocal cord paralysis due to rheumatoid arthritis. *Harefuah*, 146(2), 92-4.

[35] Takakura, K., Hirakawa, S., Kudo, K., Mori, M., Kitano, T., & Noguchi, T. (2005). Cricoarytenoid arthritis diagnosed after tracheostomy in a rheumatoid arthritis patient. *Masui*, 54(6), 690-3.

[36] Yonemoto, N., Nagahata, T., Nishimura, T., Kato, H., Kitaguchi, K., & Furuya, H. (2005). Difficult airway management during emergency tracheostomy in a patient with severe rheumatoid arthritis. *Masui*, 54(1), 39-41.

[37] Tarnowska, C., Amernik, K., Matyja, G., Brzosko, I., Grzelec, H., & Burak, M. (2004). Fixation of the crico-arythenoid joints in rheumatoid arthritis--preliminary report. *Otolaryngol Pol*, 58(4), 843-9.

[38] Ylitalo, R., Heimbürger, M., & Lindestad, P. A. (2003). Vocal fold deposits in autoimmune disease--an unusual cause of hoarseness. *Clin Otolaryngol Allied Sci*, 28(5), 446-50.

[39] Eckel, H. E., Wittekindt, C., Klussmann, J. P., Schroeder, U., & Sittel, C. (2003). Management of bilateral arytenoid cartilage fixation versus recurrent laryngeal nerve paralysis. *Ann Otol Rhinol Laryngol*, 112(2), 103-8.

[40] Jol, J.A., van Deelen, G.W., & Dinant, H.J. (1997). Sore throat in rheumatoid arthritis: 2 patients with cricoarytenoid arthritis. *Ned Tijdschr Geneeskd*, 141(32), 1567-70, 0028-2162.

[41] Miller, F. R., Wanamaker, J. R., Hicks, D. M., & Tucker, H. M. (1994). Cricoarytenoid arthritis and ankylosing spondylitis. *Arch Otolaryngol Head Neck Surg*, 120(2), 214-6.

[42] Daver, L., Toussirot, E., & Acquaviva, P. C. (1994). Severe laryngeal involvement in rheumatoid arthritis requiring permanent tracheostomy. *Rev Rhum Ed Fr*, 61(7-8), 550-3, 1169-8330.

[43] Okuda, Y., Takasugi, K., Imai, A., Hashimoto, F., Kondo, Y., Hatinota, M., et al. (1992). Cricoarytenoid joint involvement in rheumatoid arthritis. *Ryumachi*, 32(3), 245-51.

[44] Guerra, L. G., Lau, K. Y., & Marwah, R. (1992). Upper airway obstruction as the sole manifestation of rheumatoid arthritis. *J Rheumatol*, 19(6), 974-6, 0315-162X.

[45] Bolten, W. (1991). The cricoarytenoid joint in chronic polyarthritis. *Z Rheumatol*, 0340-1855, 50(1), 1-5.

[46] Dockery, K. M., Sismanis, A., & Abedi, E. (1991). Rheumatoid arthritis of the larynx: the importance of early diagnosis and corticosteroid therapy. *South Med J*, 84(1), 95-6.

[47] Ten, Holter. J. B., Van Buchem, F. L., & Van Beusekom, H. J. (1988). Cricoarytenoid arthritis may be a case of emergency. *Clin Rheumatol*, 7(2), 288-90.

[48] Gatland, D.J., Keene, M.H., & Brookes, J.D. (1988). Cricoid necrosis in laryngeal rheumatoid arthritis. *J Laryngol Otol*, 102(3), 271-5, 0022-2151.

[49] Geterud, A., Ejnell, H., Månsson, I., Sandberg, N., Bake, B., & Bjelle, A. (1986). Severe airway obstruction caused by laryngeal rheumatoid arthritis. *J Rheumatol*, 13(5), 948-51.

[50] Ejnell, H., Bake, B., Månsson, I., Hallén, O., Sandberg, N., Geterud, A., & Bjelle, A. (1985). New mobilization and laterofixation procedure for cricoarytenoid joint ankylosis in rheumatoid arthritis. *Ann Otol Rhinol Laryngol*, 94(5 Pt 1), 442-4, 0003-4894.

[51] Jurik, A. G., Pedersen, U., & Nøorgård, A. (1985). Rheumatoid arthritis of the cricoarytenoid joints: a case of laryngeal obstruction due to acute and chronic joint changes. *Laryngoscope*, 95(7 Pt 1), 846-8, 0023-852X.

[52] Sladek, G. D., Vasey, F. B., Saraceno, C., Davis, B. J., Germain, B. F., & Espinoza, L. R. (1983). Beclomethasone dipropionate in the treatment of the rheumatoid larynx. *J Rheumatol*, 10(3), 518-9, 0315-162X.

[53] Simpson, G. T., Javaheri, A., & Janfaza, P. (1980). Acute cricoarytenoid arthritis: local periarticular steroid injection. *Ann Otol Rhinol Laryngol*, 89(6 Pt 1), 558-62, 0003-4894.

[54] Schwartz, I. S., & Grishman, E. (1980). Rheumatoid nodules of the vocal cords as the initial manifestation of systemic lupus erythematosus. *JAMA*, 244(24), 2751-2.

[55] Montgomery, W. W., & Goodman, M. L. (1980). Rheumatoid cricoarytenoid arthritis complicated by upper esophageal ulcerations. *Ann Otol Rhinol Laryngol*, 89(1 Pt 1), 6-8, 0003-4894.

[56] Chalmers, A., & Traynor, J. A. (1979). Cricoarytenoid arthritis as a cause of acute upper airway obstruction. *J Rheumatol*, 6(5), 541-2, 0315-162X.

[57] Friedman, B. A. (1975). Rheumatoid nodules of the larynx. *Arch Otolaryngol*, 101(6), 361-3.

[58] Abadir, W. F., & Forster, P. M. (1974). Rheumatoid vocal cord nodules. *J Laryngol Otol*, 0022-2151, 88(5), 473-8.

[59] Gotze, M., Andersen, R. B., Westergaard, O., & Andersen, L. A. (1973). Rheumatoid arthritis in the crico-arythenoid joints. *Ugeskr Laeger*, 136(1), 39-41.

[60] Kubiak-Socha, E. (1973). Case of rheumatoid arthritis with involvement of cricoarytenoid articulations. *Wiad Lek*, 26(11), 1067-8.

[61] De Gandt, J. B. (1969). Cricoarytenoid ankylosis. *Acta Otorhinolaryngol Belg*, 23(6), 603-11.

[62] Copeman, W. S. (1968). Rheumatoid arthritis and the crico-arytenoid joints. *Br J Clin Pract*, 22(10), 421-2.

[63] Peters, J. E., Burke, C. J., & Morris, V. H. (2011). Three cases of rheumatoid arthritis with laryngeal stridor. *Clin Rheumatol*, 30(5), 723-7.

[64] Mc Geehan, D. F., Crinnion, J. N., & Strachan, D. R. (1989). Life-threatening stridor presenting in a patient with rheumatoid involvement of the larynx. *Archives of Emergency Medicine*, 6, 274-6.

[65] Fisher, B. A., Dolan, K., Hastings, L., Mc Clinton, C., & Taylor, P. C. (2008). Prevalence of subjective voice impairment in rheumatoid arthritis. *Clin Rheumatol, 27,* 1441-3.

[66] Hilgert, E, Toleti, B, Kruger, K, & Nejedlo, I. (2008). Hoarseness Due to Bamboo Nodes in Patients with Autoimmune Diseases: A Review of Literature. *Journal of Voice,* 22(3), 343-50, 0892-1997.

[67] Lehmann, T., Nef, W., Stalder, B., Thomson, D., & Gerber, N. J. (1997). Fatal postoperative airway obstruction in a patient with rheumatoid arthritis. *Annals of the Rheumatic Diseases,* 56, 512-3.

[68] Bossingham, D. H., & Simpson, F. G. (1996). Acute laryngeal obstruction in rheumatoid arthritis. *BMJ,* 312(7026), 295-6.

[69] Segebarth, B., & Limbird, T. J. (2007). Perioperative Acute Upper Airway Obstruction Secondary to Severe Rheumatoid Arthritis. *The Journal of Arthroplasty,* 22(6), 907, 0883-5403.

[70] Hart, F. D. (1966). Complicated rheumatoid disease. *Br Med J,* 2(5506), 131-5.

[71] Kumai, Y., Murakami, D., Masuda, M., & Yumoto, E. (2007). Arytenoid adduction to treat impaired adduction of the vocal fold due to rheumatoid arthritis. *Auris Nasus Larynx,* 34(4), 545-8.

[72] Absalom, A. R., Watts, R., & Kong, A. (1998). Airway obstruction caused by rheumatoid cricoarytenoid arthritis. *Lancet,* 351(9109), 1099-100.

[73] Keenan, M. A., Stiles, C. M., & Kaufman, R. L. (1983). Acquired laryngeal deviation associated with cervical spine disease in erosive polyarticular arthritis. Use of the fiberoptic bronchoscope in rheumatoid disease. *Anesthesiology,* 58(5), 441-9.

[74] Bamshad, M., Rosa, U., Padda, G., & Luce, M. (1989). Acute upper airway obstruction in rheumatoid arthritis of the cricoarytenoid joints. *South Med J,* 82(4), 507-11.

[75] Stojanović, S. P., Zivić, Lj., Stojanović, J., & Belić, B. (2010). Total fixation of cricoarytenoid joint of a patient with rheumatoid arthritis and Hashimoto thyroiditis. *Srp Arh Celok Lek,* 138(3-4), 230-2, 0370-8179.

[76] Funk, D., & Raymon, F. (1975). Rheumatoid arthritis of the cricoarytenoid joints: an airway hazard. *Anesth Analg,* 54(6), 742-5.

[77] Pincus, T., O'Dell, J. R., & Kremer, J. M. (1999). Combination therapy with multiple disease-modifying antirheumatic drugs in rheumatoid arthritis: a preventive strategy. *Ann Intern Med,* 131, 768-74.

[78] Lipsky, P. E., van der Heijde, D. M., St, Clair. E. W., Furst, D. E., Breedveld, F. C., Kalden, J. R., et al. (2000). Infliximab and methotrexate in the treatment of rheumatoid arthritis. *N Engl J Med,* 343, 1594-602.

[79] Weinblatt, M. E., Keystone, E. C., Furst, D. E., Moreland, L. W., Weisman, M. H., Birbara, C. A., et al. (2003). Adalimumab, a fully human anti-tumor necrosis factor alpha

monoclonal antibody, for the treatment of rheumatoid arthritis in patients taking concomitant methotrexate: the ARMADA trial. *Arthritis Rheum*. 48, 35-45.

[80] Kirwan, J. R. (1995). Arthritis and Rheumatism Council Low-Dose Glucocorticoid Study Group. The effect of glucocorticoids on joint destruction in rheumatoid arthritis. *N Engl J Med*, 333, 142-6, 0028-4793.

[81] Dougados, M., Combe, B., Cantagrel, A., et al. (1999). Combination therapy in early rheumatoid arthritis: a randomised, controlled, double blind 52 week clinical trial of sulphasalazine and methotrexate compared with the single components. *Annals of the Rheumatic Diseases*, 58, 220-5.

[82] Tugwell, P., Pincus, T., Yocum, D., et al. (1995). Combination therapy with cyclosporine and methotrexate in severe rheumatoid arthritis. The Methotrexate-Cyclosporine Combination Study Group. *N Engl J Med*, 333, 137-41.

[83] Landewe, R. B., Boers, M., Verhoeven, A. C., et al. (2002). COBRA combination therapy in patients with early rheumatoid arthritis: long-term structural benefits of a brief intervention. *Arthritis and Rheumatism*, 46, 347-56.

[84] Korpela, M., Laasonen, L., Hannonen, P., et al. (2004). Retardation of joint damage in patients with early rheumatoid arthritis by initial aggressive treatment with disease-modifying anti-rheumatic drugs: five-year experience from the FIN-RACo study. *Arthritis and Rheumatism*, 50, 2072-81, 0300-9742.

[85] Koufman, J. A., & Belafsky, P. C. (2003). Infectious and Inflammatory Diseases of the Larynx. *Ballenger's Otorhinolaryngology Head and Neck Surgery, Snow J.B., Jr, Ballenger J.J.*, 1207, BC Decker Inc, 1-55009-197-2, Hamilton, Ontario.

[86] Woodson, G. E. (2007). Hoarseness and Laryngeal Paralysis. *Head and Neck Manifestations of Systemic Disease, Harris, J. P., Weisman, M. H.*, 517-525, Informa Healthcare Inc, 0-8493-4050-0, New York, USA.

[87] Brazeau-Lamontagne, L., Charlin, B., Levesque, R. Y., et al. (1986). Cricoarytenoiditis: CT assessment in rheumatoid arthritis. *Radiology*, 158(2), 463-6.

Chapter 11

Andrographolide a New Potential Drug for the Long Term Treatment of Rheumatoid Arthritis Disease

María A. Hidalgo, Juan L. Hancke,
Juan C. Bertoglio and Rafael A. Burgos

Additional information is available at the end of the chapter

http://dx.doi.org/10.5772/55642

1. Introduction

Andrographis paniculata, (Burm. f.) Wall. ex Nees, a herbaceous plant belonging to the Family Acanthaceae, is one of the most commonly used medicinal plants in the traditional systems of Unani and Ayurvedic medicines. It grows in hedge rows throughout the plains of India and is also cultivated in gardens. It also grows in many other Asian countries and is used as a traditional herbal medicine in China, Hong Kong, the Philippines, Malaysia, Indonesia, and Thailand It is an annual plant of 1-3 ft high, also known as the "king of bitters", being the aerial parts most commonly used. *A. paniculata* have shown a broad range of pharmacological effects such as inhibition of replication of the HIV virus, prevention of common cold, and antimalarial, antidiarrheal, antibacterial, antihyperglycemic effects, suppression of various cancer cells, and principally anti-inflammatory properties. Andrographolide is the major labdane diterpenoid isolated from *A. paniculata* and exhibits anti-inflammatory and anticancer activities, either *in vitro* or *in vivo* experimental models of inflammation and cancer. Several immunomodulatory responses of andrographolide have been observed in *in vitro* studies, such as reduction of iNOS, COX-2, NO, PGE2, TNF-alpha and IL-12 in macrophages and microglia. In neutrophils is able to reduce the radical oxygen species production, and Mac-1, IL-8 and COX-2 expression. In T cells, andrographolide inhibits the expression of IL-2, IFNγ and IL-6, reducing the humoral and cellular adaptive immune response. Andrographolide was able to reduce the dendritic cells maturation and their ability to present antigens to T cells. Andrographolide administered in rodents reduced the Th2 cytokine IL-4, IL-5, IL-13 and serum immunoglobulin in an ovalbumin induced asthma model. A reduction of T cells response also has been observed in experimental autoimmune encephalomyelitis and systemic lupus erythematosus mouse model. Several of immunomodulatory responses have been associated to the inhibition of Nuclear Factor-κB functions. It has been demonstrated that andrographolide inhibits the nuclear translocation of the p65 subunit of NF-κB and interferes with the NF-κB binding to the DNA. Also andrographolide can reduce NFAT function in T cells and reduce the phosphorylation of signal transducer and activator of transcription-3 (STAT3) in macrophages.

We propose the potential use of andrographolide in Rheumatoid Arthritis and other autoimmune diseases. This is supported by the fact that andrographolide exerts anti-growth and pro-apoptotic effects on human rheumatoid arthritis fibroblast- like synoviocytes, the main cellular constituent of pannus, that combined with a massive infiltration of lymphocytes and macrophages, invades and destroys the local articular structure. Recently, a prospective randomized placebo-controlled trial has suggested that *A. paniculata*, a standardized extract containing NLT 30% of andrographolide was effective for symptom relief in patients with Rheumatoid Arthritis. The use of andrographolide alone or a patented *A. paniculata* standardized extract in clinical trials shows mild and few side effects, and has the potential to be developed into a new alternative drug for Rheumatoid Arthritis treatment in the long term.

2. *Andrographis paniculata* and labdane diterpenoids

The main and most interesting biological constituent of *A. paniculata* herb (aerial part) is a group of diterpene lactones belonging to the ent-labdane class, present in both free and glycosidic forms, and named andrographolides [1, 2].

Andrographolide is the bitter principle, a colourless, neutral crystalline substance, was first isolated by Boorsma from different parts of *Andrographis paniculata* [2]. In 1911 Gorter proved that it is structurally a lactone and named it andrographolide (in the Chinese literature it is sometimes cited as andrographis B). The bitter principle has been subjected to a number of chemical investigations. The properties of the compound and its diterpenoid lactone nature, as well as its stereochemistry, conformation and crystal structure were cleared by means of infrared, x, mass spectrometry and NMR analysis. Its chemical formula corresponds to the 3,14,15,18-tetrahydroxy-5,9 H,10-labda-8(20),12-dien-16-oic acid-lactone (Figure 1). Most recently, various epimers, geometric isomers, and rearrangement products of andrographolide have been isolated and structurally characterized [3, 4]. Andrographolide, as the other diterpene lactones of *A. paniculata*, are generally extracted with $CHCl_3$/EtOH or acetone, and several methods are described in the literature to determinate its content in the plant, in commercial formulation, i.e. standardized extract and in biological samples: titration with alkalis, TLC/UV spectrophotometry and HPLC methods. The maximum content of andrographolide and related diterpenoids is in the mature leaves. It has been described that the stem contained 0.2±0.02%, seeds 0.13±0.01%; root 0.44±0.01%; and leaves 2.39±0.008% of andrographolide [5]. Regional variation in the andrographolide content was also observed. The content of andrographolide varies with the harvest season. The leaves contain more than 2% andrographolide before the plant blossoms; afterward the contents decreases to less than 0.5% [2]. The pH modifies the stability of andrographolide, and hydrolysis is extremely slow below pH 7, but considerably faster on the alkaline side, producing some structural changes. Andrographolide is sparingly soluble in water; soluble in acetone, methanol, chloroform and ether. As a water soluble andrographolide derivative, the sodium bisulfite adduct has been synthesized for medical use as an antipyretic agent.

Preclinical properties include anti-retroviral [6, 7], antiproliferative and pro-apoptotic [8, 9], anti-diabetic [10, 11], anti-angiogenic [12], anti-thrombotic [13], anti-urothelial [14], anti-leishmaniasis [15], hepatoprotective [16, 17], protective activity against alcohol-induced hepatic and renal toxicity [18], and cardioprotective [19] and anti-inflammatory [20-25] properties.

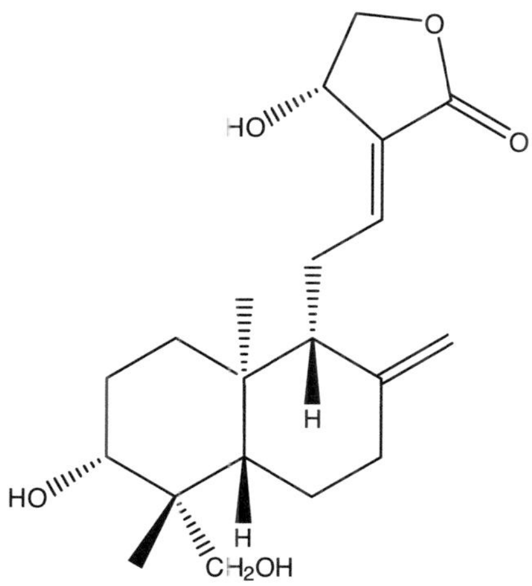

Figure 1. Chemical structure of andrographolide

2.1. Neoandrographolide

The second diterpene isolated from *A. paniculata* was the minor non-bitter constituent neoandrographolide, which was first described by Kleipool in 1952. The structure of neoandrographolide (Figure 2) was described as a diterpene glucoside and its amount in the plant is around 0.5-1%. The main preclinical effects are anti-inflammatory [23, 26, 27], chemosensitizer [28], anti-herpes-simplex virus [7] and antioxidant [29].

2.2. Minor labdane diterpenes

Afterwards, more than 20 other diterpene lactones, both glycosylated and not, have been described. The most important among them, characterized by Balmain and Connolly in 1973, are: 14-deoxy-11,12- didehydroandrographolide, withan average content in the leaf of 0.1%, 14-deoxyandrographolide (0.02%), 14-deoxy-11-oxoandrographolide (0.12%) (Figure 2) [3]. In other hand has been described that 14-deoxy-11,12- didehydroandrographolide possess vasorelaxant and antihypertensive [30, 31], anti-herpes [7], antioxidant and hepatoprotective [32], antithrombotic [33], antiretroviral [6], and antidiabetic properties [34]. Meanwhile 14-deoxyandrographolide exert hepatoprotective [35], uterine smooth muscle relaxant [36], immunomodulator [37], platelet activating factor antagonist [38], and vasorelaxant and antihypertensive [39] effects. In addition, 14-deoxy-11-oxoandrographolide only has been reported antileishmaniasis effect [40].

Andrographiside, the 19-glucoside of andrographolide, was isolated in 1981, and only a hepatoprotective effect has been described [41].

A. paniculata contains also minor andrographolide-like compounds such as andropanoside (19-glucoside of 14-deoxy-andrographolide), or andrograpanin (3,14-dideoxy-andrographolide), which are mostly all 14-deoxy- and/or 3-deoxy-derivatives. These compounds show anti-inflammatory properties in preclinical studies [42, 43].

Isoandrographolide is present in the whole plants and has been described as a cellular differentiation inducer [3], antiproliferative [44], and cytotoxic [45] effects.

Also three salts of labdanic acids, named as magnesium andrographate, disodium andrographate and dipotassium andrographate 19-*O*-D-glucoside have been isolated hydrophylic extract from the leaf.

Since the total synthesis of andrographolide and analogues, many libraries of new derivatives have been created using andrographolide as a template with the purpose to obtain compounds with improved pharmacological profiles. Andrographolide is also a starting point for the semisynthesis of other labdane diterpenes [46-48].

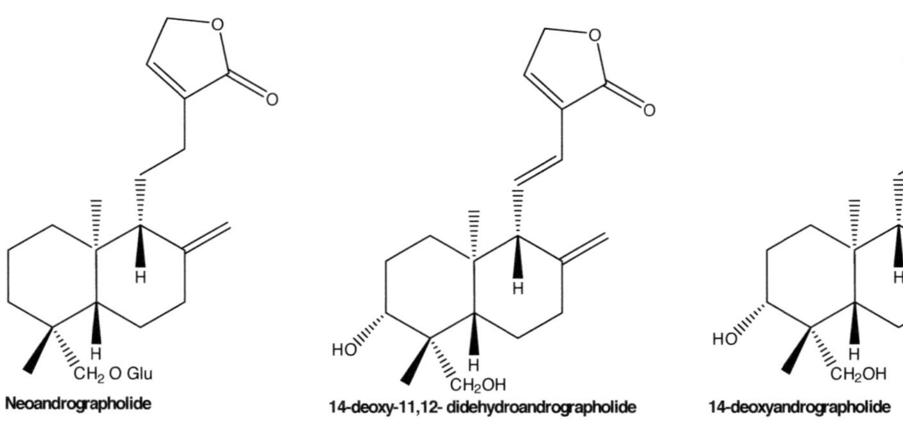

Figure 2. Chemical structure of minor labdane diterpenes isolated from *Andrographis paniculata*.

3. Anti-inflammatory and immunomodulatory effects of andrographolide *in vitro* and *in vivo*

Different preparations of *A. paniculata* administered orally reduced the pyrexia within or after 5 hrs of administration of yeast in rats [49]. On the other hand, administration of *A. panicula-*

ta (20 mg/100 g b.w.) one hour before the injection of carrageenin, reduced the edema in 65.3% in rats. The effect was comparable to oxyphenilbutazone 76.5% [2]

3.1. *In vitro* studies

Andrographolide, shows anti-inflammatory and anticancer activities in both *in vitro* and *in vivo*. The effects of andrographolide on two cells types that play an important role in the inflammatory processes, e.g. leukocyte (neutrophils, macrophages and T-cells) and endothelial cells, demonstrates the ability of this compound to reduce the expression and production of pro-inflammatory mediators.

Several *in vitro* studies show that andrographolide reduces the production of the oxygen radical superoxide anion and hydrogen peroxide, as well as the adhesion induced by chemoattractant in isolated neutrophils [50, 51]. Other antecedents describe a reduction of the expression of cyclooxygenase-2 (COX-2), inducible enzyme producing prostaglandins, in a human model of neutrophils [21]. In mouse peritoneal macrophages, andrographolide reduces the production stimulated by lipopolysaccharide (LPS) of two important cytokines that participate in the amplification and activation of the inflammatory process, the cytokines tumoral necrosis factor TNFα and granulocyte macrophage colony-stimulating factor (GM-CSF). The inhibition of the release of these cytokines by andrographolide was compared to the synthetic glucocorticoid dexamethasone, showing andrographolide to have a similar effect as dexamethasone, but with a lower potency [24, 52]. Also, the effect of andrographolide on the cellular chemotaxis, a response that allows the movement of inflammatory cells to the injured tissue, show that it reduces the chemotactic migration of macrophage induced by C5a, which may contribute to its anti-inflammatory activity [53]. In local or systemic inflammatory disorders there is an enhanced formation of nitric oxide (NO) following the expression of inducible nitric oxide synthase (iNOS). The inhibition of NO formation may have therapeutic benefit in patients with inflammatory diseases as Rheumatoid Arthritis [54]. Thus, andrographolide reduces the LPS-induced iNOS and COX-2 expression in RAW264.7 macrophages [55, 56]. Additionally, andrographolide may have an effect on inflammation-mediated neurodegeneration, since it reduces the production of reactive oxygen species (ROS), TNFα, NO and prostaglandin E2 in microglia, the counterpart of macrophages in the brain [25]. Andrographolide reduces the *in vitro* activation of human and murine T-cells, T-cells proliferation, interleukin-2 (IL-2) and IFNγ production [57-60].

Interaction of leukocyte-endothelium plays a key role in the initiation and maintenance of inflammation, being the adhesion molecule ICAM-1 important in mediating leukocyte adhesion, arrest and transmigration to the inflammatory site. In this respect, certain antecedents show that andrographolide reduces the adhesion of HL-60 cells onto human vein endothelial cells (HUVEC) and the expression of TNFα-induced ICAM-1 [61, 62]. In addition, andrographolide reduces the endothelial cell proliferation, migration and invasion, suggesting a role in angiogenesis [63]. Moreover, andrographolide reduces the growth factor deprivation-induced apoptosis in endothelial cells [64].

The therapeutic potential of andrographolide for the treatment of rheumatoid arthritis has been suggested by using of human rheumatoid arthritis fibroblast-like synoviocytes (RAFLSs) as a cellular model. Andrographolide exerts anti-proliferative and pro-apoptotic effects in RAFLSs, with G0/G1 cell cycle arrest, increases the expression of cell-cycle inhibitors p21 and p27 and reduces cyclin-dependent kinase 4 [65].

3.2. *In vivo* studies

The anti-inflammatory activity of andrographolide has been studied in diverse *in vivo* inflammatory diseases models.

Earlier studies with andrographolide show that it inhibited carrageenin, kaolin and nistatin-induced paw oedema. Moreover, andrographolide p.o. significantly inhibited the weight of granuloma induced by cotton pellets, and decreased the edema in adjuvant-induced arthritis (0.1-0.4% dead *Mycobacterium tuberculosis* suspension). Andrographolide (300 mg/kg) also inhibited dye leakage in acetic acid-induced vascular permeability. It was devoided of any ulcerogenic effect on the stomach in acute and chronic studies in rats. These effects were dose dependent, but inferior to phenylbutazone. Other diterpenic lactones, have shown to possess antipyretic effect in rabbits and rats with fever induced by 2-4-dinitrophenol. The potency was: 14-deoxy-11,12-didehydroandrographolide > deoxyandrographolide, and neoandrographolide > andrographolide [66].

In a model of ovalbumin-induced asthma in mice the intra-peritoneal administration of 30 mg/kg andrographolide reduces the levels of TNFα and GM-CSF (92 and 65 %, respectively) in bronchoalveolar fluid, and the accumulation of lymphocytes and eosinophils, supporting a potential use in asthma. Andrographolide also reduced the Th2 cytokine IL-4, IL-5, IL-13 and serum immunoglobulin [20, 52].

Andrographolide also is helpfulness in the reduction of the symptoms of a mice experimental autoimmune encephalomyelitis (EAE), an animal model of human Multiple Sclerosis, by inhibiting T-cell and antibody responses directed to myelin antigens [59]. Similarly, in another model of autoimmune disease, the administration of andrographlide reduces the susceptibility, prevents the symptoms and reduces anti-nuclear antibodies and kidney damage of systemic lupus erythematous [67, 68].

The potential effect of andrographolide on rheumatoid arthritis could involve angiogenesis inhibition. In fact, the development of new vessels, is important process that might facilitate the incoming of inflammatory cells into the synovium and, therefore, stimulate the pannus formation. [69]. In a model of induction of angiogenesis in C57BL/6 mice, andrographolide reduced the serum levels of cytokines of IL-1β, IL-6, TNFα and GM-CSF, the angiogenic factor VEGF and the NO production. Additionally, it is observable an increase of the levels of anti-angiogenic factors TIMP-1 and IL-2 [12]. Andrographolide also suppresses breast tumor growth, which correlates with the inhibition of the pro-angiogenic molecules OPN and VEGF, in the NOD/SCID mice model [70].

4. Anti-inflammatory molecular mechanisms of andrographolide

All immunomodulatory effects of andrographolide have been attributed to modulation of different intracellular mediators, however three main mechanisms are commonly described. A first anti-inflammatory mechanism involved in the reduction of COX-2 expression by andrographolide in neutrophils comprises the modulation of the NF-κB pathway. The NF-κB is a family of transcription factors that regulate the expression of a large number of pro-inflammatory genes, such as COX-2, iNOS, TNF-alpha, IL-8 or IL-1, that are involved in the pathogenesis of Rheumatoid Arthritis. The activation of NF-κB compromises two main routes: the canonical and alternative pathways. The canonical NF-κB signaling pathway is the most important one. Inflammatory receptor activation results in IκB kinase (IKK) activation, and the IKK complex phosphorylate the IκB protein, leading to its polyubiquitination. The ubiquitinated IκB is degraded via 26S proteasome, thereby exposing the nuclear localization signal on NF-κB dimer and inducing nuclear translocation. The alternative NF-κB pathway has been implicated in lymphoid organogenesis and B cell development, and is based in the processing of p100 NF-κB by IKKα, resulting in release of the p52 NF-κB bound to RelB [71].

Andrographolide reduces the luciferase activity controlled by NF-κB and inhibits the DNA binding of NF-κB induced by chemoattractants, however not affecting IκB degradation [21]. The detailed mechanism of DNA binding inhibition indicates that andrographolide form a covalent adduct with reduced cysteine 62 of p50 subunit NF-κB, which block the binding of NF-κB to DNA [72]. The NF-κB pathway inhibition by andrographolide has been described in different cells involving in inflammatory processes such as endothelial cells [62], monocytes [73], bronchial epithelial cells [20], and dendritic cells [58].

A second mechanism describes an inhibitory effect of andrographolide on iNOS and COX-2 expression in macrophages, attributable to the modulation of transcription factors AP-1 and STAT3. AP-1 and STAT3, which are important for the production of pro-inflammatory cytokines such as IL-1β, IL-6 and IL-10, plays a major role in Rheumatoid Arthritis. It has been reported an overexpression of activated STAT3 and high DNA binding activity of AP-1 in synovial tissue from patients with Rheumatoid Arthritis [74, 75]. In fact, andrographolide reduced the LPS-induced AP-1 DNA-binding activities, and also decreased the STAT3 phosphorylation, which is crucial for nuclear translocation and DNA binding [56]. Thus, andrographolide may also be contributing to reduce the inflammatory process in rheumatoid arthritis via AP-1 and/or STAT3 modulation.

A third mechanism involves the interference of the transcription factor Nuclear Factor of Activated T cells (NFAT) induced by andrographolide in T-cells. The interference of NFAT activation by andrographolide is related to the increase of andrographolide-induced JNK phosphorylation, which controls the export of NFAT from nucleus [57].

In addition to the immunomodulatory andrographolide mechanism described above, there are several cellular pathways, such as PI3K/Akt and ERK1/2 pathways, involved in the anti-inflammatory effect of andrographolide and in the pathogenesis of the Rheumatoid Arthritis

[76]. The PI3 kinase pathway, is activated by TNF-α and IL-1, within fibroblastic synovial cells, and can activate the transcription factors NF-κB and AP-1 [77]. Also, the participation of the ERK1/2 MAPK in the initiation and progression of rheumatoid arthritis suggest that ERK inhibitors may emerge as a new therapeutic tool. The use of an ERK inhibitor in the animal model of collagen-induced arthritis suppressed the antigen-specific activation of T cells [78]. *In vitro*, andrographolide reduced the Akt phosphorylation in macrophages, HUVEC and microglia, and decreased the ERK1/2 phosphorylation in macrophages, suggesting that the signaling pathways PI3K/Akt and ERk1/2 may be associated to its anti-inflammatory effect [24, 61, 79]. Additionally, andrographolide also have the ability to reduce ERK1 and ERK5 phosphorylation [57].

In the following figure we propose the main anti-inflammatory effects of andrographolide that include the inhibition of several intracellular signaling pathways (Figure 3).

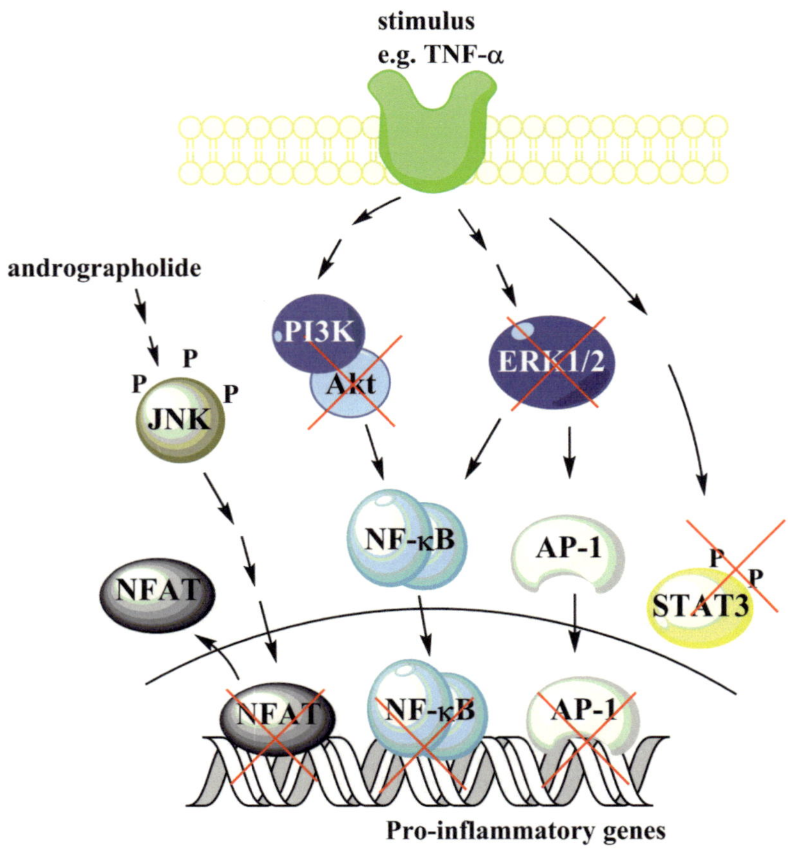

Figure 3. Proposed molecular mechanism of andrographolide in inflammation. Andrographolide shows inhibitory effect (x) on the PI3K/Akt pathway, ERK1/2 MAPK, NF-κB, NFAT, AP-1 and STAT3, and increases the JNK phosphorylation.

http://dx.doi.org/10.5772/55642

5. Effect of andrographolide on rheumatoid arthritis

5.1. Efficacy of an Andrographis paniculata composition (Paractin®) for the relief of rheumatoid arthritis symptoms: A prospective randomized placebo-controlled trial

In a prospective, double blind against placebo controlled clinical trial with chronic active Rheumatoid arthritis, the effect of a standardized patented *A. paniculata* extract (Paractin®) administration to 60 patients during 14 weeks in the reduction of symptoms and signs was studied. Each patient received either a tablet containing 30 mg of andrographolide or a placebo 3 times a day. The demographic characteristic of the patients is shown in table 2.

	Treatment groups	
	Placebo	**Active drug**
Number of patients	28	30
Age (mean years) (min-max)	44.82 (13-63)	47.1 (20-70)
Years with diagnosed (min-max)	6.5 (0.7-22.3)	6.7 (0.7-44.5
BMI (Kg/m^2) (min-max)	30.0 (19.7-41.4)	29.2 (18.3-44.5)
Height (m) (min-max)	1.52 (1.30-1.75)	1.51 (1.38-1.59)
Weight (kg) (min-max)	69.9 (43.0-106.0)	67.2 (39.5-100.0)
Intake of NSAIDs, n (%)	17 (60.7%)	18 (60.0%)

Table 1. Demographic characteristics of Rheumatoid Arthritis patients included in the double blind study of A. paniculata standardized extract (modified from Burgos et al., 2009).

The results of the study show a significant reduction at the end of the treatment in tender joint, number of swollen joints, total grade of swollen joint, number of tender joints, total grade of swollen joints, total grade of tender joints HAQ 0.52 and SF36 (two health questionnaires) within the group treated with the active drug when comparing day 0 against week 14 (figure 4). The effect was associated to a reduction of rheumatoid factor, IgA, and C4. The study concludes that the drug was significantly effective in reducing symptoms and serological parameters of the disease and therefore useful as natural complement in the treatment of Rheumatoid Arthritis [80].

The clinical efficacy of *A. paniculata* could be explained by the anti-inflammatory properties of andrographolide. Andrographolide present in the extract is a potent inhibitors of NF-κB [21], a transcription factor linked to pro-inflammatory expression of several proteins such as COX-2, iNOS, and TNF-α, IL-6. Since NF-κB is involved in the pathogenesis of Rheumatoid Arthritis and other rheumatoid conditions [81], we hypothesized that *A. paniculata* extract tablets (Paractin®) can reduce inflammatory symptoms, signs, serological parameters in these patients. In fact, the clinical findings suggest that the *A. paniculata* formulation may have an additional therapeutical effect over Prednisone and MTX in reducing pain and inflammatory clinical symptoms during treatment period. The beneficial effect in reducing pain and other

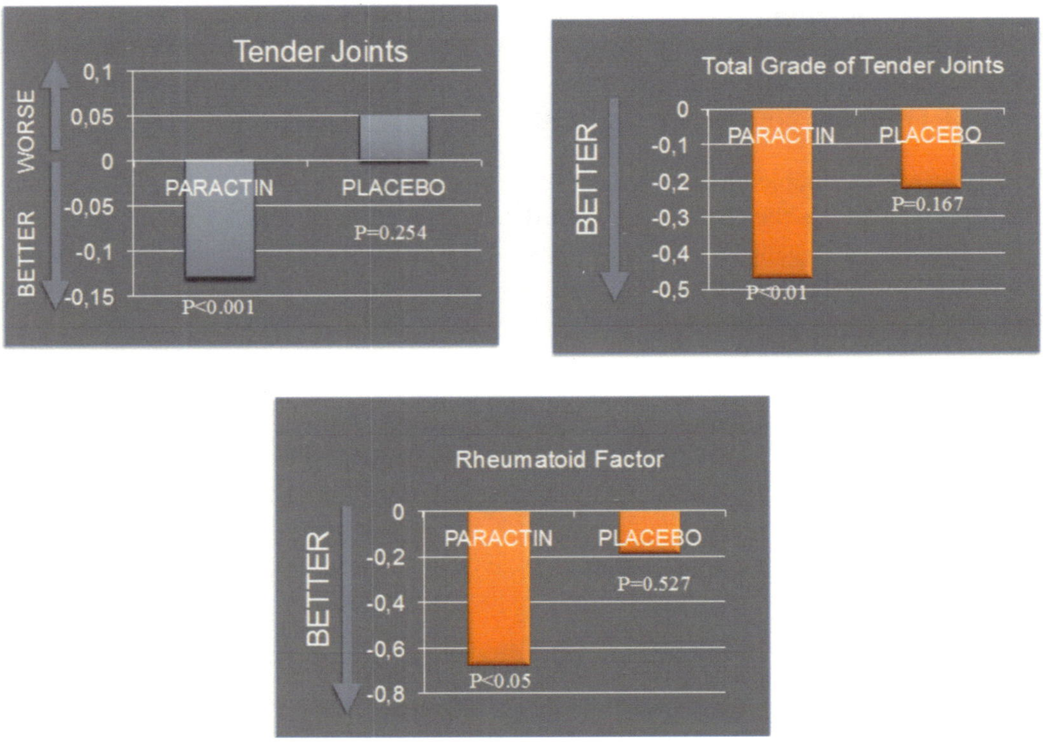

Figure 4. Effect of *A. paniculata* extract (Paractin®) on tender joints, total grade of tender joints and rheumatoid factor [80].

inflammatory symptoms with the *A. paniculata* formulation could be associated to the high standardization of total andrographolides (NLT 30%) in the extract considering. This is closely associated with the inhibition of COX-2 [21] and the reduction of PGE2 production [25], one of the main mechanisms for the control of inflammation and pain in Rheumatoid Arthritis by NSAIDs [82]. The dose of Andrographolide used in the present study was around 1.2 mg per kg. It has been reported that 1mg/kg reaches a steady state plasma concentration of 1.9 μM [83], a concentration able to reduce the PGE2 production [25]. Moreover, in patients treated with *A. paniculata* extract a decrease of rheumatoid factor (RF), creatine kinase, hemoglobin, IgA and IgM were observed. A correlation between RF titers and clinical disease activity has been reported widely [84]. RF titers decrease with methotrexate, suggesting an indirect link with disease activity [85]. Andrographolide can reduce the TNFα production in macrophages, an effect that could be associated with the reduction of auto-antibodies. It is known that a reduction of TNFα can diminish significantly the RF levels [86]. The ability of andrographolide to reduce antibody titer has also been demonstrated in other autoimmune diseases such as experimental autoimmune encephalomyelitis and lupus (see above). A reduction of immunoglobulin, such as IgM and IgA, could also be beneficial in long-term treatment because there is a positive correlation between the grade of cartilage damage in active Rheumatoid Arthritis [87] and decrease of RF. Moreover, treatment with DMARDs reduces the level of IgM and IgA in patients affected with Rheumatoid Arthritis [85]. We propose that *A. paniculata* could be useful in decreasing the radiological progression in long-term treatments of Rheumatoid Arthritis patients. In support of this, andrographolide reduces NFAT activity, a transcription factor linked with bone erosion [88]. In MC3T3, a murine osteoblast cell line, we observed that andrographolide is able to induce differentiation and calcium mineralization, via expression of COX2 (Burgos et al., data unpublished).

On the other hand, no side effects were observed, indicating that *A. paniculata* treatment was safe, non-toxic, and well tolerated. In the literature, side effects associated with *A. paniculata* or andrographolide, administered in higher doses (4-6mg/kg), have caused isolated cases of allergic reactions, tiredness, headache, pruritus/rash, diarrhea, nausea, metallic taste, bitter taste, dry tongue, eyes sensitive to light, decreased short- term memory, dizziness, heartburn, tender lymph nodes, and lymphadenopathy [89]. None of these effects were observed in Rheumatoid Arthritis patients after 14 weeks of treatment [80].

Despite, the fact that was no difference between *A. paniculata* and placebo treatment after 14 weeks, the intragroup analysis showed a significant decrease of clinical symptoms and serological parameters in the *A. paniculata* group. This effect could become more evident in a long term administration of the drug and follow up Rheumatoid Arthritis patients for several years.

5.2. Monotherapy with an *Andrographis paniculata* standardized extract (Paractin®) for the symptomatic relief of different chronic rheumatoid conditions: A prospective case report and long term follow up

5.2.1. Background

Presently, there is no specific or etiological cure for Rheumatoid Arthritis and these other rheumatoid conditions as well, and treatment aims to limit joint damage, prevent loss of function, and decrease pain. Therapies used for these purposes include nonsteroidal anti-inflammatory drugs, disease-modifying anti-rheumatic drugs (DMARDs), and corticosteroids. The American College of Rheumatology (ACR) Guidelines recommends the administration of DMARD within 3 months of diagnosis and methotrexate (MTX) as the standard treatment in monotherapy or in combination with other DMARDs [90]. MTX, as a standard therapy, induces significant improvement in the number of tender and swollen joints, pain, and functional status, in addition to physician and patient global assessment. The onset of MTX- induced improvement is generally within 3 months in the majority of patients who will eventually respond, and a plateau in the response is often reached after 6 to 12 months. However, as an anti-metabolic agent, MTX may cause adverse events such as cytopenia, serious infections, liver damage and muco-cutaneous problems. The long term use of MTX is associated with prevalence of significant liver enzymes in aprox. 13% of the patients and 3.7% of the patients discontinue MTX permanently for liver toxicity [91]

Considering that in the clinical study in patients with Rheumatoid arthritis there was a significant decrease in the group with *A. paniculata* in the symptoms over time (after 14 weeks) on the progression of the diseases, it was proposed that long term treatment could demonstrate a mayor therapeutic response similar to other DMARs treatment. We report six case reports, with different rheumatoid arthritis conditions, that support the fact that *A. paniculata* standardized extract reduces symptoms of chronic joint pain, stiffness and serological inflammatory parameters in a prospective individual case controlled follow up study over a period of 42 months.

5.2.2. Intervention

The drug of botanical origin used for the treatment of these cases is a patented (US patent *8084495*) standardized extract of *A. paniculata* known as Paractin®, manufactured and distributed by Herbal Powers (USA). Paractin® contains andrograpolide NLT 30%, neoandrographolide NLT 0.2% and deoxyandrographolide NLT 3%. Paractin® was supplied directly for this study and stored according to the instructions of the manufacturer. The batch number for the *A. paniculata* extract used in this study was PAR-070801-2. A secondary and identical batch was retained (N° 20050520) and kept at Herbal Powers. Each tablet contained 150 mg of the extract. During all duration of this treatment, two tablets were given before meals three times a day. This dosage regimen was determined in previous preclinical and clinical trials with the pure compound and other commercially available *A. paniculata* extracts [80, 83]. The content of these compounds was evaluated by HPLC using reference standards as described elsewhere [92].

5.2.3. Patients and method

The group consisted of 6 (five adults and one pediatric) patients, 3 male and 3 female, all with a long history of active diseases as shown in Table 2.

Patient	Sex	Age at Diagnosis Year. "0"	Diagnosis	Prevalence of Disease (Years)	Duration of Treatment (Months)
1	Female	51	Rheumatoid Arthritis	6	50
2	Male	36	Rheumatoid Spondylitis	7	50
3	Female	15	Rheumatoid Arthritis/Vasculitis	3	48
4	Female	39	Psoriatic Arthritis	15	60
5	Male	67	Rheumatoid Arthritis/ Serositis	8	38
6	Male	34	Psoriatic Arthritis/ Erythroderma	4	40

Table 2. Antecedents of patients treated with *Andrographis paniculata* standardized extract (Paractin®)

All patients were individually recruited and controlled by their treating physician from the Hospital Regional de Valdivia, Unit of Rheumatology in the city of Valdivia, Chile and complying confirmed diagnosis of Rheumatoid Arthritis conditions before they were enrolled. They all signed a written informed consent, including the one pediatric case that was given

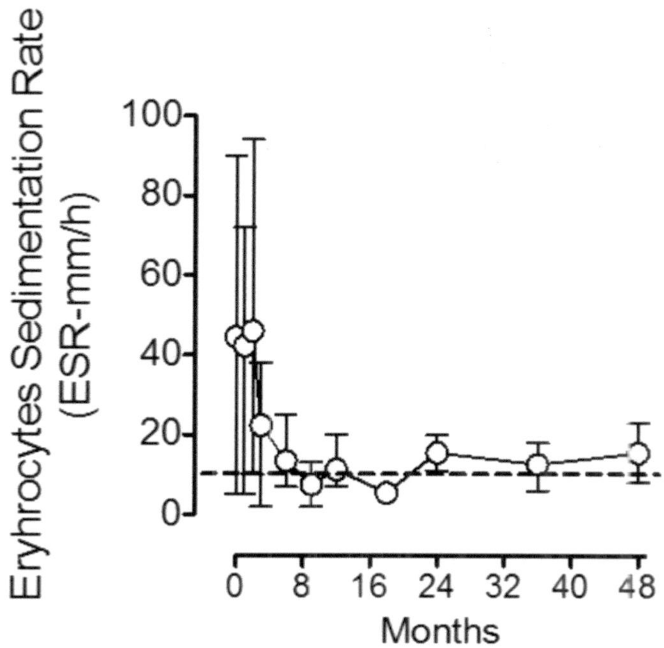

Figure 5. Erythrocyte sedimentation rate (ESR) in patients with chronic Rheumatoid Arthritis compared with ESR value at beginning of treatment. Continuous observation during 48 month. Each point represents the mean and range (maximum-minimum value). In dashed line the normal value.

consent by their parents. Advice and indications to test Paractin® was done by the rheumatologist, who requested the approval of each individual pharmacological protocol and supply of the product. The rationale and main objective was that Paractin® could reduce long term clinical symptoms and serological parameters of inflammation in these patients. Inclusion criteria were confirmed by clinical and laboratory diagnosis, that included active clinical and serological parameters of inflammation, no underlying standard treatment, poor or no response to standard treatment, or important side effects of Methotrexate and Prednisone, like in the female pediatric patient. From day 0, two tablets of Paractin® orally containing 150 mg of standardized *A. paniculata* extract (90 mg andrographolide per day) was administered during 48 month. Total withdrawal of the standard therapy was commonly decided by the treating physician and patient upon improvement observed with Paractin® treatment and informed to the investigators. All patients were controlled monthly during the first six months, then every three months thereafter at their respective place of residence and coordinated by their rheumatologist. After 24 months the treatment with Paractin® tablets, administered orally to patients with Rheumatoid Arthritis, Psoriatic Arthritis and Ankylosing spondylitis, reduced symptoms. In a similar fashion the serum immunological parameters of inflammation were reduced progressively during 48 month of Paractin® treatment.

When Paractin® was given alone; no side effects and good tolerability were observed during the complete period of administration. Only two cases reported a temporary and early and mild gastric discomfort with the tablets. Plasma biochemical parameters showed normal hematological, liver, kidney and metabolic functions. Interestingly, a moderate reactivation of joint pain and stiffness in two of the Rheumatoid arthritis patients and the one Ankylosing spondylitis patient was observed, due to an interruption of the treatment during 15, 11 and 22 days, respectively. Interestingly, these withdrawal and continuity incidents suggest that after peak and steady efficacy is reached and according to clinical and serological parameters follow up, a residual activity of the product is maintained between two and three weeks, disappearing at week four, and then recovered back again to previous status after four weeks. Also, we have so far not observed any loss of efficacy, or the need to increase dosages of the product, proving that no adaptation or refractoriness has yet been developed in this treated group. After one to five years follow up of these six rheumatologic patients, given a daily monotherapy of three Paractin® – tablets per day, we can conclude this product is well tolerated, safe and efficacious for the symptomatic relief and serological control of underlying inflammation related to their disease activity.

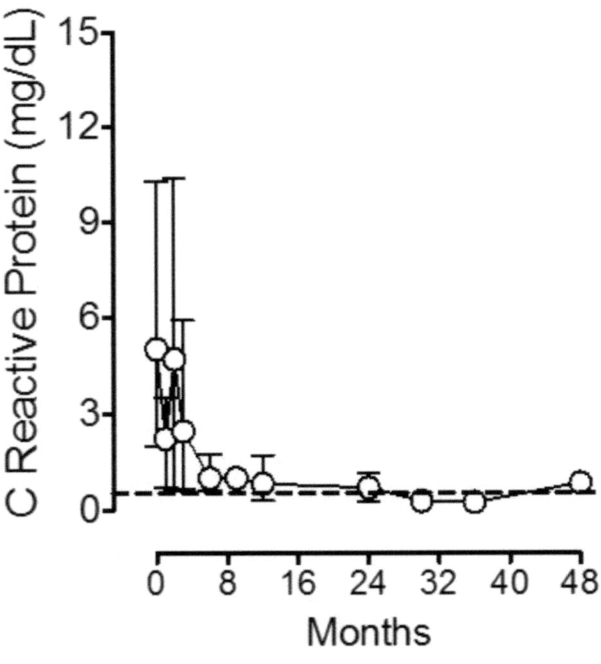

Figure 6. C Reactive protein (CRP) in patients with chronic rheumatoid disease compared with the CRP value at the beginning of treatment with Paractin®. Continuous observation during 48 months. Each point represents the mean and range (maximum-minimum value). In dashed line the normal value.

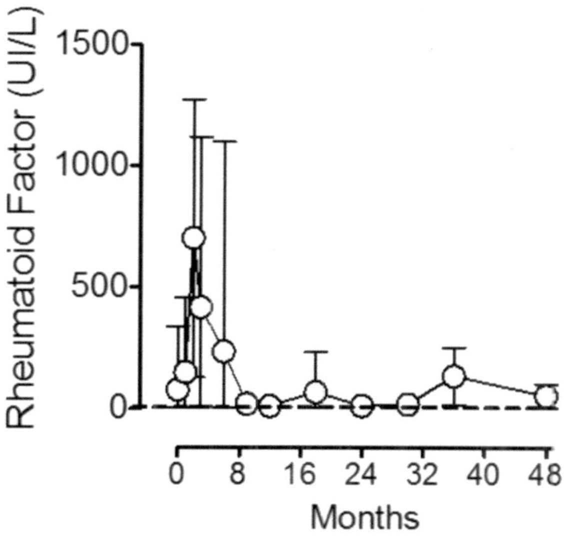

Figure 7. Rheumatoid Factor (RF) in patients with chronic rheumatoid disease treated with Paractin® during 48 month. Each point represents the mean and range (maximum-minimum value). In dashed line the normal value.

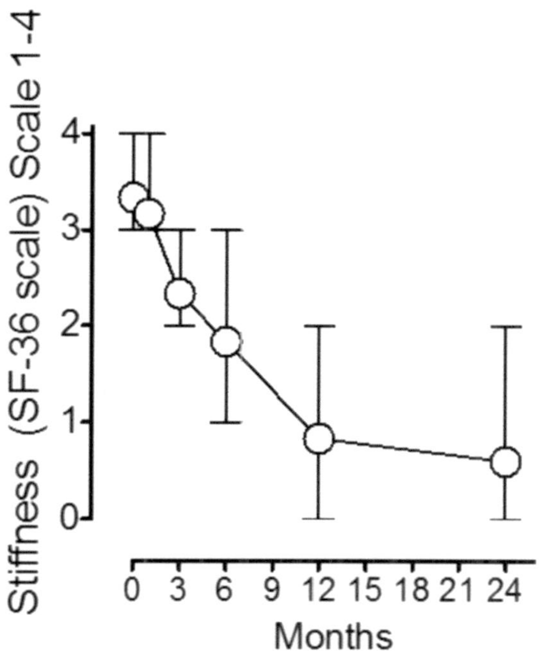

Figure 8. Variation on Rheumatologic stiffness in patients with chronic Rheumatoid Arthritis, treated with Paractin® during 24 month. Each point represents the mean and range (maximum-minimum value).

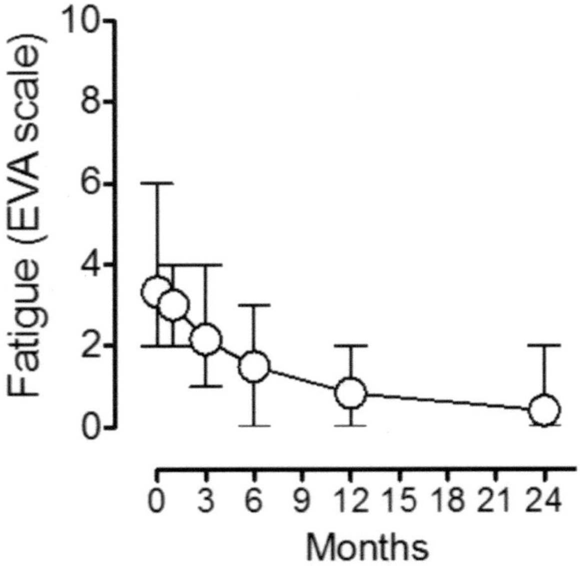

Figure 9. Effect of Paractin® on Fatigue in patients with chronic Rheumatoid Arthritis, treated during 24 month. Each point represents the mean and range (maximum-minimum value).

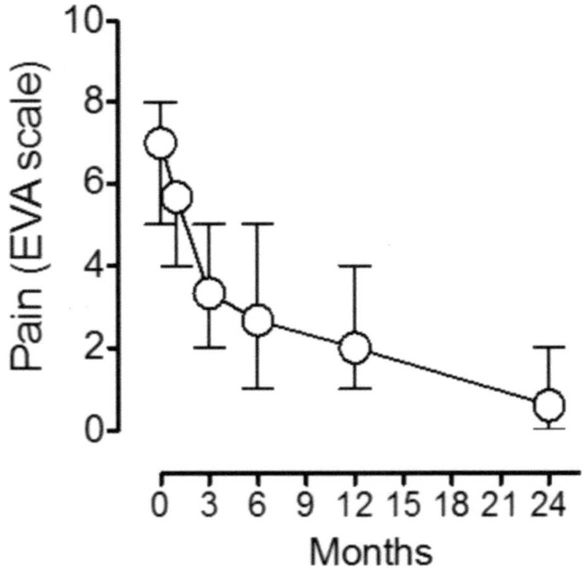

Figure 10. Effect of Paractin® on pain in patients with chronic Rheumatoid Arthritis, treated during 24 month. Each point represents the mean and range (maximum-minimum value).

6. Conclusion

Several studies describe a potent anti-inflammatory action of *Andrographis paniculata* and andrographolide. Andrographolide shows a reduction of the production of pro-inflammatory mediators, such as COX-2, iNOS and cytokines. The molecular mechanism of andrographolide implies the reduction of the activation of transcription factors as NF-κB, AP-1, STAT3 and NFAT and the inhibition of intracellular signaling pathways. *A. paniculata* standardized extract (30% andrographolide) in clinical trials showed effectiveness for symptom relief and reduce serological parameters in patients with Rheumatoid Arthritis, and the data support a long term treatment similar to other DMARDs.

Acknowledgements

FONDEF Grant DO9I1085 and DO4I1240

Author details

María A. Hidalgo[1,2], Juan L. Hancke[1,2], Juan C. Bertoglio[1,2] and Rafael A. Burgos[1,2]

1 Institute of Pharmacology and Morphophysiology, Faculty of Veterinary Science, Universidad Austral de Chile, Valdivia, Chile

2 Institute of Medicine, Faculty of Medicine, Universidad Austral de Chile, Valdivia, Chile

References

[1] Lim, J. C, Chan, T. K, Ng, D. S, Sagineedu, S. R, Stanslas, J, & Wong, W. S. Andrographolide and its analogues: versatile bioactive molecules for combating inflammation and cancer. Clin Exp Pharmacol Physiol. (2012). , 39(3), 300-10.

[2] Tang, W, & Eisenbrand, G. Chinese Drugs of Plant Origen. Berlin: Springer Verlag; (1992).

[3] Matsuda, T, Kuroyanagi, M, Sugiyama, S, Umehara, K, Ueno, A, & Nishi, K. Cell differentiation-inducing diterpenes from Andrographis paniculata Nees. Chem Pharm Bull (Tokyo). (1994). , 42(6), 1216-25.

[4] Pramanick, S, Banerjee, S, Achari, B, Das, B, & Sen, A. K. Sr., Mukhopadhyay S, et al. Andropanolide and isoandrographolide, minor diterpenoids from Andrographis paniculata: structure and X-ray crystallographic analysis. J Nat Prod. (2006). , 69(3), 403-5.

[5] Sharma, A, Lal, K, & Handa, S. S. Standardization of the indian crude drug kalmegh by high-pressure liquid-chromatographic determination of andrographolide. Phytochemical Analysis. (1992). , 3(3), 129-31.

[6] Reddy, V. L, Reddy, S. M, Ravikanth, V, Krishnaiah, P, Goud, T. V, Rao, T. P, et al. A new bis-andrographolide ether from Andrographis paniculata nees and evaluation of anti-HIV activity. Nat Prod Res. (2005). , 19(3), 223-30.

[7] Wiart, C, Kumar, K, Yusof, M. Y, Hamimah, H, Fauzi, Z. M, & Sulaiman, M. Antiviral properties of ent-labdene diterpenes of Andrographis paniculata nees, inhibitors of herpes simplex virus type 1. Phytother Res. (2005). , 19(12), 1069-70.

[8] Yang, S, Evens, A. M, Prachand, S, Singh, A. T, Bhalla, S, David, K, et al. Mitochondrial-mediated apoptosis in lymphoma cells by the diterpenoid lactone andrographolide, the active component of Andrographis paniculata. Clin Cancer Res. (2010). , 16(19), 4755-68.

[9] Zhou, J, Lu, G. D, Ong, C. S, Ong, C. N, & Shen, H. M. Andrographolide sensitizes cancer cells to TRAIL-induced apoptosis via death receptor 4 up-regulation. Mol Cancer Ther. (2008). , 53.

[10] Yu, B. C, Chang, C. K, Su, C. F, & Cheng, J. T. Mediation of beta-endorphin in andrographolide-induced plasma glucose-lowering action in type I diabetes-like animals. Naunyn Schmiedebergs Arch Pharmacol. (2008).

[11] Zhang, Z, Jiang, J, Yu, P, Zeng, X, Larrick, J. W, & Wang, Y. Hypoglycemic and beta cell protective effects of andrographolide analogue for diabetes treatment. J Transl Med. (2009).

[12] Sheeja, K, Guruvayoorappan, C, & Kuttan, G. Antiangiogenic activity of Andrographis paniculata extract and andrographolide. Int Immunopharmacol. (2007). , 7(2), 211-21.

[13] Thisoda, P, Rangkadilok, N, Pholphana, N, Worasuttayangkurn, L, Ruchirawat, S, & Satayavivad, J. Inhibitory effect of Andrographis paniculata extract and its active diterpenoids on platelet aggregation. Eur J Pharmacol. (2006).

[14] Sheeja, K, & Kuttan, G. Protective effect of Andrographis paniculata and andrographolide on cyclophosphamide-induced urothelial toxicity. Integr Cancer Ther. (2006). , 5(3), 244-51.

[15] Sinha, J, Mukhopadhyay, S, Das, N, & Basu, M. K. Targeting of liposomal andrographolide to L. donovani-infected macrophages in vivo. Drug Deliv. (2000). , 7(4), 209-13.

[16] Handa, S. S, & Sharma, A. Hepatoprotective activity of andrographolide against galactosamine & paracetamol intoxication in rats. Indian J Med Res. (1990). , 92, 284-92.

[17] Handa, S. S, & Sharma, A. Hepatoprotective activity of andrographolide from Andrographis paniculata against carbontetrachloride. Indian J Med Res. (1990). , 92, 276-83.

[18] Singha, P. K, Roy, S, & Dey, S. Protective activity of andrographolide and arabinogalactan proteins from Andrographis paniculata Nees. against ethanol-induced toxicity in mice. J Ethnopharmacol. (2007). , 111(1), 13-21.

[19] Woo, A. Y, Waye, M. M, Tsui, S. K, Yeung, S. T, & Cheng, C. H. Andrographolide upregulates cellular-reduced glutathione level and protects cardiomyocytes against hypoxia/reoxygenation injury. J Pharmacol Exp Ther. (2008). , 325(1), 226-35.

[20] Bao, Z, Guan, S, Cheng, C, Wu, S, Wong, S. H, Kemeny, D. M, et al. A novel antiinflammatory role for andrographolide in asthma via inhibition of the nuclear factor-kappaB pathway. Am J Respir Crit Care Med. (2009). , 179(8), 657-65.

[21] Hidalgo, M. A, Romero, A, Figueroa, J, Cortes, P, Concha, I. I, Hancke, J. L, et al. Andrographolide interferes with binding of nuclear factor-kappaB to DNA in HL-60-derived neutrophilic cells. Br J Pharmacol. (2005). , 144(5), 680-6.

[22] Li, J, Luo, L, Wang, X, Liao, B, & Li, G. Inhibition of NF-kappaB expression and allergen-induced airway inflammation in a mouse allergic asthma model by andrographolide. Cell Mol Immunol. (2009). , 6(5), 381-5.

[23] Parichatikanond, W, Suthisisang, C, Dhepakson, P, & Herunsalee, A. Study of anti-inflammatory activities of the pure compounds from Andrographis paniculata (burm.f.) Nees and their effects on gene expression. Int Immunopharmacol. (2010). , 10(11), 1361-73.

[24] Qin, L. H, Kong, L, Shi, G. J, Wang, Z. T, & Ge, B. X. Andrographolide inhibits the production of TNF-alpha and interleukin-12 in lipopolysaccharide-stimulated macrophages: role of mitogen-activated protein kinases. Biol Pharm Bull. (2006). , 29(2), 220-4.

[25] Wang, T, Liu, B, Zhang, W, Wilson, B, & Hong, J. S. Andrographolide reduces inflammation-mediated dopaminergic neurodegeneration in mesencephalic neuron-glia cultures by inhibiting microglial activation. J Pharmacol Exp Ther. (2004). , 308(3), 975-83.

[26] Batkhuu, J, Hattori, K, Takano, F, Fushiya, S, Oshiman, K, & Fujimiya, Y. Suppression of NO production in activated macrophages in vitro and ex vivo by neoandrographolide isolated from Andrographis paniculata. Biol Pharm Bull. (2002). , 25(9), 1169-74.

[27] Liu, J, Wang, Z. T, & Ji, L. L. In vivo and in vitro anti-inflammatory activities of neoandrographolide. Am J Chin Med. (2007). , 35(2), 317-28.

[28] Pfisterer, P. H, Rollinger, J. M, Schyschka, L, Rudy, A, Vollmar, A. M, & Stuppner, H. Neoandrographolide from Andrographis paniculata as a potential natural chemosensitizer. Planta Med. (2010). , 76(15), 1698-700.

[29] Kamdem, R. E, Sang, S, & Ho, C. T. Mechanism of the superoxide scavenging activity of neoandrographolide- a natural product from Andrographis paniculata Nees. J Agric Food Chem. (2002). , 50(16), 4662-5.

[30] Yoopan, N, Thisoda, P, Rangkadilok, N, Sahasitiwat, S, Pholphana, N, Ruchirawat, S, et al. Cardiovascular effects of 14-deoxy-11,12-didehydroandrographolide and Andrographis paniculata extracts. Planta Med. (2007). , 73(6), 503-11.

[31] Zhang, C, Kuroyangi, M, & Tan, B. K. Cardiovascular activity of 14-deoxy-11,12-didehydroandrographolide in the anaesthetised rat and isolated right atria. Pharmacol Res. (1998). , 38(6), 413-7.

[32] Akowuah, G. A, Zhari, I, Mariam, A, & Yam, M. F. Absorption of andrographolides from Andrographis paniculata and its effect on CCl(4)-induced oxidative stress in rats. Food Chem Toxicol. (2009). , 47(9), 2321-6.

[33] Thamlikitkul, V, Dechatiwongse, T, Theerapong, S, Chantrakul, C, Boonroj, P, Punkrut, W, et al. Efficacy of Andrographis paniculata, Nees for pharyngotonsillitis in adults. J Med Assoc Thai. (1991). , 74(10), 437-42.

[34] Lee, M. J, Rao, Y. K, Chen, K, Lee, Y. C, Chung, Y. S, & Tzeng, Y. M. Andrographolide and 14-deoxy-11,12-didehydroandrographolide from Andrographis paniculata attenuate high glucose-induced fibrosis and apoptosis in murine renal mesangeal cell lines. J Ethnopharmacol. (2010). , 132(2), 497-505.

[35] Roy, D. N, Mandal, S, Sen, G, Mukhopadhyay, S, & Biswas, T. Deoxyandrographolide desensitizes hepatocytes to tumour necrosis factor-alpha-induced apoptosis through calcium-dependent tumour necrosis factor receptor superfamily member 1A release via the NO/cGMP pathway. Br J Pharmacol. (2010). , 160(7), 1823-43.

[36] Burgos, R. A, Loyola, M, Hidalgo, M. A, Labranche, T. P, & Hancke, J. L. Effect of 14-deoxyandrographolide on calcium-mediated rat uterine smooth muscle contractility. Phytother Res. (2003). , 17(9), 1011-5.

[37] Naik, S. R, & Hule, A. Evaluation of immunomodulatory activity of an extract of andrographolides from Andographis paniculata. Planta Med. (2009). , 75(8), 785-91.

[38] Burgos, R. A, Hidalgo, M. A, & Monsalve, J. LaBranche TP, Eyre P, Hancke JL. 14-deoxyandrographolide as a platelet activating factor antagonist in bovine neutrophils. Planta Med. (2005). , 71(7), 604-8.

[39] Sriramaneni, R. N, Omar, A. Z, Ibrahim, S. M, & Amirin, S. Mohd Zaini A. Vasorelaxant effect of diterpenoid lactones from Andrographis paniculata chloroform extract on rat aortic rings. Pharmacognosy Res. (2010). , 2(4), 242-6.

[40] Lala, S, Nandy, A. K, Mahato, S. B, & Basu, M. K. Delivery in vivo of 14-deoxy-11-oxoandrographolide, an antileishmanial agent, by different drug carriers. Indian J Biochem Biophys. (2003). , 40(3), 169-74.

[41] Kapil, A, Koul, I. B, Banerjee, S. K, & Gupta, B. D. Antihepatotoxic effects of major diterpenoid constituents of Andrographis paniculata. Biochem Pharmacol. (1993). , 46(1), 182-5.

[42] Ji, L. L, Wang, Z, Dong, F, Zhang, W. B, & Wang, Z. T. Andrograpanin, a compound isolated from anti-inflammatory traditional Chinese medicine Andrographis panicu-

lata, enhances chemokine SDF-1alpha-induced leukocytes chemotaxis. J Cell Biochem. (2005). , 95(5), 970-8.

[43] Liu, J, Wang, Z. T, & Ge, B. X. Andrograpanin, isolated from Andrographis paniculata, exhibits anti-inflammatory property in lipopolysaccharide-induced macrophage cells through down-regulating the MAPKs signaling pathways. Int Immunopharmacol. (2008). , 38.

[44] He, X. J, Zeng, X. B, Hu, H, & Wu, Y. X. Cytotoxic biotransformed products from andrographolide by Rhizopus stolonifer ATCC 12939. Journal of Molecular Catalysis B-Enzymatic. (2010).

[45] Li, W, Xu, X, Zhang, H, Ma, C, Fong, H, Van Breemen, R, et al. Secondary metabolites from Andrographis paniculata. Chem Pharm Bull (Tokyo). (2007). , 55(3), 455-8.

[46] Suebsasana, S, Pongnaratorn, P, Sattayasai, J, Arkaravichien, T, Tiamkao, S, & Aromdee, C. Analgesic, antipyretic, anti-inflammatory and toxic effects of andrographolide derivatives in experimental animals. Arch Pharm Res. (2009). , 32(9), 1191-200.

[47] Xu, J, Huang, S, Luo, H, Li, G, Bao, J, Cai, S, et al. QSAR Studies on andrographolide derivatives as alpha-glucosidase inhibitors. Int J Mol Sci. (2010). , 11(3), 880-95.

[48] Zhou, B, Zhang, D, & Wu, X. Biological Activities and Corresponding Sar Analysis of Andrographolide and its Derivatives. Mini Rev Med Chem. (2012).

[49] Kanniappan, M, Mathuram, L. N, & Natarajan, R. A study on the antipyretic effect of chiretta (andrographis-panniculata). Indian Veterinary Journal. (1991). , 68(4), 314-6.

[50] Shen, Y. C, Chen, C. F, & Chiou, W. F. Suppression of rat neutrophil reactive oxygen species production and adhesion by the diterpenoid lactone andrographolide. Planta Med. (2000). , 66(4), 314-7.

[51] Shen, Y. C, Chen, C. F, & Chiou, W. F. Andrographolide prevents oxygen radical production by human neutrophils: possible mechanism(s) involved in its anti-inflammatory effect. Br J Pharmacol. (2002). , 135(2), 399-406.

[52] Abu-ghefreh, A. A, Canatan, H, & Ezeamuzie, C. I. In vitro and in vivo anti-inflammatory effects of andrographolide. Int Immunopharmacol. (2009). , 9(3), 313-8.

[53] Tsai, H. R, Yang, L. M, Tsai, W. J, & Chiou, W. F. Andrographolide acts through inhibition of ERK1/2 and Akt phosphorylation to suppress chemotactic migration. Eur J Pharmacol. (2004).

[54] Nagy, G, Koncz, A, Telarico, T, Fernandez, D, Ersek, B, Buzas, E, et al. Central role of nitric oxide in the pathogenesis of rheumatoid arthritis and systemic lupus erythematosus. Arthritis Res Ther. (2010).

[55] Chiou, W. F, Lin, J. J, & Chen, C. F. Andrographolide suppresses the expression of inducible nitric oxide synthase in macrophage and restores the vasoconstriction in rat aorta treated with lipopolysaccharide. Br J Pharmacol. (1998). , 125(2), 327-34.

[56] Lee, K. C, Chang, H. H, Chung, Y. H, & Lee, T. Y. Andrographolide acts as an anti-inflammatory agent in LPS-stimulated RAW264.7 macrophages by inhibiting STAT3-mediated suppression of the NF-kappaB pathway. J Ethnopharmacol. (2011). , 135(3), 678-84.

[57] Carretta, M. D, Alarcon, P, Jara, E, Solis, L, Hancke, J. L, Concha, I. I, et al. Andrographolide reduces IL-2 production in T-cells by interfering with NFAT and MAPK activation. Eur J Pharmacol. (2009).

[58] Iruretagoyena, M. I, Sepulveda, S. E, Lezana, J. P, Hermoso, M, Bronfman, M, Gutierrez, M. A, et al. Inhibition of nuclear factor-kappa B enhances the capacity of immature dendritic cells to induce antigen-specific tolerance in experimental autoimmune encephalomyelitis. J Pharmacol Exp Ther. (2006). , 318(1), 59-67.

[59] Iruretagoyena, M. I, Tobar, J. A, Gonzalez, P. A, Sepulveda, S. E, Figueroa, C. A, Burgos, R. A, et al. Andrographolide interferes with T cell activation and reduces experimental autoimmune encephalomyelitis in the mouse. J Pharmacol Exp Ther. (2005). , 312(1), 366-72.

[60] Burgos, R. A, Seguel, K, Perez, M, Meneses, A, Ortega, M, Guarda, M. I, et al. Andrographolide inhibits IFN-gamma and IL-2 cytokine production and protects against cell apoptosis. Planta Med. (2005). , 71(5), 429-34.

[61] Chen, H. W, Lin, A. H, Chu, H. C, Li, C. C, Tsai, C. W, Chao, C. Y, et al. Inhibition of TNF-alpha-Induced Inflammation by andrographolide via down-regulation of the PI3K/Akt signaling pathway. J Nat Prod. (2011). , 74(11), 2408-13.

[62] Chao, C. Y, Lii, C. K, Tsai, I. T, Li, C. C, Liu, K. L, Tsai, C. W, et al. Andrographolide inhibits ICAM-1 expression and NF-kappaB activation in TNF-alpha-treated EA.hy926 cells. J Agric Food Chem. (2011). , 59(10), 5263-71.

[63] Pratheeshkumar, P, & Kuttan, G. Andrographolide inhibits human umbilical vein endothelial cell invasion and migration by regulating MMP-2 and MMP-9 during angiogenesis. J Environ Pathol Toxicol Oncol. (2011). , 30(1), 33-41.

[64] Chen, J. H, Hsiao, G, Lee, A. R, Wu, C. C, & Yen, M. H. Andrographolide suppresses endothelial cell apoptosis via activation of phosphatidyl inositol-3-kinase/Akt pathway. Biochem Pharmacol. (2004). , 67(7), 1337-45.

[65] Yan, J, Chen, Y, He, C, Yang, Z. Z, Lu, C, & Chen, X. S. Andrographolide induces cell cycle arrest and apoptosis in human rheumatoid arthritis fibroblast-like synoviocytes. Cell Biol Toxicol. (2012). , 28(1), 47-56.

[66] Burgos, R. A, Hidalgo, M. A, Carretta, M. D, Bertoglio, J. C, Folch, H, & Hancke, J. L. Immunomodulatory activities induced by Andrographis paniculata. Govil JN, Singh VK, editors. USA: Studium Press LLC; (2009).

[67] Carreno, L. J, Riedel, C. A, & Kalergis, A. M. Induction of tolerogenic dendritic cells by NF-kappaB blockade and Fcgamma receptor modulation. Methods Mol Biol. (2011). , 677, 339-53.

[68] Kalergis, A. M, Iruretagoyena, M. I, Barrientos, M. J, Gonzalez, P. A, Herrada, A. A, Leiva, E. D, et al. Modulation of nuclear factor-kappaB activity can influence the susceptibility to systemic lupus erythematosus. Immunology. (2009). Suppl):e, 306-14.

[69] Szekanecz, Z, & Koch, A. E. Mechanisms of Disease: angiogenesis in inflammatory diseases. Nat Clin Pract Rheumatol. (2007). , 3(11), 635-43.

[70] Kumar, S, Patil, H. S, Sharma, P, Kumar, D, Dasari, S, Puranik, V. G, et al. Andrographolide Inhibits Osteopontin Expression and Breast Tumor Growth Through Down Regulation of PI3 kinase/Akt Signaling Pathway. Curr Mol Med. (2012).

[71] Vallabhapurapu, S, & Karin, M. Regulation and function of NF-kappaB transcription factors in the immune system. Annu Rev Immunol. (2009). , 27, 693-733.

[72] Xia, Y. F, Ye, B. Q, Li, Y. D, Wang, J. G, He, X. J, Lin, X, et al. Andrographolide attenuates inflammation by inhibition of NF-kappa B activation through covalent modification of reduced cysteine 62 of J Immunol. (2004). , 50.

[73] Lee, W. R, Chung, C. L, Hsiao, C. J, Chou, Y. C, Hsueh, P. J, Yang, P. C, et al. Suppression of matrix metalloproteinase-9 expression by andrographolide in human monocytic THP-1 cells via inhibition of NF-kappaB activation. Phytomedicine. (2012).

[74] Shouda, T, Yoshida, T, Hanada, T, Wakioka, T, Oishi, M, Miyoshi, K, et al. Induction of the cytokine signal regulator SOCS3/CIS3 as a therapeutic strategy for treating inflammatory arthritis. J Clin Invest. (2001). , 108(12), 1781-8.

[75] Asahara, H, Fujisawa, K, Kobata, T, Hasunuma, T, Maeda, T, Asanuma, M, et al. Direct evidence of high DNA binding activity of transcription factor AP-1 in rheumatoid arthritis synovium. Arthritis Rheum. (1997). , 40(5), 912-8.

[76] Tas, S. W, Remans, P. H, Reedquist, K. A, & Tak, P. P. Signal transduction pathways and transcription factors as therapeutic targets in inflammatory disease: towards innovative antirheumatic therapy. Curr Pharm Des. (2005). , 11(5), 581-611.

[77] Morel, J, & Berenbaum, F. Signal transduction pathways: new targets for treating rheumatoid arthritis. Joint Bone Spine. (2004). , 71(6), 503-10.

[78] Ohori, M. ERK inhibitors as a potential new therapy for rheumatoid arthritis. Drug News Perspect. (2008). , 21(5), 245-50.

[79] Chern, C. M, Liou, K. T, Wang, Y. H, Liao, J. F, Yen, J. C, & Shen, Y. C. Andrographolide inhibits PI3K/AKT-dependent NOX2 and iNOS expression protecting mice against hypoxia/ischemia-induced oxidative brain injury. Planta Med. (2011). , 77(15), 1669-79.

[80] Burgos, R. A, Hancke, J. L, Bertoglio, J. C, Aguirre, V, Arriagada, S, Calvo, M, et al. Efficacy of an Andrographis paniculata composition for the relief of rheumatoid arthritis symptoms: a prospective randomized placebo-controlled trial. Clin Rheumatol. (2009). , 28(8), 931-46.

[81] Handel, M. L, Mcmorrow, L. B, & Gravallese, E. M. Nuclear factor-kappa B in rheumatoid synovium. Localization of and p65. Arthritis Rheum. (1995). , 50.

[82] Daoud, K. F, Jackson, C. G, & Williams, H. J. Basic therapy for rheumatoid arthritis: nonsteroidal anti-inflammatory drugs. Compr Ther. (1999).

[83] Panossian, A, Hovhannisyan, A, Mamikonyan, G, Abrahamian, H, Hambardzumyan, E, Gabrielian, E, et al. Pharmacokinetic and oral bioavailability of andrographolide from Andrographis paniculata fixed combination Kan Jang in rats and human. Phytomedicine. (2000). , 7(5), 351-64.

[84] Vittecoq, O, Pouplin, S, Krzanowska, K, Jouen-beades, F, Menard, J. F, Gayet, A, et al. Rheumatoid factor is the strongest predictor of radiological progression of rheumatoid arthritis in a three-year prospective study in community-recruited patients. Rheumatology (Oxford). (2003). , 42(8), 939-46.

[85] Olsen, N. J, Teal, G. P, & Brooks, R. H. IgM-rheumatoid factor and responses to second-line drugs in rheumatoid arthritis. Agents Actions. (1991).

[86] Yazdani-biuki, B, Stadlmaier, E, Mulabecirovic, A, Brezinschek, R, Tilz, G, Demel, U, et al. Blockade of tumour necrosis factor {alpha} significantly alters the serum level of IgG- and IgA-rheumatoid factor in patients with rheumatoid arthritis. Ann Rheum Dis. (2005). , 64(8), 1224-6.

[87] He, Y, Zha, Q, Liu, D, & Lu, A. Relations between serum IgA level and cartilage erosion in 436 cases of rheumatoid arthritis. Immunol Invest. (2007). , 36(3), 285-91.

[88] Pessler, F, Dai, L, Cron, R. Q, & Schumacher, H. R. NFAT transcription factors--new players in the pathogenesis of inflammatory arthropathies? Autoimmun Rev. (2006). , 5(2), 106-10.

[89] Coon, J. T, & Ernst, E. Andrographis paniculata in the treatment of upper respiratory tract infections: a systematic review of safety and efficacy. Planta Med. (2004). , 70(4), 293-8.

[90] Guidelines for the management of rheumatoid arthritis: (2002). UpdateArthritis Rheum. 2002;, 46(2), 328-46.

[91] Salliot, C, & Van Der Heijde, D. Long-term safety of methotrexate monotherapy in patients with rheumatoid arthritis: a systematic literature research. Ann Rheum Dis. (2009). , 68(7), 1100-4.

[92] Burgos, R. A, Caballero, E. E, Sanchez, N. S, Schroeder, R. A, Wikman, G. K, & Hancke, J. L. Testicular toxicity assessment of Andrographis paniculata dried extract in rats. J Ethnopharmacol. (1997). , 58(3), 219-24.

Chapter 12

Efficacy of Nandrolone Decanoate in Treating Rheumatoid Cachexia in Male Rheumatoid Arthritis Patients

Andrew B. Lemmey, Srinivasa Rao Elamanchi, Samuele M. Marcora, Francesco Casanova and Peter J. Maddison

Additional information is available at the end of the chapter

http://dx.doi.org/10.5772/53236

1. Introduction

Rheumatoid cachexia, a consequence of chronic inflammation, is a common feature of rheumatoid arthritis (RA) [1]. It is characterised by reduced muscle mass and increased, predominantly truncal, adiposity, which in turn both contribute to physical weakness and disability [2,3]. Additionally, as in other catabolic conditions, these adverse changes in body composition exacerbate risk of falls and fracturing, contribute to impaired physical disability and reduced quality of life, and increase morbidity and mortality [e.g. 4-6]. In RA, again as in other chronic conditions, these outcomes are most marked in severe forms of cachexia where there is frank weight loss with reductions in both lean and fat mass. This overt wasting has been estimated to occur in up to 10% of RA patients and is associated with a three-fold higher mortality [7].

There is evidence that rheumatoid cachexia is established early in the course of the disease [8], and that it is resistant to antirheumatic drug treatment. This non-responsiveness to standard treatment is highlighted by the high prevalence of significant muscle wasting (approximately 67%) and the even higher incidence of obesity (approximately 80%) observed in patients with stable, controlled disease [9-13]. Despite the fact that TNF-α is considered to be a major factor driving rheumatoid cachexia, even anti-TNF treatment fails to reverse or attenuate these perturbations to body composition [8,14,15]. In fact, evidence is emerging that anti-TNF therapy increases fat mass, particularly trunk adiposity, relative to standard DMARDs [14,15]. Consequently, specific potential anabolic interventions need to be assessed as adjuncts to antirheumatic drug therapy. The most efficacious means of improving body composition and physical function in RA patients is regular, high-intensity exercise [9,10,16,17]. However, uptake of this mode of therapy is extremely low amongst RA patients [e.g. 18] as it is for the general population.

During recent years there has been a dramatic increase in the clinical use of testosterone and its synthetic derivatives, anabolic-androgenic steroids (AAS), to improve body composition; in particular, for treatment of muscle loss due to age-related sarcopenia, HIV-related muscle wasting, and hypogonadism in men [19-21]. In support of this treatment strategy, studies utilising either replacement or supraphysiologic doses of testosterone or AAS have been shown to elicit significant increases in lean/muscle mass and reductions in fat mass in healthy, young, middle-aged and old androgen-deficient men [20,21,22-29], frail elderly men [30], glucocorticoid-treated men [31], and men with heart failure [32], HIV [33-38], chronic renal failure [39-41], and COPD [42]. Surprisingly, given the profound positive effects on body composition, the effects of testosterone or AAS therapy on physical function are moderate at best [20], with many of the studies cited above failing to detect improvements in objectively or subjectively assessed function [26,28,29,37-39,41,42].

In the past, trials of testosterone or AAS in RA have mainly focused on improving bone mineral density and general wellbeing [43-45], rather than effects on body composition. Although in one controlled study [43] in which postmenopausal women with RA received 50mg nandrolone decanoate (ND) every 3 weeks for 2 years, whilst there was no effect of treatment on bone density (the primary outcome measure of the investigation), it was incidentally reported that there were significant increases in total body nitrogen and total body potassium, two proxy measures of muscle mass. However, other aspects of body composition, such as adiposity, were not assessed. Nor were the consequences of increased muscle mass on physical function investigated.

Given its anabolic effects, and its relatively reduced androgenic effects compared to testosterone (testosterone has an anabolic:androgenic ratio of 1, whereas the ratio for ND is 10 [19]), ND, an esterified form of the minimally aromatizable testosterone analog, nandrolone, would appear to be a suitable potential anabolic intervention for RA. A reduction in androgenic effects is a vital consideration when proposing potential therapies for RA as the incidence of this disease is three times higher in women than in men [46].

Thus, in the present pilot study we assessed the efficacy of 24 weeks of ND (100mg/week) administration in reversing muscle loss and decreasing fat mass in male patients with established RA. As secondary outcomes, we assessed safety and the effects on physical function of ND treatment.

http://dx.doi.org/10.5772/53236

2. Methods

2.1. Subject recruitment and eligibility

This was a randomised, placebo-controlled, double-blind trial, approved by the North West Wales NHS Research Ethics Committee. Sample size was determined by power calculations for the principal outcome variable: appendicular lean mass (ALM). This calculation was based on the results of a study conducted by our group investigating the efficacy of ND (@ 100mg/week) in increasing ALM in male haemodialysis patients [41]. Thus, we used a mean change in ALM of 1.40kg (SD = 0.46kg), assumed normal distribution, two groups, equal variance, no change in the control group, $\alpha = 0.05$, and power = 0.80. Calculations resulted in the requirement of 5 participants per group to identify a significant change in ALM. To account for potential dropouts, we aimed to recruit 12 participants per group (i.e. a total of 24 participants).

Accordingly, 24 consenting adult males with established rheumatoid arthritis from the Gwynedd Hospital Rheumatology Department were recruited into the study and randomized for treatment with either ND or placebo [41]. Eligibility criteria for subjects were: a diagnosis of RA according to the American Rheumatism Association 1987 revised criteria [47]; aged 18 years or older; functional class I or II; and stable antirheumatic drug therapy for at least 3 months. Patients were excluded if they: were cognitively impaired; had other reasons for cachexia; were taking drugs or nutritional supplements known to affect muscle mass; were engaged in regular, high intensity exercise; or had a contraindication to receiving anabolic steroids. The intervention was either 200mg nandrolone decanoate (Deca-Durabolin, Organon Laboratories Ltd., Cambridge, UK) or matched placebo (vehicle only) given by deep intramuscular injection every two weeks for 24 weeks.

2.2. Outcome measures

All study outcome measures were assessed at baseline and at 24 weeks. To monitor treatment safety, an additional blood sample was taken at 12 weeks. For each assessment, subjects presented at approximately the same time of day, fasted, and having refrained from strenuous exercise for 24 hours.

2.2.1. Body composition

Body composition was assessed by whole-body pencil-beam dual x-ray absorptiometry (DXA; Hologic, QDR1500, software version V5.72). This measurement provides estimates of total and regional lean, fat and bone masses. Subsequently, appendicular lean mass (ALM; i.e. total arms + legs soft-lean mass), a proxy measure of total body skeletal muscle mass [48], was determined [49]; relative skeletal muscle index (RSMI) was calculated (ALM (kg)/height (m)^2) [50]; and percent body fat (%BF) estimated. RSMI and %BF were then used to determine whether patients were "cachectic", "obese", and if both, "cachectic-obese", according to the definitions of Baumgartner et al. [50].

Immediately following DXA scanning, bioelectrical impedance spectroscopy (BIS; Hydra ECF/ICF 4200, Xitron Technologies, San Diego, Calif., USA) was used to estimate extracellular water (ECW), intracellular water (ICW), and total body water (TBW). Checking these is necessary since ND treatment has been associated with oedema which impairs interpretation of DXA measures of body composition.

2.2.2. Muscle strength and physical function

Maximal voluntary isometric knee extensor strength (at a fixed joint angle of 90^0) was measured by a Kin-com isokinetic dynamometer (Chattanooga, Tennessee, USA). Physical function was additionally measured by objective tests from the "Senior Fitness Test" [51]: 30-seconds sit-to-stand chair stand, the 30-seconds arm curl, and 50-foot walk. Subjective patient reported physical disability was assessed with the multidimensional Health Assessment Questionnaire [52].

2.2.3. Disease Activity and inflammation

Disease activity was evaluated by the Disease Activity Score in 28 joints (DAS28-ESR) [53], and systemic inflammation by erythrocyte sedimentation rate (ESR) and C-reactive protein (CRP) level.

2.2.4. Harms

Guidelines for reporting harms where taken from the extended CONSORT statement [54]. Proformas (templates with information completed by the lead researcher following a set pattern) were completed detailing expected adverse ND effects including androgenic effects, sodium/fluid retention, alterations to dry weight causing cramps/hypotension, haematoma at injection site, blood data including liver function tests (alanine aminotransferase (ALT), aspartate aminotransferase (AST), alkaline phosphatase (Alk Phos)), lipid profiles (total cholesterol, LDL cholesterol, HDL cholesterol, triglycerides), haemoglobin (Hb), hematocrit (Hct), and prostate specific antigen (PSA). Unexpected (not reported on medication information sheets) and serious (fatal, life threatening, or resulted in hospitalization) adverse events were collected passively as they occurred during the trial period. Decisions about whether events should be attributed to the intervention were made unblinded by the lead clinician. Decisions about whether to withdraw patients from the trial following harms were made following discussion between the patient and the lead clinician. Adverse events with ambiguous definitions were defined as follows: hypotension (fainting and concomitant low blood pressure); fluid retention (clinical signs including oedema, breathlessness, high blood pressure, and increased hydration of the lean body mass); carpal tunnel syndrome (tingling/numbness associated with medial nerve and positive Phalen's test); fitting (seizures or convulsions); heart attack (myocardial infarction), and acne and hair loss (self-reported and defined by patients). Potential drug-related adverse events such as fluid retention were monitored clinically each month of the intervention, and blood analyses i.e. liver function tests, serum lipid profile, Hb, Hct and PSA were assessed every 12 weeks. All blood analyses were performed in hospital laboratories by automated analysers using routine methods.

http://dx.doi.org/10.5772/53236

2.3. Statistical Analysis

Baseline differences between the groups were examined using multiple independent t-tests. When no difference was confirmed, treatment effects were assessed by multiple, 2-way (2x2; treatment by time (baseline and at 24 weeks)) ANOVAs. When baseline differences were revealed, the effects of ND were determined by ANCOVAs. Assumptions of sphericity were verified by Mauchly's Test, and the between subjects effect size for group was calculated as eta squared (η^2), with thresholds for small, moderate, large and very large effects set at. 01,.08,.26 and.50 respectively. Data were analysed using SPSS version 14 (Chicago, IL), and are presented as mean±SD. P values <0.05 were considered statistically significant, whilst p values from 0.05-0.10 were considered a trend.

3. Results

Of the 24 participants who were randomised, there were three dropouts in the ND group. Logistical failure meant two did not receive their injections and one developed fast atrial fibrillation after the first ND injection; the latter was thought to be unrelated to the treatment but resulted in withdrawal from treatment. The remainder (9 on ND, 12 on placebo) completed the study and provided the data used for the analysis. As shown in Table 1, there were no significant differences between the two groups at baseline in age, disease duration, functional class, DAS 28, ESR and CRP, and serum testosterone levels, and for both groups, there were no significant changes in DAS28, ESR and CRP at follow-up (data not shown). At baseline, 7 of the 9 ND subjects and 9 of the 12 placebo subjects had low serum testosterone (T) levels as defined by being below the 50th percentile for healthy males aged 60-80 years (i.e. <13.7 mmol/L) [26]. As anticipated, at 24 weeks serum concentrations of T, luteinizing hormone (LH), and follicle-stimulating hormone (FSH) were significantly reduced (p's=0.002, 0.005, 0.041, respectively) in subjects receiving ND treatment, and unchanged in those receiving placebo (data not shown). There were also no differences in serum sex hormone binding globulin (SHBG) levels between the groups at baseline (p=0.522), but in contrast to T, LH and FSH, SHBG levels were unaffected by treatment and remained similar for both groups at 24 weeks (p=0.943) (data not shown).

Variable	Nandrolone (n = 9)	Placebo (n = 12)	p value
Age	56.9 ± 12.4	64.4 ± 8.5	0.100
Disease duration (years)	9.7 ± 8.0	15.8 ± 11.4	0.270
Functional class	1.60 ± 0.52	1.70 ± 0.89	0.350
HAQ (0-3)	0.85 ± 0.64	1.18 ± 0.93	0.390
DAS 28 score	3.50 ± 1.54	5.29 ± 3.48	0.157
ESR (mm/hr)	22.11 ± 27.59	28.91 ± 26.40	0.573
CRP (mg/l)	24.33 ± 27.32	13.50 ± 6.31	0.197
Testosterone (mmol/L)	11.70 ± 6.04	11.82 ± 6.20	0.957

Table 1. Baseline characteristics of study participants. Data are presented as means ± SD.

The effects of ND on body composition are summarised in Table 2. At baseline there were no significant differences in body composition variables, and a similar proportion of subjects in the ND (6 of 9) and placebo (9 of 12) groups were initially classified as cachectic (RSMI ≤7.26kg/ m²) and/or obese (7 of 9, and 10 of 12, respectively; %BF ≥27% for males [50]). In the ND group, there were substantial mean increases in both total lean mass (TLM) and ALM (a surrogate measure of muscle mass) at 24 weeks (4.24kg and 2.39kg, respectively; i.e. 8.4% and 12.1% increases versus baseline, respectively), whereas these remained stable in the controls. ND also induced large reductions in total fat mass (FM) (mean of 2.16kg; -8.6% versus baseline) and in truncal FM (mean of 0.97kg; -7.1% versus baseline). By contrast, both mean total and truncal FM increased in the control group (by 1.93kg and 0.90kg, respectively). Thus, post intervention, percent body fat was significantly different between the two groups. Body mass increased slightly in both groups following the intervention period, but remained similar as increased muscle mass in the ND group corresponded with increased FM in the controls. As a consequence of the respective treatment effects, at 24 weeks there were reductions in the number of subjects classified as either cachectic or obese in the ND group (6 of 9 to 4/9, and 7/9 to 4/9, respectively), but not the placebo group (9/12 to 9/12, and 10/12 to 11/12, respectively).

There was no significant change in bone density for either group (data not shown).

Variable	Nandrolone (n = 9)	Placebo (n = 12)	p value
Body mass (kg)	78.45 ± 16.21	77.32 ± 11.59	0.650
Baseline	81.13 ± 15.05	79.14 ± 12.33	
Post-intervention			
Total lean mass (kg)	50.39 ± 7.39	48.65 ± 6.44	0.001
Baseline	54.63 ± 7.99	48.37 ± 6.88	0.002
Post-intervention	19.71 ± 3.64	18.54 ± 3.03	
Appendicular lean mass (kg)	22.10 ± 4.28	18.48 ± 3.10	
Baseline			
Post-intervention			
Total fat mass (kg)	25.47 ± 11.02	26.88 ± 8.50	0.005
Baseline	23.29 ± 10.26	28.81 ± 8.06	
Post-intervention			
Trunk fat mass (kg)	13.58 ± 6.06	15.13 ± 5.78	0.074
Baseline	12.61 ± 6.02	16.03 ± 4.94	
Post-intervention			
% Body fat	31.33 ± 8.41	34.44 ± 7.03	0.001
Baseline	28.20 ± 7.72	36.22 ± 6.26	
Post-intervention			

Table 2. Effects of 24 weeks of nandrolone (200mg every two weeks) or placebo on body composition in male patients with rheumatoid arthritis

As a consequence of randomization, mean objectively assessed physical function at baseline was generally significantly lower for the placebo group than for the ND group (e.g. knee extensor strength, p=0.010; chair stand test, p=0.005; arm curls, p<0.001). As expected, physical function of both groups was reduced relative to that of age- and sex-matched, sedentary, healthy individuals (i.e. mean performances in the objective measures were 31-32% less for the ND group and 47-51% less in the placebo group than the 50th percentile levels for healthy 60-64 year old males [51]). Increased muscle mass and reduced fat mass following ND treatment, however, was not accompanied by significant improvements, by ANCOVA, in knee extensor strength or performance in the 30sec chair stand or 50 foot walk tests. In contrast, a significant improvement in the arm curl test was observed in the ND group following 24 weeks treatment, albeit the effect size was only moderate (Table 3).

Variable	Nandrolone (n = 9)	Placebo (n = 12)	p value	ή²
Knee extensor strength	403.50 ± 113.99	287.96 ± 76.01	0.012	
(newtons)	420.21 ± 155.61	293.45 ± 81.78	0.622	0.014
Baseline	*360.55 ± 31.53*	*338.19 ± 26.65*		
Post-intervention				
Adjusted				
30 sec chair stand test (reps)	11.11 ± 1.96	7.83 ± 2.55	0.005	
Baseline	12.77 ± 3.23	9.25 ± 2.99	*0.873*	*0.001*
Post-intervention	*10.86 ± 0.78*	*10.68 ± 0.65*		
Adjusted				
30 sec arm curl test (reps)	14.89 ± 1.90	10.08 ± 2.57	0.001	
Baseline	16.56 ± 2.65	10.83 ± 2.41	*0.034*	*0.227*
Post-intervention	*15.27 ± 1.00*	*11.80 ± 0.82*		
Adjusted				
50 foot walk (secs)	9.50 ± 2.24	12.34 ± 3.97	0.070	
Baseline	8.22 ± 1.92	11.27 ± 2.98	*0.112*	*0.134*
Post-intervention	*9.02 ± 0.72*	*10.67 ± 0.62*		
Adjusted				

Table 3. Effects of 24 weeks of nandrolone (200mg every two weeks) or placebo on objective strength and physical function in male patients with rheumatoid arthritis. Differences between groups at baseline were tested by paired t tests. Pretest and posttest scores are presented as means ± SD. Adjusted scores (posttest scores adjusted for pretest scores) are presented in italics as means ± SEM. Differences between groups in the adjusted scores were tested by ANCOVA. Thresholds for small, moderate, large and very large effects (ή²) were set at 0.01, 0.08, 0.26 and 0.50, respectively.

ND taken fortnightly for 24 weeks at a dose of 200mg was generally well tolerated. One participant complained of mood swings which were attributed to the intervention. An increase in ECW (mean of 0.99kg; p=0.003) was associated with ND treatment but there was no change in the ECW:ICW ratio between groups following treatment (ANOVA interaction p=0.791; data not shown). Supporting this finding, no clinical indication of fluid overload was evident in the ND treated subjects. As anticipated, ND treatment elicited a significant increase in Hb (pre- vs post-treatment: 13.9 ±1.8 vs 15.9±1.4, respectively; p=0.004) and Hct (41.7 ± 5.4 vs 48.0 ± 4.2, respectively; p<0.001). ND treatment also resulted in increased levels of transaminases (p=0.002), but these remained within the normal range except in three participants in whom there was a minimal elevation of AST above normal (less than 1 SD in each case). Serum levels of total, LDL and HDL cholesterol, triglycerides and PSA remained unchanged throughout the treatment period (data not shown). No serious adverse events occurred, and no other adverse events were reported, in either group.

4. Discussion

The main finding in this randomised control trial was that 24 weeks of 100mg/week nandrolone decanoate improved body composition; with mean increases in TLM and ALM (≈4.2kg and 2.4kg, respectively, or gains of 8.4% and 12.1%, respectively, relative to baseline) accompanied by reductions in fat mass (≈2.2kg; -8.6% versus baseline) including truncal adiposity (≈1.0kg; -7.1% versus baseline). This was not unexpected since dose responsiveness of body composition to ND has been well established in healthy young and older adults and in patients with a variety of catabolic conditions [31,35,38-42,55]. The mechanism for testosterone and its synthetic analogs' effects on body composition is thought to be via enhanced differentiation of multipotent mesenchymal stem cells into the myogenic lineage and concomitant inhibition into the adipogenic lineage [56]. Such preferential differentiation results in hypertrophy of both type I and type II muscle fibres and an increase in myonuclear number [57]. This anabolic effect could potentially reduce morbidity and mortality, particularly in extreme cases of cachexia. Indeed, anabolic steroids have been used therapeutically in catabolic states such as HIV/AIDS and severe age-related sarcopenia.

However, despite the significant improvement in muscle mass in particular, there were no obvious corresponding improvements in physical function at 24 weeks. A similar observation has been made in numerous trials of ND and testosterone [26,28,29,31,37-42]. Even in healthy individuals, the dose-response relationship between anabolic steroid administration and physical functioning is not as clear as that with increased muscle mass. Indeed, in reported studies, the correlations between the increment in muscle mass and measures of strength are not particularly strong [e.g. 20,22]. It has been suggested by Sattler et al. [27] that threshold increments of 1.5kg in LBM and 0.8kg in ALM need to be achieved if improvements in physical function following testosterone treatment are to be realized. However, in our study, 7 of the 9 ND subjects exceeded both these threshold increases, yet all failed to achieve consistent improvements in function. Additionally, there was no correlation between increases in either LBM or ALM and gains in function.

Perhaps the results of our study reflect a physiological delay in adaptation following muscle hypertrophy, although it is clear that factors other than muscle size influence strength and physical function. To illustrate this, we observed substantial improvements in the same objectively assessed measures of physical function used in the current study (17-30% relative to baseline; p's = 0.027-0.001) in RA patients following 24 weeks of high intensity progressive resistance training (PRT; i.e. strength training), despite the increases in LBM and ALM (1.54kg and 1.21kg, respectively, relative to baseline) being substantially less than those observed following 24 weeks ND treatment [9]. Interestingly, in the PRT study, increases in LBM correlated significantly with gains in function – and this relationship is characteristic of anabolic exercise interventions [58]. All of which suggests that, in addition to muscle hypertrophy, neural, circulatory, endocrine and biochemical adaptations, as observed following exercise training, are prerequisites for improving strength, power and endurance. There is also evidence from both experimental animal studies and treating people with chronic catabolic disorders that physical activity is an important adjunct to anabolic steroids in improving physical functioning. Thus, the dose-response effects of ND appeared to be attenuated in inactive rat models [59], and combining ND therapy with resistance exercise training in CKD patients on haemodialysis resulted in improvements in both muscle mass and physical function [40], whereas ND alone only increased muscle mass in these patients. We would predict the same effects in people with RA.

Although our conclusions regarding the effects of ND (and testosterone therapy generally) on function are compromised by our study's lack of power, it is clear that the dose effect of testosterone and AAS on physical function is considerably less evident than that on body composition, and that the correlation between changes in muscle mass and function following treatment with either testosterone or AAS is at best moderate [20,22]. It is also notable that numerous studies which feature much larger subject numbers (i.e. up to n=120 in the treatment group) [26,28,29,37,38,42], higher doses of testosterone or ND (i.e. up to 1120 mg testosterone undecanoate/week) [26,37], and longer treatment periods (i.e. up to 3 years) [28,29,31] failed to demonstrate improved function. Interestingly, Ottenbacher et al [20] in their meta-analysis, having concluded that the effects of androgen therapy on strength in elderly men are mixed and inconclusive, also noted that reported effect sizes were smaller in trials rated as high quality than in those designated as being of lower quality.

As reported by others [26,43], ND had a negligible effect on total bone density in the current study. There was, however, a significant increase in haemoglobin, probably due largely to direct androgen stimulation of erythropoiesis. This is a well reported consequence of androgen therapy [32,60,61], and could be an additional benefit should ND be used in rheumatoid cachexia, since anaemia is a common accompaniment of this condition. ND at a dose of 200mg every two weeks for twenty four weeks appeared to be well tolerated. Mood changes in one participant were attributed to the anabolic steroid but, apart from a clinically insignificant elevation of serum transaminases, there were no serious or non-serious observed side effects. An increase in extracellular water with ND treatment was demonstrated by BIS, but there were no clinical manifestations associated with this. As previously reported [38,42,62], ND treatment reduced serum T, LH and FSH levels in our subjects. However, this effect is transient and reversible with cessation of androgenic therapy [62]. These apparently benign treatment effects are consistent with those reported by systematic reviews and meta-analyses on testosterone and AAS therapy [19,32,60,61].

We restricted recruitment of participants to males with RA to avoid the potential virilising effects of ND. However, we have observed in our studies of CKD [41] that in women in order to produce significant muscle mass increase without virilising effects, the nandrolone dose should not exceed 50mg/week.

In conclusion, we have demonstrated that male patients with established RA respond to 100mg/week ND for 24 weeks with a considerable increase in muscle mass and decrease in fat mass. However, these improvements in body composition were not accompanied by general improvements in strength or physical function, which probably requires an additional intervention such as exercise. This treatment was well tolerated and might be appropriate for extreme cases of rheumatoid cachexia.

Acknowledgements

Dr Jeremy Jones for reviewing the manuscript. Organon Laboratories Ltd., Cambridge, UK for providing the study drug and placebo.

Author details

Andrew B. Lemmey[1*], Srinivasa Rao Elamanchi[2], Samuele M. Marcora[2], Francesco Casanova[1] and Peter J. Maddison[1,2]

*Address all correspondence to: a.b.lemmey@bangor.ac.uk

1 School of Sport Health and Exercise Sciences (SSHES), Bangor University, U. K.

2 Department of Rheumatology, Gwynedd Hospital, Bangor, U. K.

References

[1] Summers, G. D., Deighton, C. M., Rennie, M. J., & Booth, A. H. (2008). Rheumatoid cachexia: a clinical perspective. *Rheumatology*, 47, 1124-31.

[2] Giles, J. T., Bartlett, S. J., Andersen, R. E., Fontaine, K. R., & Bathon, J. M. (2008). Association of body composition with disability in rheumatoid arthritis: Impact of appendicular fat and lean tissue mass. *Arthritis Rheum*, 59(10), 1407-1415.

[3] Kramer, H. R., Fontaine, K. R., Bathon, J. M., & Giles, J. T. (2012). Muscle density in rheumatoid arthritis. Associations with disease features and functional outcomes. *Arthritis Rheum*, 64(8), 2438-2450.

[4] Kotler, D. P. (2000). Cachexia. *Ann Intern Med*, 133, 622-634.

[5] Melton, L. J., Khosla, S., Crowson, C. S., O'Connor, M. K., O'Fallon, W. M., & Riggs, B. L. (2000). Epidemiology of sarcopenia. *J Am Geriatr Soc*, 48, 625-630.

[6] Morley, J. E., Baumgartner, RN, Roubenoff, R., Mayer, J., & Nair, K. S. (2001). From the Chicago meetings: Sarcopenia. *J Lab Clin Med*, 137, 231-243.

[7] Morley, J. E., Thomas, D. R., & Wilson, M. M. G. (2006). Cachexia: pathophysiology and clinical relevance. *Am J Clin Nutr*, 83, 735-743.

[8] Marcora, S. M., Chester, K. R., Mittal, G., Lemmey, A. B., & Maddison, P. J. (2006). Randomized phase 2 trial of anti-tumor necrosis factor therapy for cachexia in patients with early rheumatoid arthritis. *Am J Clin Nutr*, 84, 1463-1472.

[9] Lemmey, A. B., Marcora, S. M., Chester, K., Wilson, S., Casanova, F., & Maddison, P. J. (2009). Effects of high-intensity resistance training in patients with rheumatoid arthritis: A randomized controlled trial. *Arthritis Care Res*, 61, 1726-1734.

[10] Marcora, S. M., Lemmey, A. B., & Maddison, P. J. (2005). Can progressive resistance training reverse cachexia in patients with rheumatoid arthritis? Results of a pilot study. *J Rheumatol*, 32, 1031-1039.

[11] Marcora, S. M., Lemmey, A. B., & Maddison, P. J. (2005). Dietary treatment of rheumatoid cachexia with ß-hydroxy- ß-methylbutyrate, glutamine and arginine: a randomised controlled trial. *Clin Nutr*, 24, 442-454.

[12] Stavropoulos-Kalinoglou, A., Metsios, G., Panoulas, V. F., et al. (2009). Underweight and obese states both associate with worse disease activity and physical function in patients with established rheumatoid arthritis. *Clin Rheumatol*, 28, 439-444.

[13] Roubenoff, R., Roubenoff, R. A., Cannon, J. G., et al. (1994). Rheumatoid cachexia: cytokine-driven hypermetabolism accompanying reduced body cell mass in chronic inflammation. *J Clin Invest*, 93, 2379-2386.

[14] Metsios, G. S., Stavropoulos-Kalinoglou, A., Douglas, K. M., et al. (2007). Blockade of tumor necrosis factor alpha in rheumatoid arthritis: effects on components of rheumatoid cachexia. *Rheumatology*, 46, 1824-27.

[15] Engvall-L, I., Trengstrand, B., Brismar, K., & Hafstrom, I. (2010). Infliximab therapy increases body fat mass in early rheumatoid arthritis independently of changes in disease activity and levels of leptin and adiponectin: a randomised study over 21 months. *Arthritis Res Therapy*, 12, R197.

[16] Hakkinen, A., Hakkinen, K., & Hannonen, P. (1994). Effects of strength training on neuromuscular function and disease activity in patients with recent-onset inflammatory arthritis. *Scand J Rheumatol*, 23, 237-242.

[17] Hakkinen, A., Pakarinen, A., Hannonen, P., et al. (2005). Effects of prolonged combined strength and endurance training on physical fitness, body composition and serum hormones in women with rheumatoid arthritis and in healthy controls. *Clin Exp Rheumatol*, 23, 505-512.

[18] Sokka, T., Hakkinen, A., Kautiainen, H., et al. (2008). Physical inactivity in patients with rheumatoid arthritis: Data from twenty-one countries in a cross-sectional, international study. *Arthritis Rheum*, 59, 42-50.

[19] Evans, N. A. (2004). Current concepts in anabolic-androgenic steroids. *Am J Sports Med*, 32(2), 534-542.

[20] Ottenbacher, K. J., Ottenbacher, ME, Ottenbacher, A. J., Alfaro, Acha. A., & Ostir, G. V. (2006). Androgen treatment and muscle strength in elderly men: A meta-analysis. *J Am Geriatr Soc*, 54, 1666-1673.

[21] Vermeulen, A. (2001). Androgen replacement therapy in the aging male: a critical evaluation. *J Clin Endocrinol Metab*, 86, 2380-2390.

[22] Bhasin, S., Woodhouse, L., Casaburi, R., et al. (2001). Testosterone dose-response relationships in healthy young men. *Am J Physiol*, 281, E 1172-E1181.

[23] Bhasin, S., Woodhouse, L., Casaburi, R., et al. (2005). Older men are as responsive as young men to the anabolic effects of graded doses of testosterone on the skeletal muscle. *J Clin Endocrinol Metab*, 90, 678-688.

[24] Bhasin, S., Storer, T. W., Berman, N., Callegari, C., Clevenger, BA, Phillips, J., Bunnell, T., Tricker, R., Shirazi, A., & Casaburi, R. (1996). The effects of supraphysiologic doses of testosterone on muscle size and strength in men. *N Eng J Med*, 335, 1-7.

[25] Brodsky, L. G., Balagopal, P., & Nair, K. S. (1996). Effects of testosterone replacement on muscle mass and muscle protein synthesis in hypogonadal men- a clinical research center study. *J Clin Endocrinol Metab*, 81, 3469-3475.

[26] Emmelot-Vonk, M. H., Verhaar, H. J. J., Nakhai, Pour. H. R., Aleman, A., Lock, T. M. T. W., Ruud Bosch, J. L. H., Grobbee, D. E., & van der Schouw, Y. T. (2008). Effect of testosterone supplementation on functional mobility, cognition, and other parmeters in older men. *JAMA*, 299(1), 39-52.

[27] Sattler, F., Bhasin, S., He, J., Chou-P, C., Castaneda-Sceppa, C., Yarasheski, K., Binder, E., Schroeder, E. T., Kawakubo, M., Zhang, A., Roubenoff, R., & Azen, S. (2011). Testosterone threshold levels and lean tissue mass targets needed to enhance skeletal muscle strength and function: The HORMA Trial. *J Gerontol A Biol Sci Med*, 66A(1), 122-129.

[28] Snyder, P. J., Peachy, H., Hannoush, P., Berlin, J. A., Loh, L., Lenrow, D. A., Holmes, J. H., Dlewati, A., Santanna, J., Rosen, C. J., & Strom, B. L. (1999). Effect of testosterone treatment on body composition and muscle strength in men over 65 years of age. *J Clin Endocrinol Metab*, 84, 2647-2653.

[29] Sreekumaran, Nair. K., Rizza, R. A., O'Brien, P., Dharariya, K., Short, K. R., Nehra, A., Vittone, J. L., Klee, G. G., Basu, A., Basu, R., Cobelli, C., Toffolo, G., Dalla, Man. C., Tindall, D. J., Melton, L. J. III, Smith, G. E., Khosla, S., & Jensen, MD. (2006). DHEA in elderly women and DHEA or testosterone in elderly men. *N Engl J Med*, 355, 1647-1659.

[30] Srinivas-Shankar, . U., Roberts, S. A., Connolly, M. J., O'Connell, M. D. L., Adams, J. E., Oldham, J. A., & Wu, F. C. W. (2010). Effects of testosterone on muscle strength, physical function, body composition, and quality of life in intermediate-frail and frail elderly men: A randomized, double-blind, placebo-controlled study. *J Clin Endocrinol Metab*, 95, 639-650.

[31] Crawford, B. A. L., Liu, P. Y., Kean, M. T., Bleasel, J. F., & Handelsman, D. J. (2003). Randomized placebo-controlled trial of androgen effects on muscle and bone in men requiring long-term systematic glucocorticoid treatment. *J Clin Endocrinol Metab*, 88, 3167-3176.

[32] Toma, M., Mc Alister, F. A., Coglianese, E. E., Vidi, V., Vasaiwala, S., Bakal, J. A., Armstrong, P. W., & Ezekowitz, J. A. (2012). Testosterone supplementation in heart failure. A meta-analysis. *Circ Heart Fail*, 5, 315-321.

[33] Bhasin, S., Storer, T. W., Asbel-Sethi, N., et al. (1998). Effects of testosterone replacement with a non-genital, transdermal system: Androderm in human immunodeficiency virus-infected men with low testosterone levels. *J Clin Endocrinol Metab*, 129, 3155-3162.

[34] Bhasin, S., Storer, T. W., Javanbakht, M., Berman, N., Yarasheski, K. E., Phillips, J., Dike, M., Sinha-Hikim, I., Shen, R., Hays, R. D., & Beall, G. (2000). Testosterone replacement and resistance exercise in HIV-infected men with weight loss and low testosterone levels. *JAMA*, 283, 763-770.

[35] Gold, J., High, H., & Li, Y. (1996). Safety and efficacy of nandrolone decanoate for treatment of wasting in patients with HIV-infection. *AIDS*, 10, 745-752.

[36] Grinspoon, S., Corcoran, C., Askari, H., et al. (1998). Effects of androgen administration in men with the AIDS wasting syndrome: a randomized, double-blind, placebo-controlled trial. *Ann Intern Med*, 129, 18-26.

[37] Knapp, P. E., Storer, T. W., Herbst, K. L., Singh, A. B., Dzekov, C., Dzekov, J., La Valley, M., Zhang, A., Ulloor, J., & Bhasin, S. (2008). Effects of a supraphysiological dose of testosterone on physical function, muscle performance, mood, and fatigue in men with HIV-associated weight loss. *Am J Physiol Endocrinol Metab*, 294, E1135-1143.

[38] Storer, T. W., Woodhouse, L. J., Sattler, F., Singh, A. B., Schroeder, E. T., Beck, K., Padero, M., Mac, P., Yarasheski, K. E., Geurts, P., Willemsen, A., Harms, M. K., & Bhasin, S. (2005). A randomized, placebo-controlled trial of nandrolone decanoate in human immunodeficiency virus-infected men with mild to moderate weight loss with recombinant human growth hormone as active reference treatment. *J Clin Endocrinol Metab*, 90, 4474-4482.

[39] Johansen, K. L., Mulligan, K., & Schambelan, M. (1999). Anabolic effects of nandrolone decanoate in patients receiving dialysis: a randomized controlled trial. *JAMA*, 281, 1275-1281.

[40] Johansen, K. L., Painter, P. L., Sakkas, G. K., Gordon, P., Doyle, J., & Shubert, T. (2006). Effects of resistance exercise training and nandrolone decanoate on body composition and muscle function among patients who receive hemodialysis: a randomized controlled trial. *J Am Soc Nephrol*, 17, 2307-2314.

[41] Macdonald, J. H., Marcora, S. M., Jibani, M. M., Kumwenda, M. J., Ahmed, W., & Lemmey, A. B. (2006). Nandrolone decanoate as anabolic therapy in chronic kidney disease: a randomized phase II dose-finding study. *Nephron Clin Pract*, 106, 125-135.

[42] Creutzberg, E. C., Wouters, E. F. M., Mostert, R., Pluymers, R. J., & Schols, A. M. W. J. (2003). A role for anabolic steroids in the rehabilitation of patients with COPD? A double-blind, placebo-controlled, randomized trial. *Chest*, 124, 1733-1742.

[43] Bird, H. A., Burkinshaw, L., Pearson, D., et al. (1987). Controlled trial of nandrolone decanoate in the treatment of rheumatoid arthritis in postmenopausal women. *Ann Rheum Dis*, 46, 237-243.

[44] Booij, A., Biewenger-Booij, C. M., Huber-Bruning, O., et al. (1996). Androgens as adjuvant treatment in postmenopausal female patients with rheumatoid arthritis. *Ann Rheum Dis*, 55, 811-886.

[45] Hall, G. M., Larbre, J. P., Spector, T. D., Perry, L. A., & Da Silva, J. A. (1996). A randomized trial of testosterone therapy in males with rheumatoid arthritis. *Br J Rheumatol*, 35, 568-573.

[46] Tobon, G. J., Youinou, P., & Saraux, A. (2010). The environment, geo-epidemiology, and autoimmune disease: rheumatoid arthritis. *Autoimmun Rev*, 9, A 288-292.

[47] Arnett, F. C., Edworthy, S. M., Bloch, D. A., et al. (1988). The American Rheumatism Association 1987 revised criteria for the classification of rheumatoid arthritis. *Arthritis Rheum*, 31, 315-324.

[48] Kim, J., Wang, Z., Heymsfield, S. B., Baumgartner, RN, & Gallagher, D. (2002). Total-body skeletal muscle mass: estimation by a new dual-energy X-ray absorptiometry method. *Am J Clin Nutr*, 76, 378-383.

[49] Fuller, N. J., Laskey, MA, & Elia, M. (1992). Assessment of the composition of major body regions by dual-energy X-ray absorptiometry (DEXA), with special reference to limb muscle mass. *Clin Physiol*, 12, 253-266.

[50] Baumgartner, R. N., Koehler, K. M., Gallagher, D., Romero, L., Heymsfield, S. B., Ross, R. R., et al. (1999). Epidemiology of sarcopenia among the elderly in New Mexico. *Am J Epidemiol*, 147, 755-763.

[51] Rikli, R. E., & Jones, C. J. (2001). Senior fitness test manual. *Champaign: Human Kinetics*.

[52] Pincus, . T., Swearingen, C., & Wolfe, F. (1999). Toward a multidimensional Health Assessment Questionnaire (MDHAQ): assessment of advanced activities of daily liv-

ing and psychological status in the patient-friendly health assessment questionnaire format. *Arthritis Rheum*, 42, 2220-2230.

[53] van Gestel, A. M., Haagsma, C. J., & van Riel, P. L. (1998). Validation of rheumatoid arthritis improvement criteria that include simplified joint counts. *Arthritis Rheum*, 41, 1845-1850.

[54] Ioannidis, J. P., Evans, S. J., Gotzsche, P. C., O'Neill, R. T., Altman, D. G., Schulz, K., & Moher, D. (2004). Better reporting of harms in randomized trials: an extension of the CONSORT statement. *Ann Intern Med*, 141, 781-788.

[55] Hartgens, F., Van Marken, Lichtenbelt. W., Ebbing, S., Vollaard, N., Rietjens, G., & Kuipers, H. (2001). Body composition and anthropometry in bodybuilders: regional changes due to nandrolone decanoate administration. *Int J Sports Med*, 22, 235-241.

[56] Bhasin, S., & Jasuja, R. (2009). Selective androgen receptor modulators (SARMs) as function promoting therapies. *Curr Opin Clin Nutr Metab Care*, 12(3), 232-240.

[57] Sinha-Hikim, I., Artaza, J., Woodhouse, L., et al. (2002). Testosterone-induced increase in muscle size in healthy young men is associated with muscle fiber hypertrophy. *Am J Physiol Endocrinol Metab*, 283, E154-E164.

[58] Kraemer, W. J., Fleck, S. J., & Evans, W. J. (1996). Strength and power training: physiological mechanisms of adaptation. *Exerc Sport Sci Rev*, 24, 363-397.

[59] Gayan-Ramirez, G., Rollier, H., Vanderhoydonc, F., Verhoeven, G., Gosselink, R., & Decramer, M. (2000). Nandrolone decanoate does not enhance training effects but increases IGF-I mRNA in rat diaphragm. *J Appl Physiol*, 88, 26-34.

[60] Bhasin, S., Woodhouse, L., & Storer, T. W. (2003). Androgen effects on body composition. 13. *Growth Hormone & IGF Res*, S 63-S71.

[61] Fernandez-Balsells, M. M., Murad, M. H., Lane, M., Lampropulos, J. F., Albuquerque, F., Mullan, R. J., Agrwal, N., Elamin, M. B., Gallegos-Orozco, J. F., Wang, A. T., Erwin, P. J., Bhasin, S., & Montori, V. M. (2010). Adverse effects of testosterone therapy in adult men: a systematic review and meta-analysis. *J Clin Endocrinol Metab*, 95(6), 2560-2575.

[62] Bijlsma, J. W., Duursma, S. A., Thijssen, , et al. (1982). Influence of nandrolone decanoate on the pituitary-gonadal axis in males. *Acta Endocrinol*, 101, 108-112.

Chapter 13

Role of Cysteine Cathepsins in Joint Inflammation and Destruction in Human Rheumatoid Arthritis and Associated Animal Models

Uta Schurigt

Additional information is available at the end of the chapter

http://dx.doi.org/10.5772/53710

1. Introduction

Destruction of bone and articular cartilage during pathogenesis of rheumatoid arthritis (RA) is caused by increased activity of a huge panel of proteases, which are secreted by several cell types of arthritic joint. Besides matrix metalloproteases (MMPs), the papain-like cysteine proteases (clan CA, family C1) have been identified as proteases potentially involved in cartilage and bone destruction as well as in immune response during inflammatory arthritis. Several clinical studies demonstrated that expression and activity of different cysteine cathepsins have been increased frequently in synovial membranes and fluids from RA patients. However, the exact roles of papain-like cysteine proteases have not been fully understood yet. Therefore, their contribution to joint inflammation and destruction has been investigated by *in vivo* and *in vitro* experiments in the last decades of arthritis research. This chapter focuses on cysteine cathepsins K, B, L, and S - the best-studied members of the papain-like protease family in arthritic diseases - in order to understand better their impact on inflammatory arthritis in respect to their collagenolytic activities as well as to their contributions to immune response. Latest results about the impact of cysteine cathepsins in different animal models for RA are discussed comprehensively. Furthermore, a short excursion to cathepsin V (= cathepsin L2) - an exclusively human cathepsin L-like cysteine cathepsin - and its impact on autoimmune disease progression is included in this review. The chapter clarifies that cathepsins K and S are attractive targets for the development of new highly specific anti-arthritis drugs.

2. Cysteine cathepsins

Cathepsins are a heterogeneous group of proteases. Originally, the name cathepsin was used for proteases with the highest activity in a slightly acidic environment as found in the lysosomes. The name cathepsin originates from greek "kathepsein" (= to digest). Today, the cathepsin family consists of at least 15 members and can be subdivided by their catalytic mechanism into three distinct groups: serine proteases (cathepsin A and G), aspartat proteases (cathepsin D and E), and cysteine proteases (cathepsins B, C, F, H, K, L, O, S, V, W, and X). Most cathepsins reside in endosomal/lysosomal compartment and are thus termed lysosomal cathepsins (except cathepsins E and G). Caused by this localization, cathepsins were initially considered as intracellularly active enzymes responsible for the non-specific bulk proteolysis in the acidic environment of the endosomal/lysosomal compartment, where they degrade intracellular and endocytosed extracellular proteins. However, this view has changed rapidly in the last years and there is a strong experimental evidence that cathepsins have huge panel of highly specialized functions [1, 2]. The cysteine cathepsins are characterized by the presence of a cysteine residue at their active site and are highly homologue to papain - a cysteine protease isolated originally from papaya fruit (*Carica papaya*). Therefore they are termed papain-like cysteine proteases and together with the parent protease papain they are classified in clan CA family C1 in "MEROPS – the peptidase database" [3]. Cysteine cathepsins are expressed by viruses, plants, primitive parasites, invertebrates, and vertebrates [4]. They play pivotal roles in chronic diseases (e.g. RA, cancer) as well as in infectious diseases (e.g. malaria, leishmaniasis) [2, 4, 5, 6]. Cysteine cathepsins are transported to the lysosomes via a specific mannose-6-phosphate receptor pathway, which explains the primary lysosomal localization [7]. Mature proteolytically active cathepsins are released after activation by removal of the N-terminal propeptide at the low pH of the lysosomes. The papain-like cysteine protease family contains both enzymes with endo- and exopeptidase activities. Cathepsin B is an endo- and an exopeptidase [3, 8]. It also acts as a peptidyl-dipeptidase [9]. Cysteine cathepsins K, L (= L1), S, and V (= L2) are endopeptidases [3]. The stability and activity of papain-like cysteine cathepsins depend on the acidic pH prevailing in lysosomes [2]. The functions of these enzymes may be altered with changes in pH and their cellular localization [2].

3. Cell types and tissues in arthritic joints

RA is an autoimmune disease with unknown etiology. The immune system of RA patients produces autoantibodies against components of their own extracellular matrix (ECM) in diarthrodial synovial joints (e.g. against collagens) [10]. This effectively leads the immune system to attack and finally to destroy - together with synovium-/pannus-associated cells - the articular cartilage and the bone in arthritic joints during disease progression. The diarthrodial synovial joint consists of highly specialized connective tissues (bone, hyaline cartilage, synovial tissue etc.) and a fibrous capsule (Figure 1). Bone is composed approximately to 70% of inorganic, mainly mineral compound called hydroxyapatite, 20% of organic material, mainly type I collagen, and 10% water [11]. Morphologically two types of bone can be distinguished: porous trabecular bone, also known as spongy bone, and dense cortical bone, also known as compact bone. Osteoclasts are bone-demineralizing and -degrading cells, which are also responsible for bone resorption and type I collagen degradation during normal physiological bone turnover (Figure 1). They are large multinucleated cells that express tartrate-resistant phosphatase (TRAP), calcitonin receptors, and cathepsin K [12]. Osteoclasts are able to acidify an isolated area between the cell and bone matrix, which is named resorption lacuna. Active acidification of bone by osteoclasts results in demineralization of bone, solubilization of mineral components, and finally an uncovering/liberalization of matrix collagens. In addition, it provides an acidic environment for secreted cathepsin K for optimal proteolytic activity. Bone resorption occurs at the contact site between the osteoclast and the bone, the so called ruffled border. Minerals of bone are solubilized due to the secretion of acids, which depends on the activity of carbonic anhydrase and proton pumps of osteoclasts. The degradation of organic matrix of bone (mainly type I collagens) occurs probably due to the activity of lysosomal cysteine proteases, other lysosomal hydrolases, and collagenases of MMP family secreted by osteoclasts. So far cathepsins B, K, and L could also be detected in osteoclasts [13, 14, 15, 16, 17, 18]. Articular cartilage (= hyaline cartilage) covers articulating bone surfaces in diarthrodial joints. Cartilage is composed of water (65 - 85%) and a solid phase, consisting of 15 - 20% type II collagen, 3 - 10% large aggregating molecules of proteoglycan, which are called aggrecans, and various other types of collagen [19]. The synovial membrane (or synovium) is the soft tissue between the articular capsule and the joint cavity of diarthrodial synovial joints. The word "synovium" is related to the word "synovial" (= synovial fluid), which is the clear, viscid, lubricating fluid secreted by synovial fibroblasts of synovial membrane (Figure 1). Continuous inflammation of synovium during RA pathogenesis leads to membrane expansion by hyperproliferation of activated synovial fibroblasts. Such arthritic synovial fibroblasts are infiltrated by mononuclear cells (e.g. T helper (Th) cells, B cells, macrophages) and form finally, together with these infiltrates, the so called invasive pannus tissue, which is characterized by an increased protease expression.

In advanced RA, arthritic synovial fibroblasts are the main source of destructive proteinases (e.g. MMPs and cathepsins) mediating pannus invasion of bone and articular cartilage. Additionally pannus-infiltrating macrophages contribute after their activation to joint degradation by increased cytokine and protease expression. Expression of cathepsins B, K, L, and S by different cell types of synovium of RA patients was detected [20, 21, 22]. Professional antigen presenting cells (APC) in arthritic joints are dendritic cells, B cells, and macrophages. Cathepsins B, L, and S contribute to antigen presentation in APCs [23]. Furthermore, B cells are responsible for producing autoantibodies. Studies of Th cell-secreted cytokine spectrum led to the classification of RA as a Th1-like disease [24]. This cell population, predominantly producing gamma interferon (IFNγ) and interleukin-2 (IL-2), stimulates protease overexpression in synovial fibroblasts and macrophages in pannus tissue. In contrast, Th2 cells, predominantly producing IL-4 and IL-10, are rarely found in arthritic joints. Anyway, both Th1 and Th2 cells can stimulate MMP expression in arthritic synovial fibroblasts by secretion of macrophage migration inhibitory factor [25]. Tumor necrosis factor alpha (TNFα) is considered as the main proinflammatory cytokine in the pathogenesis of RA [26]. It is produced by Th1 cells, synovial monocytes/macrophages, synovial fibroblasts, lymphocytes, and osteoblasts. TNFα can stimulate osteoclast formation in pannus tissue. Furthermore, TNFα appears to influence the distribution of osteoclast precursor cells in the body by increasing their influx from the bone marrow into synovium. TNFα also had a stimulating effect on secretion of procathepsin B by human arthritic synovial fibroblasts [27].

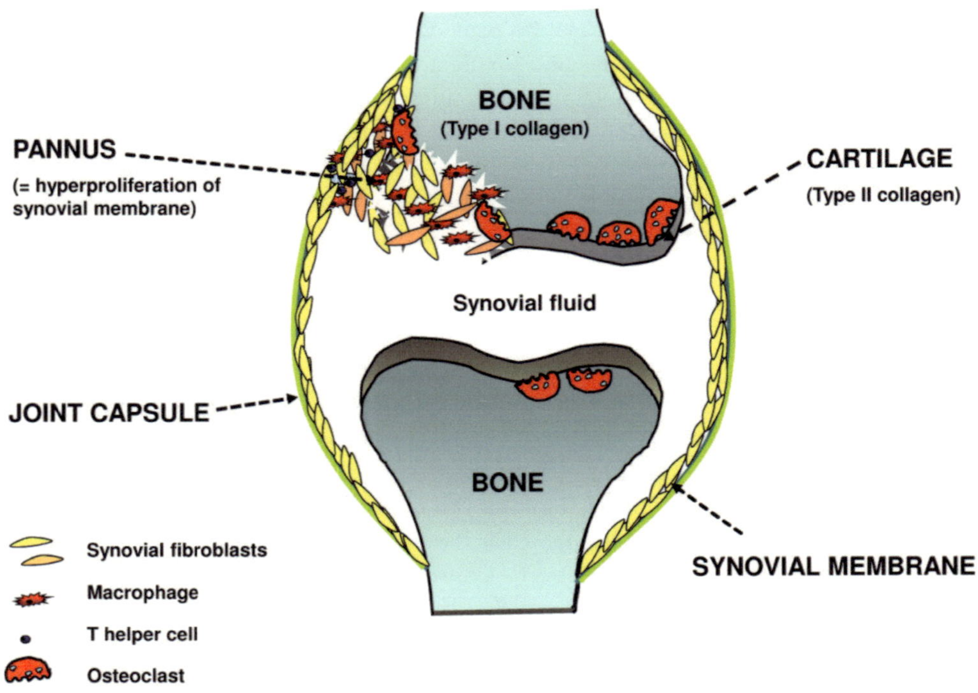

Figure 1. Organization of a diarthrodial synovial joint

4. Type I and type II collagens

One hallmark of human RA is the proteolytic degradation of collagens in ECM of affected joints. The ECM is the material between the cells in tissues of multicellular organisms. It provides structural framework of bone and articular cartilage of joints and is responsible for their resistance to pressure, torsion, and tension. Articular cartilage and bone contain specialized ECM components (collagens, elastin, proteoglycans etc.), which give diarthrodial joints strength and structural qualities. Collagens - the structural main components in joints - are extracellular matrix molecules used by cells for structural integrity and with a variety of other functions. About 28 different collagens have been identified in mammals and humans [28]. The typical mature collagen molecule consists of three single collagen polypeptide chains, so called alpha (α) chains, which coil into a helical molecule [28]. The different types of collagen are formed from a combination of more than 45 distinct collagen α polypeptide chains [28]. In the triple helical regions of collagens, termed Col domains, every third animo acid is glycine (gly) organized in as repeating peptide triplets of gly-X-Y [28]. In this triplet, X often is proline, and Y frequently is 4-hydroxyproline [28]. Col domains of each α chain are flanked by non-helical (non-gly-X-Y) regions, termed NC domains [28, 29]. In contrast, the telopeptides - the NC domains - of collagens have not the repeating gly-X-Y structure and do not adopt triple helical conformation. Telopeptides account for 2% of the collagen α chain and are essential for fibril formation [29]. Triple helical molecules aggregate spontaneously and form covalent cross-links among themselves to form collagen fibrils [29]. Both, the Col and the NC domains of collagen molecules are immunogenic [30]. Bone organic matrix contains predominantly type I collagen (90%). Type II collagen is the molecular principal compound of mammalian and human articular collagen, but additionally collagens III, VI, IX, X, XI, XII, and XIV contribute to composition of ECM of cartilage [31]. Type I and type II collagens, together with the other extracellular matrix molecules, are degraded during physiological processes (e.g. morphogenesis, growth, wound healing, physiological bone turnover) but also during pathological processes (e.g. cancer, RA).

5. Collagenolytic activities of papain-like cysteine proteases

Native collagens are highly resistant to proteolytic degradation due to their rigid and compact structure. However, hydrolysis of non-helical collagen telopeptides by proteases leads to depolymerization of the fibrillar collagen network, whereas cleavage within the triple helix results in depolymerization and denaturation of native triple helical collagen molecule. Only few proteases with collagenase activity have the capacity to initiate the cleavage of native triple helical collagens. Collagenases are enzymes that catalyze the hydrolysis of peptide bonds in triple helical regions of collagen. In contrast, denatured collagens (= gelatin) lost the triple helical structure and they are readily degraded by multiple proteinases (= gelatinases). Gelatinases are proteolytic enzymes hydrolyzing denatured collagen (= gelatin).

The exact mechanisms of collagen degradation have been not completely understood yet. Historically, MMPs have been considered as the main players of ECM degradation. This was justified by their membrane association or extracellular localization, their neutral pH optimum, and their ability to degrade structural extracellular proteins such as collagens, elastin, and proteoglycans. MMPs are members of a subfamily of proteases, which includes collagenases (MMP-1, -8, -13, and -18), stromelysins (MMP-3, -7, -10, -11, and -12), gelatinases (MMP-2 and -9), and membrane type MMPs (MT-MMPs: MMP-14, -15, -16, and -17). The collagenases among the MMPs are able to initiate degradation of native triple helical collagens. However, results of various studies have suggested that also other proteases must degrade ECM components. Especially, the papain-like cysteine cathepsins were supposed to contribute to collagen cleavage that occurs at acidic pH, in particular in collagen cleavage mediated by osteoclasts.

The investigation of tissue-degrading enzyme expression in synovial membrane, synovial fluid, and serum of RA patients is of particular interest in arthritis research, because elevations of analysed protease imply an impact on RA pathogenesis. The contribution of papain-like cysteine proteases to bone and cartilage destruction in RA was supposed, because several clinical studies showed that cysteine cathepsins were increasingly expressed and highly active in clinical samples from RA patients. Elevated levels of cysteine cathepsins B, L, S were detected in synovial fluids and in different cell types from patients with RA [32, 33, 34, 35]. Furthermore, it was shown, that cathepsins B and L were expressed in the synovial membrane shortly after symptom onset what implies that the potential for joint destruction exists at a very early stage in the course of the disease [36]. An enhanced transcription of cathepsin B in synovial cells from RA patients was detected [37]. Cathepsin B and L activities were detected in synovial membranes of RA patients [38]. Macrophages abundant in chronic RA subchondral bone lesions were characterized by high cathepsin L expression and an involvement of this protease in bone and cartilage destruction was supposed [39]. Furthermore, it was suggested that cathepsins B and L expressed by chondrocytes are involved in cartilage destruction during arthritis [40]. Cathepsin K was elevated in the serum of RA patients [41].

However, first direct experimental evidence supporting the role of papain-like cysteine proteases in bone resorption was provided by showing that specific inhibitors for different cysteine cathepsins and broad spectrum cysteine cathepsin inhibitors decreased bone resorption by osteoclasts [14, 16, 42, 43, 44]. The inhibition of lysosomes with cathepsin K-specific inhibitors led to an accumulation of undigested material within the endosomal/lysosomal compartment of osteoclasts [45]. Additionally, invasiveness of synovial fibroblasts from RA patients into cartilage both *in vitro* and *in vivo* in the SCID mouse coimplantation model was reduced after treatment with ribozymes cleaving specifically cathepsin L mRNA and therefore decreasing the synthesis of this cysteine protease [46].

Finally, *in vitro* analyses of collagenolytic activities helped to clarify the contribution of these individual cysteine cathepsins to physiological and pathological cartilage and bone degradation. Cleavage of soluble type I and type II collagen *in vitro* has been reported for cathepsins B, K, L, S, and V [47, 48, 49, 51, 59, 63] (Table 1). However, it is notable that latter proteases have only gelatinolytic activities and additionally contribute to unspecific cleavage of telopeptides of collagens [50]. Native triple helical type I and type II collagens are resistant to proteolysis by cathepsins B, L, S, and V. Although these cathepsins have not the capacity to cleave triple helical collagen, they attack their telopeptides, which are involved in intra- and intermolecular links [29]. This attack by cysteine cathepsin - similar to MMP-9 highly expressed in osteoclast - may destabilize the fibril collagen helices and therefore may contribute to joint destruction. Cathepsin L is the cysteine protease hitherto considered to have the highest telopeptidase and gelatinase activity among the papain-like cysteine proteases. Despite its own limited proteolytic activity, cathepsin B is able to proteolytically activate collagenase that mediates triple helical collagen cleavage [64].

http://dx.doi.org/10.5772/53710

Protease	Proteolytic activities		Cartilage- and bone-related phenotypes of protease-deficient mice	Investigation of protease-deficient mice in animal models for RA
	Collagenase activity	Gelatinase activity		
Cathepsin B	No	Yes [47, 48, 49]	No phenotypes reported	Antigen-induced arthritis: [personal communication by author] No differences to arthritic wild-type mice
Cathepsin K	Yes [50]	Yes [51]	Osteopetrotic phenotype in long bones, trabelular and cortical bone mass is increased, higher brittleness of bone [52, 53, 54, 55, 56]	hTNFtg mice: [57] Reduction of osteoclast-dependent cartilage and bone destruction Adjuvant arthritis: [58] Reduction in pro-inflammatory Th17 cells number by suppression of toll-like receptor 9 signaling in dendritic cells is responsible for attenuated arthritis
Cathepsin L	No	Yes [47, 48, 49, 51, 59]	Decrease in trabecular bone volume [60]	Antigen-induced arthritis: [61] Impairment of Th cell response, reconstitution by expression of human cathepsin V in thymus
Cathepsin S	No	Yes [47]	No phenotypes reported	Collagen-induced arthritis [62] Milder arthritis by impairment of antigen-presentation
Cathepsin V	No	Yes [63]	Not expressed in mice	

Table 1. Summary of proteolytic activities of individual cysteine cathepsins, the resulting phenotypes of protease-deficient mice, and the clinical outcome of these mice in animal models for human RA

However, only cathepsin K is able to cleave native type I collagen within the triple helical domain [50] (Table 1). This unique proteolytic activity is caused by the formation of an oligomeric complex between cathepsin K molecules and extracellular matrix-resident glycosaminoglycans [65]. However, in the absence of this complex, monomeric cathepsin K exhibits only the telopeptide cleavage capability and lacks this collagenase activity like the other papain-like cysteine cathepsins [50, 66]. To control the collagenase activity of cathepsin K by disruption of the glycosaminoglycan/cathepsin K complex or by prevention of its formation may open possibilities to develop new drugs to reduce bone destruction in RA. Cathepsin K was originally identified as an osteoclast-specific lysosomal protease. It is highly expressed and active in osteoclasts associated with bone surface and is secreted in resorption lacuna [15, 67]. The importance of cathepsin K for bone resorption has been demonstrated by cathepsin K inhibition studies with cathepsin K antisense oligodeoxynucleotides [68]. It has been shown that cathepsin K is capable to cleave type II collagen within the helical region of N-terminus, a unique capacity of this protease among papain-like cysteine proteases [69]. Therefore, inhibition of cathepsin K has been suggested to also play a pivotal role in protection of cartilage degradation during RA. Furthermore, cathepsin K is a critical protease in synovial fibroblast-mediated collagen degradation [70]. In contrast to MMPs with neutral or near-neutral pH optimum, cathepsin K is able to degrade the organic matrix in an acidic microenviroment. This acidic "collagenase" cleaves both triple-helical type I and type I collagen, the major structural components of the extracellular matrix of articular cartilage and bone. In contrast to collagenases (MMPs -1, -8, -13, -18), which cleave collagen creating typical ¼ C-terminal and ¾ N-terminal fragment, cathepsin K can cleave triple helical type I collagen at multiple sites resulting in a more complex degradation pattern [50, 69].

6. Phenotypes of cysteine cathepsin-deficient mice

Phenotyping is one of the first analytical steps after generation of gene knock out mice. Cartilage and bone phenotypes would be expected in cysteine cathepsin-deficient mice, if these proteases would contribute to physiological cartilage and bone turnover. Mice deficient in cysteine cathepsins B, K, L, and S were generated in the last years [52, 53, 54, 55, 62, 71, 72]. Cathepsin V is expressed exclusively in humans. No phenotypes of the bone or articular cartilage have been reported so far for cathepsin B-, and S-deficient mice (Table 1). In contrast, the bone phenotype in cathepsin K-deficient mice is very strong [52, 53, 54, 55, 56] (Table 1). Therefore, cathepsin K is possibly the most important proteolytic enzyme of osteoclasts in the papain-like cysteine protease family. Cathepsin K-deficient mice partially reflect the phenotype of pycnodysostosis, a human hereditary disease [52, 73]. The name "pycnodysostosis" appropriately describes this disease as formation of abnormally dense (greek: pykno) bone. The late 19th century French poster artist Henri de Toulouse-Lautrec (1864 - 1901) was the most prominent pycnodysostosis patient [74]. Therefore, this disease is sometimes referred as Toulouse-Lautrec syndrome. Cathepsin K mutations in patients with pycnodysostosis result in a total loss or inactivity of cathepsin K, which causes abnormal degradation of bone matrix proteins such as type I collagen [75]. Pycnodysostosis is characterized by a variable clinical appearance that includes short stature, open fontanelles, partial or total aplasia of the terminal phalanges, a predisposition to bone fractures, osteopetrosis, and an increased roentgenographic density of the entire skeleton [73, 74, 76, 77]. Cathepsin K-deficient mice are phenotypically characterized by an osteopetrotic phenotype in long bones - especially in distal femur - and lumbar vertebrae [52, 53, 54, 55, 56]. The trabecular and cortical bone mass is increased in cathepsin K-deficient mice compared with their wild-type littermates [55]. The bones of cathepsin K-deficient mice show a higher brittleness [53]. However, the osteopetrosis of pycnodysostosis patients seems to be more severe than that of cathepsin K-deficient mice and some of the skeletal changes seen in pycnodysostosis patients, such as retardation, phalangeal deformities, or delayed suture closure in the skull, have not been reported in cathepsin K-deficient mice [52, 53, 54, 55]. However, other clinical symptoms of pycnodysostosis as for instance the accumulation of undigested collagen fibrils in lysosomes of osteoclasts and fibroblasts are described for cathepsin K-deficient mice [45, 70, 73]. The lack of cathepsin K decreases the rate of osteoclast-mediated bone resorption but does not completely inhibit this process [52, 55]. The number of osteoclasts was significantly increased in trabecular bone of cathepsin K-deficient mice compared to wild-type controls, probably to compensate the inefficient bone degradation [54]. A cartilage phenotype of cathepsin K-deficient mice has not been reported. Furthermore, and in strong contrast to cathepsin K-deficient mice, cathepsin L knock out mice revealed a decrease in trabecular bone volume [60] (Table 1). This reduction in bone mass may suggest that cathepsin L is involved in endochondral ossification [60]. This effect was reduced after ostrogen withdrawal by ovariectomy [60].

7. Animal models of RA

The use of animal models allows *in vivo* investigation of single aspects, as for instance inflammation, antigen presentation, and joint destruction during the complex pathogenesis of inflammatory arthritis. Additionally, animal models have been applied to evaluate potential anti-arthritis drugs for clinical use. RA models are relatively easy to use, produce reproducible results, and are of short duration [78, 79, 80, 81]. They feature many of the clinical symptoms of the human disease. The most important difference between animal models of RA and human RA is the disease progression rate. It is much faster in animal models of RA than in the human disease. Therefore, animal models of inflammatory arthritis are characterized primarily by an acute inflammatory response and only a weak chronification of disease. Anyway, investigation of inflammatory arthritis with test animals is important for the understanding of specific aspects in pathogenesis of human RA. Especially the investigation of cysteine cathepsin-deficient or -transgenic mice in such models as well as the application of specific inhibitors in arthritic animals enables the understanding of the contribution of individual proteases to the disease outcome. Animal models for human RA can be classified into induced and spontaneous models [82]. It is important to select the right animal model for RA to address a specific scientific question. The repertory of animal models of RA includes among others adjuvant arthritis, antigen-induced arthritis (AIA), collagen-induced arthritis (CIA), and human TNF-transgenic (hTNFtg) mice [78, 80, 81, 82]. Each of these animal models only reflects a few of the clinical aspects of the human disease. Therefore, the exact knowledge of all clinical aspects, disease progression rate, and the contribution of individual cell types to inflamed joints to disease outcome is fundamental to understand the *in vivo* functions of investigated proteases or the *in vivo* effects of applied cysteine cathepsin-specific drugs. The latter is especially important because papain-like cysteine proteases not only directly contribute to ECM degradation in arthritic joints but also to local and systemic immune response. Several cysteine cathepsins are involved in antigen presentation and inflammatory pathways [23, 58]. First experimental results in animal models for RA with cysteine cathepsin-deficient and -transgenic mice have been helpful to understand the impact of these proteases on joint inflammation and destruction *in vivo*.

TNFα plays a central role in pathophysiology of RA [26, 83]. This was confirmed by the development of transgenic mice that overexpress human TNFα [81, 84]. The phenotype of hTNFtg mice validated the theory that TNFα is the apex of pro-inflammatory cascade in RA. In this simple mouse model for RA the investigators utilized a targeting vector that contained a genomic fragment encoding the entire human TNFα gene in which the ARE-containing 3`UTR was replaced with the 3`UTR from β-globin gene [81, 84]. This mutation resulted in a chronic overexpression of TNFα mRNA. hTNFtg mice develop spontaneously an erosive symmetrical polyarthritis with histopathological features of inflammation and bone destruction similar to human RA [81, 84]. Early symptoms of disease in hTNFtg mice after spontaneous onset are infiltration with polymorphonuclear cells, lymphocytes, and synovial hyperplasia [81]. Pannus formation, destruction of fibrous tissue, as well as massive articular cartilage and subchondral bone destruction are additional hallmarks of the late stage of arthritis in hTNFtg mice [81, 84]. The bone surface of hTNFtg mice is covered by multinucleated TRAP+ osteoclasts, interposed between the bone surface and the "erosive" front of the synovium [81, 84]. The process of bone destruction is mediated exclusively by osteoclasts because c fos-deficient hTNFtg mice completely lacking osteoclasts were fully protected against bone destruction [85]. This absence of osteoclasts alters TNF-mediated arthritis from a destructive to a nondestructive arthritis [85]. Taken together, the hTNFtg mouse model is especially interesting to investigate the impact of an individual protease to osteoclast-dependent bone resorption during inflammatory arthritis. The investigation of cathepsin K-deficient hTNFtg mice for instance confirmed that cathepsin K is a protease secreted by osteoclasts that has a very high impact to bone destruction [57] (Table 1). Unexpectedly it was also demonstrated that cathepsin K is important but not essential for osteoclast-dependent bone resorption in hTNFtg mouse model for RA [57]. The bone destruction in cathepsin K-deficient hTNFtg mice was only reduced about 50% [57]. Therefore, other proteases, especially MMPs might contribute to subchondral bone destruction process. The MMP activity detected in cathepsin K-deficient osteoclasts might be a compensatory mechanism [57]. Consequently, strategies to prevent arthritic osteoclast-dependent bone destruction cannot be restricted to a selective inhibiton of cathepsin K activity. The detected impairment of synovium-derived osteoclast formation might be partially responsible for the significant reduction in the area of bone erosion in cathepsin K-deficient hTNFtg mice [57]. A clinical case of the onset of an erosive psoriatic arthritis in a "cathepsin K activity-deficient" pycnodysostosis patient was recently reported [86]. This "experiment of nature" supported the idea that cathepsin K in humans is also not essential for osteoclast-mediated bone degradation during inflammatory arthritis [86]. Nevertheless, cathepsin K plays a pivotal role in arthritis. Transgenic mice, overexpressing cathepsin K, become spontaneously susceptible to inflammatory arthritis characterized by synovitis, synovial hyperplasia, fibrosis, and subsequently in degradation of articular cartilage and bone [87].

Rat adjuvant arthritis is an experimental model of polyarthritis that has been widely used for preclinical drug testing. In rats it is induced by a single dosis of Freund`s adjuvant, containing *Mycobacterium tuberculosis* [79, 80]. Arthritis develops in around 10 - 45 days after induction and generally subsides after one month [80]. The hallmarks of this model are a reliable onset of robust polyarticular inflammation with infiltration of joints with mono- and polymorphonuclear cells, pannus formation, and marked bone resorption [79, 80]. The cartilage destruction is relatively mild in comparison to the observed inflammation and bone destruction [79]. The mechanism of arthritis development after immunization with complete Freund`s adjuvant is unknown. Activation of APCs was supposed to contribute to arthritis onset. The enzymatic activity of cathepsin B correlated positively with the severity of joint destruction and inflammation in rat adjuvant-induced arthritis [88]. Oral administration of a vinyl sulfone cysteine cathepsin-specific inhibitor reduced the signs of inflammation and tissue destruction in this animal model probably by direct local effects and attenuation of MHC-dependent antigen-presentation [88]. Oral administration of fluoromethyl ketones in rats with adjuvant-induced arthritis inhibited at least cysteine cathepsins B and L, and resulted in a reduction of articular cartilage and bone destruction [89]. Adjuvant arthritis can also be investigated in mice. Induction of adjuvant arthritis in cathepsin K-deficient mice demonstrated clearly that cathepsin K plays, besides its role in osteoclast-mediated bone destruction, a critical role in toll-like receptor 9 signaling in dendritic cells [58]. The suppression of this signal pathway by cathepsin K deficiency resulted in attenuated induction of pro-inflammatory Th17 cells, without affecting the antigen-presenting ability of dendritic cells [58] (Table 1). In addition, pharmacological inhibition using cathepsin K-specific inhibitors resulted in the reduction of inflammation in joints [58]. Furthermore, cathepsin B and L activities were strongly increased in chondrocytes and cells of the inflamed synovium of rats, which developed an arthritis induced by the synthetic adjuvant CP20961 [90].

Collagen-induced arthritis (CIA) is an experimental autoimmune disease that can be elicited in susceptible strains of rodents (rat und mouse) and non-human primates by immunization with type II collagen of several species the major constituent of articular cartilage [78, 80]. Susceptibility to CIA is restricted to mouse strains with MHC class II types I-A^q and I-A^r [78, 80]. The immune response to type II collagen is characterized by the stimulation of collagen-specific T cells and the production of high titers of collagen-specific antibody [78]. Hallmarks of polyarthritic CIA are synovitis, infiltration of joint with polymorphonuclear and mononuclear cells, pannus formation, erosion of cartilage and bone, and fibrosis [78, 80]. In mice, immunization with bovine, chick or rat type II collagens usually leads to a relatively acute form of arthritis [80]. Papain-like cysteine proteases contribute to disease progression in the CIA arthritis model. Cathepsin K expression is upregulated in murine CIA [91]. Pharmacological inhibition of the proteolytic activity of cathepsin K in murine CIA reduced the destruction of bone and cartilage within arthritic joints [92]. Additionally, the severity of CIA in DBA/1 mice was decreased by fluoroketone inhibitors, which inhibit specifically cathepsin B and L [89]. Cathepsin S-deficient mice develop a diminished CIA probably caused by influences of cathepsin S to late stages of Li degradation in APCs and influencing the peptide repertoire displayed by MHC class II molecules [62] (Table 1). Therapeutic applications of a highly selective and oral available cathepsin S inhibitor reduced significantly the disease score in arthritic CIA mice [93]. The development of further new cathepsin S-specific inhibitors may be useful in treatment of human RA and other autoimmune diseases. Interestingly, the development of highly selective activity-based probes to monitor cathepsin S activity and their successful application in murine zymosam-induced arthritis was reported [94]. These active site probes open the possibility to investigate the *in vivo* roles of cathepsin S in CIA and other RA models more precisely and to monitor the bioavailability of cathepsin S-specific inhibitors in therapeutical trials with arthritic animals.

The antigen-induced arthritis (AIA) can be induced in mice, rats, and rabbits following intra-articular injection of a protein antigen (e.g. methylated bovine serum albumin) into the knee joint of animals that have been previously immunized with the same antigen [80]. The histopathological appearance of AIA has similarities to human RA, including synovial lining layer hyperplasia, perivascular infiltration with lymphocytes and plasma cells, lymphoid follicles, pannus formation, and cartilage erosion [80]. Bone erosion in this arthritis model is relatively week [61, 95]. The AIA is strict Th cell-dependent as shown with depletion experiments with anti CD4 antibodies [96]. Depletion of CD25+ regulatory T cell resulted in an increase of disease severity [95]. In contrast to RA, the AIA is a monoarticular disease that affects only treated joints [80]. Anyway, susceptibility to AIA is not MHC class II-restricted and this makes this model useful for studies with transgenic and gene-deficient mice on different genetic backgrounds [80]. So far the investigated cysteine cathepsins play no or unexpected roles in this RA model. At least the contribution of these proteases to antigen presentation and therefore an alteration in disease outcome was expected because Th1/Th2 balance was influenced by cathepsin L- and B-specific inhibitors applied in *Leishmania*-infected and ovalbumine-immunized mice [43, 97, 98, 99]. However, cathepsin B-deficient mice did not show any difference in disease outcome compared to wild-type mice (unpublished data by author) (Table 1). In addition, no significant upregulation at mRNA level of cathepsin B was detected during time course of AIA [100]. The severity of AIA was decreased in cathepsin L-deficient mice [61]. Clinical outcome in this mice was characterized by decreased inflammation, reduction in cartilage and bone destruction, as well as diminished cellular and humoral immune responsiveness [61] (Tabel 1). Both, Th1 and Th2 cell responses were impaired in arthritic cathepsin L-deficient mice [61]. Interestingly this effect was not caused by local activity of cathepsin L in the arthritic joint, which correlated with only slight local upregulation of cathepsin L in arthritic knee joints in the acute phase and no increase in expression during chronic phase of AIA [100]. In fact the attenuation of AIA in cathepsin L-deficient mice was caused by an impaired positive selection of conventional disease promoting CD4+ Th cells in thymus and a unchanged development of the protective CD25+/FOXP3+ regulatory T cells compartment [61, 101]. Experimentally it could be further clearly demonstrated that transgenic expression of human cathepsin L-like protease cathepsin V in thymic epithelium of cathepsin L-deficient mice reconstituted all parameters by normalization of the ratio of regulatory to conventional T cells [61, 101] (Tabel 1). Therefore, human cathepsin V - the syntenic orthologous proteases of mouse cathepsin L - is clearly involved in Th cell positive selection in the thymus. This influence of cathepsin V on Th cell compartment development might further explain that genetic polymorphisms of cathepsin V are associated with human autoimmune diseases such as diabetes type 1 and myasthenia gravis [102]. In future studies it would be highly attractive to investigate whether cathepsin V polymorphisms are associated with the incidence and clinical outcomes in patients with RA.

As described above cysteine cathepsin-specific inhibitors were applied successfully in several animal models of human RA [58, 88, 89, 92, 93]. The reduction of disease severity was observed. The proteolytic activities of cysteine cathepsins, which contribute directly to joint destruction by collagen degradation as well as indirectly by modulation of the immune response, were inhibited. However, the exact understanding of the contribution of cysteine cathepsins to immune response will be very critically to avoid severe side effects in patients. Potential consequences of systemic application of cathepsin S- and K-specific inhibitors for the outcome of other human chronic and infectious diseases must be critically discussed. Cell type-specific delivery of inhibitors should become a key aspect in arthritis research in future. Osteoclast-specific delivery of cathepsin K-specific inhibitors for instance could be an interesting strategy to avoid joint destruction by inhibition of the collagenolytic activities without interfering with systemic immune response.

8. Summary

Several papain-like cysteine cathepsins are able to cleave type I and type II collagen and therefore contribute to direct joint destruction. Additionally, they play roles in antigen presentation and development of Th cell compartment. Especially cathepsin K with its unique collagenase activity has a great impact to bone degradation in inflammatory arthritis and plays a crucial role in inflammatory processes. In addition, cathepsin S is a key player in antigen-presentation during arthritis. At least cathepsin K and S are attractive targets for the development of new anti-arthritic drugs.

Author details

Uta Schurigt

Address all correspondence to: uta.schurigt@uni-wuerzburg.de

Institute of Molecular Infection Biology (IMIB), University of Wuerzburg, Wuerzburg, Germany

References

[1] Reinheckel T, Deussing J, Roth W, Peters C. Towards specific functions of lysosomal cysteine peptidases: phenotypes of mice deficient for cathepsin B or cathepsin L. Biol Chem 2001; 382: 735-41.

[2] Turk V, Stoka V, Vasiljeva O, Renko M, Sun T, Turk B, Turk D. Cysteine cathepsins: from structure, function and regulation to new frontiers. Biochim Biophys Acta 2012; 1824: 68-88.

[3] MEROPS. The Peptidase Database. http://merops.sanger.ac.uk

[4] Otto HH, Schirmeister T. Cysteine Proteases and Their Inhibitors. Chem Rev 1997; 97: 133-172.

[5] Mottram JC, Coombs GH, Alexander J. Cysteine peptidases as virulence factors of *Leishmania*. Curr Opin Microbiol 2004; 7: 375-81.

[6] Mason SD, Joyce JA. Proteolytic networks in cancer. Trends Cell Biol 2011; 21: 228-37.

[7] Hasilik A, Wrocklage C, Schroder B. Intracellular trafficking of lysosomal proteins and lysosomes. Int J Clin Pharmacol Ther 2009; 47 Suppl 1: S18-33.

[8] Musil D, Zucic D, Turk D, Engh RA, Mayr I, Huber R, Popovic T, Turk V, Towatari T, Katunuma N, et al. The refined 2.15 A X-ray crystal structure of human liver cathepsin B: the structural basis for its specificity. EMBO J 1991; 10: 2321-30.

[9] Aronson NN, Jr., Barrett AJ. The specificity of cathepsin B. Hydrolysis of glucagon at the C-terminus by a peptidyldipeptidase mechanism. Biochem J 1978; 171: 759-65.

[10] Rowley MJ, Nandakumar KS, Holmdahl R. The role of collagen antibodies in mediating arthritis. Mod Rheumatol 2008; 18: 429-41.

[11] Antoine SE, Child AM, Nicholson RA, Pollard AM. The biochemistry and microbiology of buried human bone, in ralation to dietary reconstruction. Circaea 1992; 9: 65-79.

[12] Faust J, Lacey DL, Hunt P, Burgess TL, Scully S, Van G, Eli A, Qian Y, Shalhoub V. Osteoclast markers accumulate on cells developing from human peripheral blood mononuclear precursors. J Cell Biochem 1999; 72: 67-80.

[13] Sazaki T, Ueno-Matsuda E. Cystein-proteinase localization in osteoclasts: An immunocytochemical study. Cell Tissue Res 1993; 271: 177-179.

[14] Rifkin BR, Vernillo AT, Kleckner AP, Auszmann JM, Rosenberg LR, Zimmerman M. Cathepsin B and L activities in isolated osteoclasts. Biochem Biophys Res Commun 1991; 179: 63-9.

[15] Kamiya T, Kobayashi Y, Kanaoka K, Nakashima T, Kato Y, Mizuno A, Sakai H. Fluorescence microscopic demonstration of cathepsin K activity as the major lysosomal cysteine proteinase in osteoclasts. J Biochem 1998; 123: 752-9.

[16] Kakegawa H, Nikawa T, Tagami K, Kamioka H, Sumitani K, Kawata T, Drobnic-Kosorok M, Lenarcic B, Turk V, Katunuma N. Participation of cathepsin L on bone resorption. FEBS Lett 1993; 321: 247-50.

[17] Goto T, Yamaza T, Tanaka T. Cathepsins in the osteoclast. J Electron Microsc (Tokyo) 2003; 52: 551-8.

[18] Goto T, Tsukuba T, Kiyoshima T, Nishimura Y, Kato K, Yamamoto K, Tanaka T. Immunohistochemical localization of cathepsins B, D and L in the rat osteoclast. Histochemistry 1993; 99: 411-4.

[19] Choi JA, Gold GE. MR imaging of articular cartilage physiology. Magn Reson Imaging Clin N Am 2011; 19: 249-82.

[20] Hou WS, Li W, Keyszer G, Weber E, Levy R, Klein MJ, Gravallese EM, Goldring SR, Bromme D. Comparison of cathepsins K and S expression within the rheumatoid and osteoarthritic synovium. Arthritis Rheum 2002; 46: 663-74.

[21] Justen HP, Grunewald E, Totzke G, Gouni-Berthold I, Sachinidis A, Wessinghage D, Vetter H, Schulze-Osthoff K, Ko Y. Differential gene expression in synovium of rheumatoid arthritis and osteoarthritis. Mol Cell Biol Res Commun 2000; 3: 165-72.

[22] Kaneko M, Tomita T, Nakase T, Ohsawa Y, Seki H, Takeuchi E, Takano H, Shi K, Takahi K, Kominami E, Uchiyama Y, Yoshikawa H, Ochi T. Expression of proteinases and inflammatory cytokines in subchondral bone regions in the destructive joint of rheumatoid arthritis. Rheumatology (Oxford) 2001; 40: 247-55.

[23] Honey K, Rudensky AY. Lysosomal cysteine proteases regulate antigen presentation. Nat Rev Immunol 2003; 3: 472-82.

[24] Miossec P, van den Berg W. Th1/Th2 cytokine balance in arthritis. Arthritis Rheum 1997; 40: 2105-15.

[25] Schurigt U, Pfirschke C, Irmler IM, Huckel M, Gajda M, Janik T, Baumgrass R, Bernhagen J, Brauer R. Interactions of T helper cells with fibroblast-like synoviocytes: up-regulation of matrix metalloproteinases by macrophage migration inhibitory factor from both Th1 and Th2 cells. Arthritis Rheum 2008; 58: 3030-40

[26] Feldmann M. The cytokine network in rheumatoid arthritis: definition of TNF alpha as a therapeutic target. J R Coll Physicians Lond 1996; 30: 560-70.

[27] Huet G, Flipo RM, Colin C, Janin A, Hemon B, Collyn-d'Hooghe M, Lafyatis R, Duquesnoy B, Degand P. Stimulation of the secretion of latent cysteine proteinase activity by tumor necrosis factor alpha and interleukin-1. Arthritis Rheum 1993; 36: 772-80.

[28] Gordon MK, Hahn RA. Collagens. Cell Tissue Res 2010; 339: 247-57.

[29] Kadler KE, Holmes DF, Trotter JA, Chapman JA. Collagen fibril formation. Biochem J 1996; 316 (Pt 1): 1-11.

[30] Lynn AK, Yannas IV, Bonfield W. Antigenicity and immunogenicity of collagen. J Biomed Mater Res B Appl Biomater 2004; 71: 343-54.

[31] Eyre D. Collagen of articular cartilage. Arthritis Res 2002; 4: 30-5

[32] Ikeda Y, Ikata T, Mishiro T, Nakano S, Ikebe M, Yasuoka S. Cathepsins B and L in synovial fluids from patients with rheumatoid arthritis and the effect of cathepsin B on the activation of pro-urokinase. J Med Invest 2000; 47: 61-75

[33] Lenarcic B, Gabrijelcic D, Rozman B, Drobnic-Kosorok M, Turk V. Human cathepsin B and cysteine proteinase inhibitors (CPIs) in inflammatory and metabolic joint diseases. Biol Chem Hoppe Seyler 1988; 369 Suppl: 257-61.

[34] Gabrijelcic D, Annan-Prah A, Rodic B, Rozman B, Cotic V, Turk V. Determination of cathepsins B and H in sera and synovial fluids of patients with different joint diseases. J Clin Chem Clin Biochem 1990; 28: 149-53.

[35] Hashimoto Y, Kakegawa H, Narita Y, Hachiya Y, Hayakawa T, Kos J, Turk V, Katunuma N. Significance of cathepsin B accumulation in synovial fluid of rheumatoid arthritis. Biochem Biophys Res Commun 2001; 283: 334-9.

[36] Cunnane G, FitzGerald O, Hummel KM, Gay RE, Gay S, Bresnihan B. Collagenase, cathepsin B and cathepsin L gene expression in the synovial membrane of patients with early inflammatory arthritis. Rheumatology (Oxford) 1999; 38: 34-42.

[37] Trabandt A, Gay RE, Fassbender HG, Gay S. Cathepsin B in synovial cells at the site of joint destruction in rheumatoid arthritis. Arthritis Rheum 1991; 34: 1444-51.

[38] Solau-Gervais E, Zerimech F, Lemaire R, Fontaine C, Huet G, Flipo RM. Cysteine and serine proteases of synovial tissue in rheumatoid arthritis and osteoarthritis. Scand J Rheumatol 2007; 36: 373-7.

[39] Iwata Y, Mort JS, Tateishi H, Lee ER. Macrophage cathepsin L, a factor in the erosion of subchondral bone in rheumatoid arthritis. Arthritis Rheum 1997; 40: 499-509.

[40] Maciewicz RA, Wotton SF. Degradation of cartilage matrix components by the cysteine proteinases, cathepsins B and L. Biomed Biochim Acta 1991; 50: 561-4.

[41] Skoumal M, Haberhauer G, Kolarz G, Hawa G, Woloszczuk W, Klingler A. Serum cathepsin K levels of patients with longstanding rheumatoid arthritis: correlation with radiological destruction. Arthritis Res Ther 2005; 7: R65-70.

[42] Delaisse JM, Eeckhout Y, Vaes G. *In vivo* and *in vitro* evidence for the involvement of cysteine proteinases in bone resorption. Biochem Biophys Res Commun 1984; 125: 441-7.

[43] Katunuma N, Matsunaga Y, Matsui A, Kakegawa H, Endo K, Inubushi T, Saibara T, Ohba Y, Kakiuchi T. Novel physiological functions of cathepsin B and L on antigen processing and osteclastic bone resorption. Advan. Enzyme Regul. 1998; 38: 235-251.

[44] Hill PA, Buttle DJ, Jones SJ, Boyde A, Murata M, Reynolds JJ, Meikle MC. Inhibition of bone resorption by selective inactivators of cysteine proteinases. J Cell Biochem 1994; 56: 118-30.

[45] Everts V, Hou WS, Rialland X, Tigchelaar W, Saftig P, Bromme D, Gelb BD, Beertsen W. Cathepsin K deficiency in pycnodysostosis results in accumulation of non-digested phagocytosed collagen in fibroblasts. Calcif Tissue Int 2003; 73: 380-6.

[46] Schedel J, Seemayer CA, Pap T, Neidhart M, Kuchen S, Michel BA, Gay RE, Muller-Ladner U, Gay S, Zacharias W. Targeting cathepsin L (CL) by specific ribozymes de-

creases CL protein synthesis and cartilage destruction in rheumatoid arthritis. Gene Ther 2004; 11: 1040-7.

[47] Maciewicz RA, Etherington DJ. A comparison of four cathepsins (B, L, N and S) with collagenolytic activity from rabbit spleen. Biochem J 1988; 256: 433-40.

[48] Delaisse JM, Ledent P, Vaes G. Collagenolytic cysteine proteinases of bone tissue. Cathepsin B, (pro)cathepsin L and a cathepsin L-like 70 kDa proteinase. Biochem J 1991; 279 (Pt 1): 167-74.

[49] Garnero P, Ferreras M, Karsdal MA, Nicamhlaoibh R, Risteli J, Borel O, Qvist P, Delmas PD, Foged NT, Delaisse JM. The type I collagen fragments ICTP and CTX reveal distinct enzymatic pathways of bone collagen degradation. J Bone Miner Res 2003; 18: 859-67.

[50] Garnero P, Borel O, Byrjalsen I, Ferreras M, Drake FH, McQueney MS, Foged NT, Delmas PD, Delaisse JM. The collagenolytic activity of cathepsin K is unique among mammalian proteinases. J Biol Chem 1998; 273: 32347-52.

[51] Nosaka AY, Kanaori K, Teno N, Togame H, Inaoka T, Takai M, Kokubo T. Conformational studies on the specific cleavage site of type I collagen (alpha-1) fragment (157-192) by cathepsins K and L by proton NMR spectroscopy. Bioorg Med Chem 1999; 7: 375-9.

[52] Saftig P, Hunziker E, Wehmeyer O, Jones S, Boyde A, Rommerskirch W, Moritz JD, Schu P, von Figura K. Impaired osteoclastic bone resorption leads to osteopetrosis in cathepsin-K-deficient mice. Proc Natl Acad Sci U S A 1998; 95: 13453-8.

[53] Li CY, Jepsen KJ, Majeska RJ, Zhang J, Ni R, Gelb BD, Schaffler MB. Mice lacking cathepsin K maintain bone remodeling but develop bone fragility despite high bone mass. J Bone Miner Res 2006; 21: 865-75.

[54] Kiviranta R, Morko J, Alatalo SL, NicAmhlaoibh R, Risteli J, Laitala-Leinonen T, Vuorio E. Impaired bone resorption in cathepsin K-deficient mice is partially compensated for by enhanced osteoclastogenesis and increased expression of other proteases via an increased RANKL/OPG ratio. Bone 2005; 36: 159-72

[55] Gowen M, Lazner F, Dodds R, Kapadia R, Feild J, Tavaria M, Bertoncello I, Drake F, Zavarselk S, Tellis I, Hertzog P, Debouck C, Kola I. Cathepsin K knockout mice develop osteopetrosis due to a deficit in matrix degradation but not demineralization. J Bone Miner Res 1999; 14: 1654-63.

[56] Pennypacker B, Shea M, Liu Q, Masarachia P, Saftig P, Rodan S, Rodan G, Kimmel D. Bone density, strength, and formation in adult cathepsin K (-/-) mice. Bone 2009; 44: 199-207.

[57] Schurigt U, Hummel KM, Petrow PK, Gajda M, Stockigt R, Middel P, Zwerina J, Janik T, Bernhardt R, Schuler S, Scharnweber D, Beckmann F, Saftig P, Kollias G, Schett G, Wiederanders B, Brauer R. Cathepsin K deficiency partially inhibits, but does not

prevent, bone destruction in human tumor necrosis factor-transgenic mice. Arthritis Rheum 2008; 58: 422-34.

[58] Asagiri M, Hirai T, Kunigami T, Kamano S, Gober HJ, Okamoto K, Nishikawa K, Latz E, Golenbock DT, Aoki K, Ohya K, Imai Y, Morishita Y, Miyazono K, Kato S, Saftig P, Takayanagi H. Cathepsin K-dependent toll-like receptor 9 signaling revealed in experimental arthritis. Science 2008; 319: 624-7.

[59] Kirschke H, Kembhavi AA, Bohley P, Barrett AJ. Action of rat liver cathepsin L on collagen and other substrates. Biochem J 1982; 201: 367-72.

[60] Potts W, Bowyer J, Jones H, Tucker D, Freemont AJ, Millest A, Martin C, Vernon W, Neerunjun D, Slynn G, Harper F, Maciewicz R. Cathepsin L-deficient mice exhibit abnormal skin and bone development and show increased resistance to osteoporosis following ovariectomy. Int J Exp Pathol 2004; 85: 85-96.

[61] Schurigt U, Eilenstein R, Gajda M, Leipner C, Sevenich L, Reinheckel T, Peters C, Wiederanders B, Brauer R. Decreased arthritis severity in cathepsin L-deficient mice is attributed to an impaired T helper cell compartment. Inflamm Res 2012; 61: 1021-9.

[62] Nakagawa TY, Brissette WH, Lira PD, Griffiths RJ, Petrushova N, Stock J, McNeish JD, Eastman SE, Howard ED, Clarke SR, Rosloniec EF, Elliott EA, Rudensky AY. Impaired invariant chain degradation and antigen presentation and diminished collagen-induced arthritis in cathepsin S null mice. Immunity 1999; 10: 207-17.

[63] BRENDA. The Comprehensive Enzyme Information System. http://www.brenda-enzymes.org/php/result_flat.php4?ecno=3.4.22.43

[64] Eeckhout Y, Vaes G. Further studies on the activation of procollagenase, the latent precursor of bone collagenase. Effects of lysosomal cathepsin B, plasmin and kallikrein, and spontaneous activation. Biochem J 1977; 166: 21-31.

[65] Li Z, Hou WS, Bromme D. Collagenolytic activity of cathepsin K is specifically modulated by cartilage-resident chondroitin sulfates. Biochemistry 2000; 39: 529-36.

[66] Li Z, Hou WS, Escalante-Torres CR, Gelb BD, Bromme D. Collagenase activity of cathepsin K depends on complex formation with chondroitin sulfate. J Biol Chem 2002; 277: 28669-76.

[67] Bromme D, Okamoto K. Human cathepsin O2, a novel cysteine protease highly expressed in osteoclastomas and ovary molecular cloning, sequencing and tissue distribution. Biol Chem Hoppe Seyler 1995; 376: 379-84.

[68] Inui T, Ishibashi O, Inaoka T, Origane Y, Kumegawa M, Kokubo T, Yamamura T. Cathepsin K antisense oligodeoxynucleotide inhibits osteoclastic bone resorption. J Biol Chem 1997; 272: 8109-12.

[69] Kafienah W, Bromme D, Buttle DJ, Croucher LJ, Hollander AP. Human cathepsin K cleaves native type I and II collagens at the N-terminal end of the triple helix. Biochem J 1998; 331 (Pt 3): 727-32.

[70] Hou WS, Li Z, Gordon RE, Chan K, Klein MJ, Levy R, Keysser M, Keyszer G, Bromme D. Cathepsin K is a critical protease in synovial fibroblast-mediated collagen degradation. Am J Pathol 2001; 159: 2167-77.

[71] Deussing J, Roth W, Saftig P, Peters C, Ploegh HL, Villadangos JA. Cathepsins B and D are dispensable for major histocompatibility complex class II-mediated antigen presentation. Proc Natl Acad Sci U S A 1998; 95: 4516-21.

[72] Roth W, Deussing J, Botchkarev VA, Pauly-Evers M, Saftig P, Hafner A, Schmidt P, Schmahl W, Scherer J, Anton-Lamprecht I, Von Figura K, Paus R, Peters C. Cathepsin L deficiency as molecular defect of furless: hyperproliferation of keratinocytes and pertubation of hair follicle cycling. FASEB J 2000; 14: 2075-86.

[73] Gelb BD, Shi GP, Chapman HA, Desnick RJ. Pycnodysostosis, a lysosomal disease caused by cathepsin K deficiency. Science 1996; 273: 1236-8.

[74] McKiernan M. Henri de Toulouse-Lautrec medical examination, Rue des Moulins (1894): North wall fresco, lower panel 5.398 m x 13.716 m. Detroit Institute of Arts, Detroit, USA. Occup Med (Lond) 2009; 59: 366-8.

[75] Xue Y, Cai T, Shi S, Wang W, Zhang Y, Mao T, Duan X. Clinical and animal research findings in pycnodysostosis and gene mutations of cathepsin K from 1996 to 2011. Orphanet J Rare Dis 2011; 6: 20.

[76] Edelson JG, Obad S, Geiger R, On A, Artul HJ. Pycnodysostosis. Orthopedic aspects with a description of 14 new cases. Clin Orthop Relat Res 1992; 263-76.

[77] Fratzl-Zelman N, Valenta A, Roschger P, Nader A, Gelb BD, Fratzl P, Klaushofer K. Decreased bone turnover and deterioration of bone structure in two cases of pycnodysostosis. J Clin Endocrinol Metab 2004; 89: 1538-47.

[78] Brand DD, Kang AH, Rosloniec EF. The mouse model of collagen-induced arthritis. Methods Mol Med 2004; 102: 295-312.

[79] Bendele A, McComb J, Gould T, McAbee T, Sennello G, Chlipala E, Guy M. Animal models of arthritis: relevance to human disease. Toxicol Pathol 1999; 27: 134-42.

[80] Williams RO. Rodent models of arthritis: relevance for human disease. Clin Exp Immunol 1998; 114: 330-2.

[81] Li P, Schwarz EM. The TNF-alpha transgenic mouse model of inflammatory arthritis. Springer Semin Immunopathol 2003; 25: 19-33.

[82] Cuzzocrea S. Characterization of a novel and spontaneous mouse model of inflammatory arthritis. Arthritis Res Ther 2011; 13: 126.

[83] Geiler J, Buch M, McDermott MF. Anti-TNF treatment in rheumatoid arthritis. Curr Pharm Des 2011; 17: 3141-54.

[84] Keffer J, Probert L, Cazlaris H, Georgopoulos S, Kaslaris E, Kioussis D, Kollias G. Transgenic mice expressing human tumour necrosis factor: a predictive genetic model of arthritis. EMBO J 1991; 10: 4025-31.

[85] Redlich K, Hayer S, Ricci R, David JP, Tohidast-Akrad M, Kollias G, Steiner G, Smolen JS, Wagner EF, Schett G. Osteoclasts are essential for TNF-alpha-mediated joint destruction. J Clin Invest 2002; 110: 1419-27.

[86] Ainola M, Valleala H, Nykanen P, Risteli J, Hanemaaijer R, Konttinen YT. Erosive arthritis in a patient with pycnodysostosis: an experiment of nature. Arthritis Rheum 2008; 58: 3394-401.

[87] Morko J, Kiviranta R, Joronen K, Saamanen AM, Vuorio E, Salminen-Mankonen H. Spontaneous development of synovitis and cartilage degeneration in transgenic mice overexpressing cathepsin K. Arthritis Rheum 2005; 52: 3713-7.

[88] Biroc SL, Gay S, Hummel K, Magill C, Palmer JT, Spencer DR, Sa S, Klaus JL, Michel BA, Rasnick D, Gay RE. Cysteine protease activity is up-regulated in inflamed ankle joints of rats with adjuvant-induced arthritis and decreases with *in vivo* administration of a vinyl sulfone cysteine protease inhibitor. Arthritis Rheum 2001; 44: 703-11.

[89] Esser RE, Angelo RA, Murphey MD, Watts LM, Thornburg LP, Palmer JT, Talhouk JW, Smith RE. Cysteine proteinase inhibitors decrease articular cartilage and bone destruction in chronic inflammatory arthritis. Arthritis Rheum 1994; 37: 236-47.

[90] Meijers MH, Koopdonk-Kool J, Meacock SC, Van Noorden CJ, Bunning RA, Billingham ME. Cysteine proteinase activity in the development of arthritis in an adjuvant model of the rat. Agents Actions 1993; 39 Spec No: C219-21.

[91] Ibrahim SM, Koczan D, Thiesen HJ. Gene-expression profile of collagen-induced arthritis. J Autoimmun 2002; 18: 159-67.

[92] Svelander L, Erlandsson-Harris H, Astner L, Grabowska U, Klareskog L, Lindstrom E, Hewitt E. Inhibition of cathepsin K reduces bone erosion, cartilage degradation and inflammation evoked by collagen-induced arthritis in mice. Eur J Pharmacol 2009; 613: 155-62.

[93] Baugh M, Black D, Westwood P, Kinghorn E, McGregor K, Bruin J, Hamilton W, Dempster M, Claxton C, Cai J, Bennett J, Long C, McKinnon H, Vink P, den Hoed L, Gorecka M, Vora K, Grant E, Percival MD, Boots AM, van Lierop MJ. Therapeutic dosing of an orally active, selective cathepsin S inhibitor suppresses disease in models of autoimmunity. J Autoimmun 2011; 36: 201-9.

[94] Caglic D, Globisch A, Kindermann M, Lim NH, Jeske V, Juretschke HP, Bartnik E, Weithmann KU, Nagase H, Turk B, Wendt KU. Functional *in vivo* imaging of cysteine cathepsin activity in murine model of inflammation. Bioorg Med Chem 2011; 19: 1055-61.

[95] Frey O, Petrow PK, Gajda M, Siegmund K, Huehn J, Scheffold A, Hamann A, Radbruch A, Brauer R. The role of regulatory T cells in antigen-induced arthritis: aggra-

vation of arthritis after depletion and amelioration after transfer of CD4+CD25− T cells. Arthritis Res Ther 2005; 7: R291-301.

[96] Pohlers D, Nissler K, Frey O, Simon J, Petrow PK, Kinne RW, Brauer R. Anti-CD4 monoclonal antibody treatment in acute and early chronic antigen-induced arthritis: influence on T helper cell activation. Clin Exp Immunol 2004; 135: 409-15.

[97] Maekawa Y, Himeno K, Katunuma N. Cathepsin B-inhibitor promotes the development of Th1 type protective T cells in mice infected with *Leishmania major*. J Med Invest 1997; 44: 33-9.

[98] Onishi K, Li Y, Ishii K, Hisaeda H, Tang L, Duan X, Dainichi T, Maekawa Y, Katunuma N, Himeno K. Cathepsin L is crucial for a Th1-type immune response during Leishmania major infection. Microbes Infect 2004; 6: 468-74.

[99] Zhang T, Maekawa Y, Sakai T, Nakano Y, Ishii K, Hisaeda H, Dainichi T, Asao T, Katunuma N, Himeno K. Treatment with cathepsin L inhibitor potentiates Th2-type immune response in *Leishmania major*-infected BALB/c mice. Int Immunol 2001; 13: 975-82.

[100] Schurigt U, Stopfel N, Huckel M, Pfirschke C, Wiederanders B, Brauer R. Local expression of matrix metalloproteinases, cathepsins, and their inhibitors during the development of murine antigen-induced arthritis. Arthritis Res Ther 2005; 7: R174-88.

[101] Sevenich L, Hagemann S, Stoeckle C, Tolosa E, Peters C, Reinheckel T. Expression of human cathepsin L or human cathepsin V in mouse thymus mediates positive selection of T helper cells in cathepsin L knock-out mice. Biochimie 2010; 92: 1674-80.

[102] Viken MK, Sollid HD, Joner G, Dahl-Jorgensen K, Ronningen KS, Undlien DE, Flato B, Selvaag AM, Forre O, Kvien TK, Thorsby E, Melms A, Tolosa E, Lie BA. Polymorphisms in the cathepsin L2 (CTSL2) gene show association with type 1 diabetes and early-onset myasthenia gravis. Hum Immunol 2007; 68: 748-55.